Coronavirus Disease-19 (COVID-19): A Perspective of New Scenario

(Volume 2)

Coronavirus Disease-19 (COVID-19): Different Models and Treatment Strategies

Edited by

Kamal Niaz

Department of Pharmacology and Toxicology
Faculty of Bio-Sciences, Cholistan University of Veterinary and Animal Sciences
Bahawalpur-63100
Pakistan

&

Muhammad Farrukh Nisar

Department of Physiology and Biochemistry
Faculty of Bio-Sciences, Cholistan University of Veterinary and Animal Sciences (CUVAS)
Bahawalpur-63100
Pakistan

Coronavirus Disease-19 (COVID-19): A Perspective of New Scenario

(Volume 2)

COVID-19: Different Models and Treatment Strategies

Editors: Kamal Niaz & Muhammad Farrukh Nisar

ISBN (Online): 978-1-68108-907-2

ISBN (Print): 978-1-68108-908-9

ISBN (Paperback): 978-1-68108-909-6

need for a court order if at any point you breach any terms of this License Agreement. In no event will any delay or failure by Bentham Science Publishers in enforcing your compliance with this License Agreement constitute a waiver of any of its rights.

3. You acknowledge that you have read this License Agreement, and agree to be bound by its terms and conditions. To the extent that any other terms and conditions presented on any website of Bentham Science Publishers conflict with, or are inconsistent with, the terms and conditions set out in this License Agreement, you acknowledge that the terms and conditions set out in this License Agreement shall prevail.

Bentham Science Publishers Ltd.
Executive Suite Y - 2
PO Box 7917, Saif Zone
Sharjah, U.A.E.
Email: subscriptions@benthamscience.org

BENTHAM SCIENCE

CONTENTS

FOREWORD

According to World Health Organization, 122 million cases and over 2.69 million deaths of coronavirus disease-2019 (COVID-19) pandemic have impacted nearly every region of the globe. The pandemic has a huge global economic influence, and successfully fighting against COVID-19 needs efforts. Newly emerging respiratory diseases such as Severe Acute Respiratory Syndrome-coronavirus (SARS-CoV), Middle East Respiratory Syndrome (MERS), and severe acute respiratory syndrome-coronavirus-2 (SARS-CoV-2) posing a serious threat to the human population and reported in the years 2003, 2012, and 2019, respectively. Furthermore, SARS-CoV-2 new strains shocked the world due to genetic mutation over time.

This book is very relevant and consists of two key modules. The first module provides clear information regarding different animals and cell line models and differentiation from other respiratory diseases. The second part focuses on therapeutic agents (antivirals, natural compounds, ultraviolet radiation, herbal remedies, blood plasma, stem cell therapy, and vaccines. It will give step-by-step awareness to the scholars about SARS-CoV-2. Basic and advanced knowledge about the disease is arranged into clear and easy-to-read chapters for general readers, scholars, and molecular biology teachers, making this book a valuable and thorough guide for all.

Prof. Dr. Zahir Shah
University of Chitral
Chitral
Khyber Pakhtunkhwa
Pakistan

PREFACE

Coronavirus disease-19 (COVID-19) is a complex disease that causes illnesses ranging from mild to severe respiratory problems. It is caused by a novel coronavirus severe acute respiratory syndrome coronavirus-2 (SARS-CoV-2), an enveloped, positive-sense, and single-stranded RNA (+ssRNA) virus that belongs to the coronavirus family. It has a fast-spreading potential worldwide, which leads to high death cases regardless of lows death rates. Yet, there are no animal models or specific drugs for disease prevention and/or treatment. Therefore, it is highly demanded to identify the known drugs and test them as a possible therapeutic approach. In this critical situation, one or more of these drugs may represent the only option to treat or reduce the severity of the disease until a specific drug or vaccine is developed and approved. A wide variety of therapeutics have been explored to treat COVID-19, initially suggested for other diseases and already established safety profiles, and approved by the Food and Drug Administration (FDA). Such treatments are referred to by the World Health Organization (WHO) as repurpose medications. Still, there are many ongoing clinical trials regarding the safety and effectiveness of repurposing immune-therapeutics to mitigate the symptoms of COVID-19.

In this book volume-2 proposal, we consolidate the various animal models and treatment strategies widely used for the global emergency of COVID-19. Since SARS-CoV-2 is the closest to SARS-CoV and MERS-CoV, the approaches brought here will be similar and/or varying with a slight degree. It is cleared that in the last 17-18 years, this is the third outbreak of the same coronavirus with a small mutation that shock the whole world. The chapters in this book should be prioritized as up-to-date literature of techniques used in the study SARS-CoV-2 and will act as a suitable reference if any such wary appear soon.

The 2nd volume of the proposed book proposal has been classified into Part IV: Models for SARS-CoV-2 and Part V: Treatment Strategies for SARS-CoV-2. With the emergence of new coronavirus variants, epidemiology, different host tropism permits a thorough analysis of their evolution and acquired adaptability to their host. The 1st volume already discussed the entry, epidemiology, genetic alteration, and diagnostic approaches. In the 2nd volume, part IV, we have planned to describe chapter-wise models used in COVID-19. No studies are complete without animal models closely related to human physiology to replicate the disease and observe the pathology conditions as in human cases. Such animal models play a vital role in virus pathogenesis and prepare a therapeutic immune response. Here describe bio-engineered transgenic mouse model inserting with specific genes, or CRISPR-Case9 gene-editing tool has been used previously for SARS-CoV and MERS-CoV. The chapter will deal with culture techniques or cell lines for COVID-19-also histopathology of COVID-19, essential proteins that up or down-regulate SARS-CoV-2. The last chapter of this part will describe other diseases having similar signs and symptoms and their differentiation. In the last part of the book proposal, part V, chapters will deal with therapeutic approaches to attenuate SARS-CoV-2 as there is no specific treatment available to date, just symptomatic therapy. However, scientists will elucidate effective antiviral drugs in clinical trials, phytochemicals, photomedicine such as ultraviolet A & B, homemade remedies, blood plasma transfusion, stem cell therapy, and computational approaches *in vivo* and *in vitro* trials.

This book will appear as a baseline for academicians, scientists, and health professionals as still, research is going to overcome this outbreak of COVID-19, the novelty of best animal models, and find an effective treatment. However, just a single book proposal like this wouldn't have flourished without enthusiasm and determined publishers' and investigators' strength to take time from their busy schedule and subsidize on time.

We thank the whole investigators who contributed, directly and indirectly, to bring it to reality.

Kamal Niaz
Department of Pharmacology and Toxicology
Faculty of Bio-Sciences, Cholistan University of Veterinary and Animal Sciences
Bahawalpur-63100
Pakistan

&

Muhammad Farrukh Nisar
Department of Physiology and Biochemistry
Faculty of Bio-Sciences, Cholistan University of Veterinary and Animal Sciences
(CUVAS)
Bahawalpur-63100
Pakistan

List of Contributors

Abdullah	Department of Pharmacy, University of Malakand, Chakdara Dir Lower, KPK, Pakistan
Ahmad Farooq	Department of Biological Sciences, International Islamic University, Islamabad, Pakistan
Aadil Javed	Department of Biotechnology, Graduate School of Natural and Applied Sciences, Ege University, Bornova, Izmir, Turkey
Abhinav Anand	School of Pharmaceutical Sciences, Lovely Professional University, Phagwara, Punjab, PIN- 144 411, India CT Institute of Pharmaceutical Sciences, CT Group of Institutions, Shahpur, Jalandhar, Punjab, PIN- 144 020, India
Amjad Islam Aqib	Department of Medicine, Faculty of Veterinary Science, Cholistan University of Veterinary and Animal Sciences, Bahawalpur, Pakistan
Amna Ahmad	Faculty of Veterinary Science, University of Agriculture, Faisalabad, Pakistan
Ahmed Abdelmajed Alkhodary	Ministry of Health, Gaza Governorates, Palestine International Centre for Casemix and Clinical Coding, Faculty of Medicine, National University of Malaysia, Kuala Lumpur, Malaysia
Afshan Shafi	Department of Food Science and Technology, MNS University of Agriculture, Multan, Pakistan
Ahmad Uddin	Drug Discovery Research Centre, Southwest Medical University, Luzhou, China
Devesh Tewari	School of Pharmaceutical Sciences, Lovely Professional University, Phagwara, Punjab, PIN- 144 411, India
Faisal Siddique	Department of Microbiology, Faculty of Veterinary Science, Cholistan University of Veterinary and Animal Sciences (CUVAS), Bahawalpur, Pakistan
Firasat Hussain	Department of Microbiology, Faculty of Veterinary Science, Cholistan University of Veterinary and Animal Sciences, Bahawalpur, Pakistan
Fazlullah Khan	Department of Allied Health Sciences, Bashir Institute of Health Sciences, Bharakahu, Islamabad, Pakistan
Ihtisham Ulhaq	Department of Biosciences, COMSATS University Islamabad (CUI), 45550, Pakistan
Iqra Muzammil	Department of Clinical Medicine and Surgery, University of Agriculture, Faisalabad, Pakistan
Ismail Shah	Department of Pharmacy, Garden Campus, Abdul Wali Khan University, Mardan, Pakistan
Iyad Ibrahim Shaqura	Department of Health Management and Economics, School of Public Health, Tehran University of Medical Sciences, Tehran, Iran Ministry of Health, Gaza Governorates, Palestine

Kamal Niaz	Department of Pharmacology & Toxicology, Faculty of Bio-Sciences, Cholistan University of Veterinary and Animal Sciences, Bahawalpur-63100, Pakistan
Kashif Akram	Department of Food Sciences, Faculty of Bio-Sciences, Cholistan University of Veterinary and Animal Sciences, Bahawalpur, Pakistan
Kashif Rahim	Department of Microbiology, Faculty of Veterinary Science, Cholistan University of Veterinary and Animal Sciences (CUVAS), Bahawalpur, Pakistan
Laiba Hassan	Department of Microbiology, The University of Haripur, Haripur, Pakistan
Maqsood ur Rehman	Department of Pharmacy University of Malakand, Chakdara Dir Lower, Cholistan University of Veterinary & Animal Sciences, Pakistan
Muhammad Mazhar Munir	Department of Pharmacology & Toxicology, Faculty of Bio-Sciences, Cholistan University of Veterinary & Animal Sciences, Bahawalpur, Pakistan
Muhammad Mazhar Ayaz	Department of Parasitology, Faculty of Veterinary Science, Cholistan University of Veterinary and Animal Sciences, Bahawalpur, Pakistan
Muhammad Ibrar	Department of Allied Health Sciences, Iqra University Peshawar, Swat Campus, KPK, Pakistan
Muhammad Farrukh Nisar	Department of Physiology and Biochemistry, Faculty of Bio-Sciences, Cholistan University of Veterinary and Animal Sciences (CUVAS), Bahawalpur, Pakistan
Muhammad Yasir Waqas	Department of Physiology and Biochemistry, Faculty of Bio-Sciences, Cholistan University of Veterinary and Animal Sciences (CUVAS), Bahawalpur, Pakistan
Muhammad Ali Syed	Department of Microbiology, The University of Haripur, Haripur, Pakistan
Mohammad Ejaz	Department of Microbiology, The University of Haripur, Haripur, Pakistan
Muhammad Ali Syed	Department of Microbiology, The University of Haripur, Haripur, Pakistan
Navneet Khurana	School of Pharmaceutical Sciences, Lovely Professional University, Phagwara, Punjab, PIN- 144 411, India
Neha Sharma	School of Pharmaceutical Sciences, Lovely Professional University, Phagwara, Punjab, PIN- 144 411, India
Ovais Sideeq	School of Medicine, Tehran University of Medical Sciences (TUMS), Tehran, Iran
Qaisar Tanveer	Institute of Pharmacy, Physiology and Pharmacology, University of Agriculture, Faisalabad, Pakistan
Qudratullulah	Department of Surgery, Faculty of Veterinary Science, Cholistan University of Veterinary and Animal Sciences (CUVAS), Bahawalpur, Pakistan
Sana Muzammal	Department of Mathematics, National College of Business Administration and Economics, Sub-Campus Bahawalpur, Pakistan
Shaukat Hussain Munawar	Department of Pharmacology and Toxicology, Faculty of Bio-Sciences, Cholistan University of Veterinary and Animal Sciences (CUVAS), Bahawalpur, Pakistan

Sonali Bajaj	School of Pharmaceutical Sciences, Lovely Professional University, Phagwara, Punjab, PIN- 144 411, India
Tapan Behl	Chitkara College of Pharmacy, Chitkara University, Punjab, India
Tean Zaheer	Department of Parasitology, University of Agriculture, Faisalabad, Pakistan
Zahid Manzoor	Department of Pharmacology & Toxicology, Faculty of Bio-Sciences, Cholistan University of Veterinary & Animal Sciences, Bahawalpur, Pakistan

Part I: Models for COVID-19

CHAPTER 1

Genetically Engineered Mouse Models for COVID-19

Aadil Javed[1,*], **Kamal Niaz**[2] and **Ovais Sideeq**[3]

[1] *Department of Biotechnology, Graduate School of Natural and Applied Sciences, Ege University, Bornova, Izmir, Turkey*

[2] *Department of Pharmacology & Toxicology, Faculty of Bio-Sciences, Cholistan University of Veterinary and Animal Sciences, Bahawalpur-63100, Pakistan*

[3] *School of Medicine, Tehran University of Medical Sciences (TUMS), Tehran, Iran*

Abstract: Previous severe acute respiratory syndrome-coronavirus (SARS-CoV) outbreaks resulted in a cohort of preclinical studies that utilized various mice models for determining the pathogenesis of the infection, including the viral replication, spread, and mortality of the disease. Such studies have provided a framework upon which new investigations have been launched for understanding the outbreak of new coronavirus disease-19 (COVID-19) causing viral agents and their interaction with the host and its body. Recent investigations showed that the previous SARS-CoV and the recently discovered severe acute respiratory syndrome-coronavirus-2 (SARS-CoV-2) both require the spike S protein to enter the host cell upon infection the binding with the receptors on the surface of the cells. The viral entry also requires proteases from the host cells. Since there are key similarities between the structure of the viruses and the construct of the viral transmission along with the spread inside the host's body in animal models. They were developed for the previous viral agent. The disease can be emulated or manipulated to bring forth novel investigations leading to key data that can broaden the sphere of COVID-19 studies being conducted. There are several different options to choose the right animal model for the question being raised in the experimental design with the pathogenesis of COVID-19. This chapter focused on the already established animal models for other coronavirus outbreaks and some of the strategies that can be exploited to develop new animal models. For COVID-19, research aimed at targeting the therapy or basic investigations for understanding cellular or organ level mechanisms involved in the disease.

Keywords: COVID-19, Knockout, Mouse models, SARS-CoV-2, Transgenic.

* **Corresponding author Aadil Javed:** Department of Biotechnology, Graduate School of Natural and Applied Sciences, Ege University, Bornova, Izmir, Turkey. E-mail: adiljaved313@hotmail.com

Kamal Niaz & Muhammad Farrukh Nisar (Eds.)

INTRODUCTION

In December 2019, a novel coronavirus outbreak was reported in Wuhan, China which caused a pandemic and is an ongoing public health concern worldwide [1]. The disease known as coronavirus disease-19 (COVID-19) is caused by the novel severe acute respiratory syndrome-coronavirus-2 (SARS-CoV-2), which leads to deadly pneumonia and severe health issues related to lung damage [2]. The genomic properties of the viral agent responsible for the local epidemic in China were timely shared across the scientific community. Since then, a valiant effort to combat the disease and understanding the agent responsible for the pandemic has been ongoing. Across the world, millions of people have been affected by the pandemic leading to a change in lifestyle globally [3 - 5]. The diverse scientific community took upon understanding the pandemic and the viral agent responsible for the COVID-19 from the get-go during the earlier days of the pandemic in 2020 [6]. Millions of people have been infected, and hundreds of thousands of people have lost their lives due to the COVID-19 pandemic outbreak [7]. Various attempts have been reported to classify the epidemiological features of the pandemic, including the case fatality rate, reproduction number, and recovery rate. To date, it is being assumed that various factors that affect the rigorous testing and other socio-economic factors hamper any progress in determining the true features of the pandemic [8 - 13].

The SARS-CoV-2 virus belonging to the *Coronaviridae* family of the virus has been studied extensively due to the urgency of pandemics. The vaccine development approaches have been challenging so far, and various mouse models have been utilized for understanding different aspects of the physiology of this novel coronavirus. Previously, the Middle East Respiratory Syndrome (MERS) and SARS candidates for vaccines were evaluated in the different mouse models [14, 15]. The clinical features, including the pathogenesis of the coronavirus, can be studied in great detail upon the development of animal models that can efficiently mimic the properties of the disease. For this purpose, numerous models have been developed in animals such as hamsters, guinea pigs, mice, cats, and rabbits, *etc*., [16 - 20]. The major receptor of SAR-CoV is angiotensin-converting enzyme 2 (ACE2) and is utilized to develop transgenic mouse models containing the human ACE2 gene [21]. *Rhesus macaques* were the first animal model for vaccine development against MERS-CoV, showing the symptoms of the infections as seen in clinical patients [22]. Golden Syrian hamsters were also used as animal models for establishing the vaccine candidate's safety and viral pathogenesis for different strains of SARS-CoV [19]. NSP16 CoV attenuated vaccine development approaches utilized mice as well [23]. Developing animal models, MERS-CoV had several drawbacks due to the inefficiency of the virus being replicated in the respiratory system. Therefore, new approaches like gene targeting paved the way for demonstrating modified models containing genes of interest or lack thereof for more naturalized infectivity of the virus, *e.g.,* human DPP4 transgenic mice [24]. Clustered regularly interspaced short palindromic repeats and associated protein 9 (CRISPR-Cas9) the system has been efficiently employed for developing mouse models that are engineered to get infected by the virus and show high replication [25, 26]. Small animals like rabbits and mice are used to develop mouse models specific for a particular infection such as SAR-CoV-2 for various reasons, including efficacy, cost issues, and manipulation approaches. There is still much work that is needed to better understand the behavior of COVID-19 and transgenic animal models can efficiently smoothen the process of understanding due to ease in receptor identification, protection, pathogenesis models and immune response studies [15, 27]. Various applications and interference points for different types of mouse models in understanding or combating SARS have been depicted in Fig. (**1**). The aim of this chapter is to summarize the well-known animal models that can be used for coronavirus along with some of the strategies that can be exploited to develop new animal models for COVID-19 as a model to target the therapy or basic investigations the underline molecular mechanisms involved in the disease.

Emerging Role of CRISPR/Cas9

In molecular diagnostics, CRISPR, and the Cas protein-containing CRISPR-Cas systems, have advanced the process of functional research. Since its discovery almost 30 years ago, the field of genome editing using CRISPR systems has been revolutionized [28]. In clinical sciences and modern molecular biology approaches, CRISPR-Cas9 systems are routinely applied for targeting the cells of mammalian origin involving gene editing methodology [29]. Such approaches have been utilized to detect Zika virus and methicillin-resistant *Staphylococcus aureus* along with nucleic acid detection-based diagnosis procedures that use RNA-guided or RNA-targeting CRISPR-Cas systems [30 - 32]. In the wake of the COVID-19 pandemic of 2020, CRISPR-Cas13 approached for diagnostic applications are being considered [33]. The potential for this technology is deemed as tremendous, as described by Xiang *et al.* [34]. A fast and accurate method for detecting SARS-CoV-2 is the need for the hour, and SHERLOCK protocols can provide the scientific community an approach that has huge potential in this area. A recently reported DETECTR assay for the detection of SARS-CoV-2 *via* employing CRISPR leads to a 95% positive prediction along with a 100% negative prediction agreement in a real-time RT-PCR [35]. Genome-wide CRISPR screens were employed to determine the therapeutic targets for COVID-19. Apart from already established protease cathepsin and receptor ACE2, SWI/SNF chromatin complex proteins that comprise the transforming growth factor-beta (TGF-β) signaling network were also identified using the technology [36]. The protocol for designing a transgenic mouse model for SARS-CoV-2 that conforms to the CRISPR-Cas9 technology has also been reported recently [37]. Such models can successfully provide representativeness of the infection with tissue specificity of the human genes as well [37].

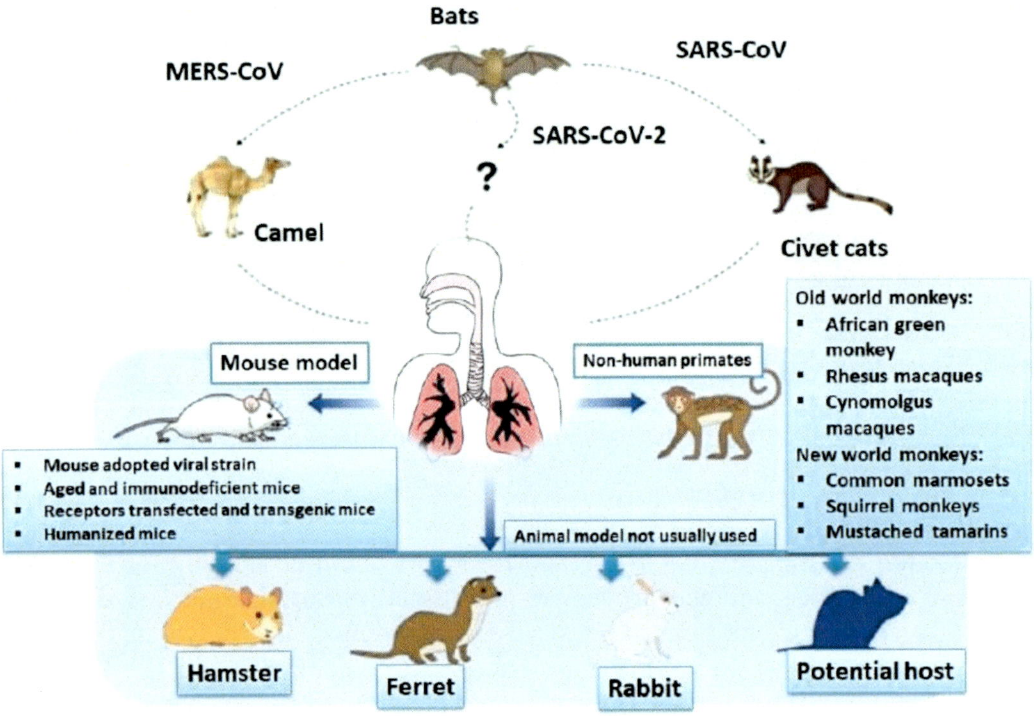

Fig. (1). Experimental animals of SARS-CoV, MERS-CoV, and SARS-CoV-2. The coronaviruses with high infectivity and pathogenicity break the species barrier and infect humans in the past two decades. Besides NHP, mice, hamsters, ferrets, and rabbits, the other possible natural hosts might be able to support the studies of coronavirus infection, pathogenesis, and drug discovery.

Human ACE2 Expression

A carboxypeptidase named ACE2, which is encoded by the gene ACE2 resides on chromosome Xp22. It gives rise to a type I type transmembrane protein containing an extracellular N-terminal domain with carboxypeptidase which is heavy, and a short C-terminal domain having a cytoplasmic tail intracellularly [38, 39]. The SARS-CoV binding site in ACE2 is present on the N-terminal peptidase domain [40]. Cellular ACE2 manifests in either soluble or membrane-bound form and is usually expressed in pneumocytes and enterocytes located in the small intestine [41]. Vascular endothelial cells located in the heart, brain, and kidneys also exhibit ACE2 expression [42, 43]. The major site of infection for the coronavirus, especially SARS-CoV, is the respiratory tract. In human airway epithelia and lung parenchyma, ACE2 is expressed and is considered the receptor for these coronaviruses. SARS-CoV also seemed to infect the differentiated epithelial cells more than undifferentiated cells as the differentiated epithelia are reported to have higher expression of ACE2 receptor *via* SARS S protein [44].

ACE2 gene in humans produces the protein receptor that is identified by SARS coronaviruses, including SARS-CoV and NL63, along with the novel SARS-CoV-2 virus that caused the pandemic of 2020 [45]. *In vitro* studies suggest that SARS-CoV infection correlates with the expression of the ACE2 receptor. The variations or mutations in the ACE2 sequence lead to a reduced association or linkage between the spike protein on the SARS-CoV or NL63 with the ACE2 receptor [40, 46]. It has been concluded that the severity, susceptibility, or even the symptoms of SARS-CoV-2 infection is dependent on the expression of the receptor ACE2. Recently, ACE2 expression levels from single-cell RNA-sequencing experiments concluded that Asian males show higher expression of the receptor [47]. However, more studies need to be conducted to profile a linkage with ethnicities based on ACE2 expression and COVID-19 epidemiological features. The overall function of ACE2 in different populations and the genetic background correlations, are yet to be understood in detail [48]. A systematic analysis of variants of ACE2 (coding region variants) that can influence the expression pattern has been performed. The genetic analysis from microarray data showed that the East Asian populations have a higher allelic frequency of different eQTL variants associated with higher expression of ACE2. More studies on the pilot data need to be performed in other populations to report concrete evidence related to receptor and virus spike protein [49].

ACE2 Knockout Mouse for Acute respiratory Distress Syndrome (ARDS) Investigation

Major causes of death resulting from SARS include acute lung injury along with ARDS. ACE2 knockout mice are reported to be protected from infections by SARS [50]. Moreover, studies showing data from knockout ACE2 receptors have depicted that the spike protein of the virus can cause the downregulation of the ACE2 expression and ACE2 being involved in the protection of lungs from acute injury of the lungs [50, 51]. The introduction of recombinant ACE2 protein can reduce ARDS in mice due to the angiotensin and renin pathway [51]. Moreover, knockout ACE2 mice have been reported to be more prone to impaired lung functionality and exacerbated fibrosis of the lung along with reduced exercise capacity when compared with wild-type mice [52]. In another investigation, knockout ACE2 mice depicted an increased level of lung edema, increased vascular permeability and demonstrated severe lung disease [51].

On the one hand, knockout ACE2 shows severe lung disease, the introduction of recombinant ACE leads to elevated symptoms related to ARDS [53]. It can be deduced from the studies on knockout ACE2 models that ACE2 is a key factor involved in the pathogenesis of SARS viruses and could be the most promising target for therapy that does not include the immunization procedures that can target ARDS. Based on the data obtained through knockout studies, recombinant human ACE2 studies showed promising results in improving the pulmonary circulatory hemodynamics and arterial hypoxemia associated with ARDS [54]. ACE2 knockout mice are known to be resistant to SARS infection as the viral titers determined from the knockout model were a hundred thousand folds lower than the wild-type mice lungs [50].

K18-hACE2 Transgenic Mouse

Coronaviruses, especially those that cause SARS, infect many animal species, including ferrets, mice, cynomolgus, hamsters, and rhesus macaques, among others [55]. Apart from different types of coronaviruses available for studies that demonstrate the infectivity comparable to human coronaviruses. The clinical disease that arises from infection by the SARS-CoV is difficult to replicate in animals in terms of clinical signs and severity as observed in the patients. To determine the vaccine efficacy along with the overall pathogenesis of SARS-CoV, a reproducible and equivalent animal model is the need of the hour that can mimic the immune response in the host as well. Transgenic models are preferred to overcome this drawback, *e.g.,* hACE2 transgenic mice, which show overexpression of the receptor ACE against the SARS-CoV [56]. Since mACE2 does not bind as efficiently with the virus as hACE2. Therefore hACE2 is the specific target for generating transgenic mice. Moreover, the expression of ACE2 being higher in transgenic hACE2 mice also result in a severe disease upon infection with the SARS-CoV in the epithelia of mice [57]. pK18-hACE2 transgenic mice were generated by cloning into pCR2.1-TOPO vector the amplified hACE2 coding sequence from IMAGE consortium clone ID 5243048. The final construct for generating transgenic mice contained a promoter and intron for human cytokeratin 18 (K18 gene) and the enhancer sequence obtained from the alfalfa mosaic virus upstream to the hACE2 coding sequence. Besides, 2 exons and 1 intron of K18 along with polyA signal tail were included for bringing higher specificity towards the epithelia in terms of selective translation in the downstream sequence [57, 58]. For the final generation of the mice, the transgene was injected into pronuclei of the fertilized mice eggs (C57BL/6J) for embryo generation and validated by PCR specific for transgene primers. In one of the recent reports, the SARS-CoV-2 viral agent responsible for the COVID-19 pandemic (one of the earlier isolates) was infected in transgenic hACE2 mice for determining the pathogenicity of the novel SARS-CoV-2 in hACE2 mice [59]. As a result of this experimental infection, the mice lost weight and demonstrated interstitial pneumonia, known as the clinical signs of COVID-19 [59, 60]. Specific immunoglobulins (IgG) targeting SARS-CoV-2 were also observed in the lungs of transgenic hACE2 mice along with virus replication. More studies are needed to determine the immune response against the infection in these animals.

TMPRSS2 Knockout Mouse for Viral Entry and Pathogenesis Studies

Coronavirus fusion glycoproteins which are also known as spike proteins, are cleaved by transmembrane protease serine-type 2 (TMPSS2) belongs to a family of transmembrane serine protease type II. Thus activates the spike protein resulting in the fusion of the cell-virus membrane to facilitate the next step of infection further; the entry of the virus in the host cell [61 - 63]. There are reports which suggest that TMPRSS2 knockout mice are resistant to severe outcomes from infection by the influenza virus. At the same time, higher expression of this gene leads to severe outcomes after infection with the influenza virus [64, 65]. Mice deficient in TMPRSS2 are reported to have shown a reduced loss of weight and replication of viral agents in the lungs. It spreads the virus in the airways of the animals when infected with SARS-CoV and MERS-CoV [61]. The viral entry of coronaviruses and influenza viruses depends critically on TMPRSS2 as the viral protein interacts and binds with ACE2 localized in the epithelia. Viral protein is cleaved by special proteases such as TMPRSS2 to activate the process of internalization of the virus, leading to the next phases of the infection [66]. SARS-CoV-2 and other coronaviruses and influenza viruses require TMPRSS2 to activate the virus and its entry into the host cell for carrying the infection [62, 67, 68]. Therefore, TMPRSS2 can be placed at the center of the pathogenesis of COVID-19 and other pandemics of the past [69].

Since it has been established that TMPRSS2 is vital for entry of SARS-CoV-2 and involved in the dysregulation of ACE2. Therefore, it has been hypothesized by various accounts that it can play a vital role in preventing the critical circumstances of COVID-19 disease if used in a well-defined elaborated therapeutic strategy [70]. TMPRSS2 mediated entry of the SARS-CoV-2 can be inhibited by the serine protease inhibitor known as camostat mesylate [71, 72]. The envelope and plasma membrane fusion between SARS-CoV-2 mediated by TMPRSS2 and ACE2 can also be inhibited by nafamostat mesylate showing 10-times more efficacy than the camostat mesylate [73]. TMPRSS2 is now considered one of the most promising candidates as a therapeutic target for COVID-19. TMPRSS2 knockout mice model study indicated that the influenza virus entry into the cell is inhibited compared to wild-type mice, further implying the role of TMPRSS2 in regulating the pathogenesis of viruses as the crucial step of viral entry inhibition can lead to reduced mortality [74]. TMPRSS2 knockout mouse model can be generated in C57BL/6 Embryonic Stem Cells (ESCs) usually obtained from KOMP (knockout Mouse Project) repository. It is followed by injection of ESCs into blastocyst for generating chimeric mice, followed by male and female mice for creating homologous genotype [61, 75]. The viral kinetics observed in the lungs of TMPRSS2 knockout mice upon infection by SARS-CoV were reduced along with a reduced weight loss upon infection. Moreover, the inflammatory cytokine and chemokine response usually associated with such infections were also observed to be weakened in TMPRSS2 knockout mice [61]. For SARS-CoV-2 experimental infections in mice models, more studies need to be performed to understand the underlying mechanisms of the inflammation-mediated responses and immune responses generated *via* infections that lead to severe clinical circumstances of COVID-19 disease.

STAT1 Knockout Mouse for Studying Pneumonia and Antiviral Strategies

Signal transducer and activator of transcription 1 (STAT1) is considered one of the STAT family members of proteins involved in the signaling responses of the innate immune system. The signaling works by cytokines or growth factors that elicit response inside the cells, leading to phosphorylation of these proteins by the kinases associated with certain receptors, further causing the translocation of these proteins to the nucleus. One of the most important cytokine-mediated signalings in immune responses caused by viruses is interferon receptor signaling, which requires STAT1 responses [76]. The severe cases of COVID-19 show a cytokine storm phenotype, which is considered to be caused by SARS-CoV-2 nsp3 due to the de-mono-ADP-ribosylation of STAT1. It further highlights the importance of STAT1 as a therapeutic target in the precarious times of the COVID-19 pandemic [77]. A group of cytokines known as type 1 interferons (IFN-1) having further subtypes is known to be secreted by different cells like dendritic cells when pattern recognition receptors (PRRs) recognize the viral antigens or components [78]. IFN-1 is considered the first type of cytokine produced and released upon infection by a viral agent.

Interferon gets fixated upon interferon-α/β receptor (IFNAR), transcription factors including STAT1 are phosphorylated, leading to their translocation to the nucleus, further causing activation interferon-stimulated genes (ISGs). ISGs are known for the modulation of immune responses and signaling related to inflammatory pathways. After activation, ISGs lead to the further secretion of cytokines promoting adaptive immunity and interference with viral replication or spread and slowing down the cell's metabolism [79, 80]. Previously available IFN-1 treatment data on SARS-CoV and MERS-CoV can be valuable in determining the SARS-CoV-2 related mechanisms of pathogenesis and immune responses, as both of these viruses led to the disruption of the interferon signaling pathway. SARS-

CoV Orf6 protein has been reported to inhibit the STAT1 transport to the nucleus upon interferon response by disrupting karyopherin transport [81, 82]. Therefore, STAT1 knockout models are important in understanding the role of viral proteins and their subsequent action in determining the immune response resulting from the infection [83]. The innate immune response that leads to clearance of the SARS-CoV also requires STAT1 activity, which modulates the IFN signaling [84]. IFN deficient mice showed that these components of innate immune responses are required STAT1 deficiency to prolong the viral shedding or susceptibility, allowing for lethal infection outcomes. STAT1 deficient mice data revealed the mechanistic role of these proteins in regulating SARS-CoV pathogenesis in the lungs.

Moreover, the pathogenesis of SARS-CoV seemed to be dependent on STAT1 and not on IFN subtypes, highlighting the role of STAT1 in controlling SARS especially viral replication, wound repairing, or cell proliferation in the lethal type disease [85]. Profibrotic phenotype resulting from the lethal outcome of SARS-CoV in the lungs of STAT1 knockout mice was also reported [86]. Therefore, the role of STAT1 in clearing the SARS-CoV-2 infection cannot be avoided and can be used in determining the therapeutic strategies for lethal conditions of COVID-19 [87]. Moreover, the role of STAT1 knockout, as highlighted in studies, demonstrated the role of an innate immune response about interferon signaling, can be utilized for potential therapeutic approaches for COVID-19.

Standard Mouse Strains (BALB/c mice, C57BL/6, and 129S6)

The development of COVID-19 therapy approaches along with vaccine studies, and preclinical investigations can be performed in these mice as they are known to support the replication of viral agents (SARS-CoV and MERS). The standard mice used in laboratory research, like BALB/c mice, C57BL/6, and 129S6, demonstrate the SARS-CoV replication along with other mice models in conjunction with the experimental designs [55]. Mouse-adapted SARS-CoV-2 infection in BALB/c mice showed severe symptoms compared to young mice, showing the clinical similarities observed in human patients of COVID-19 [88, 89]. Moreover, acute lung injury models have also been developed using C57BL/6 mice, which may further understand the therapeutic agent selection against ARDS associated with the severity of COVID-19 [90]. Similarly, 126S6 mice have been used in viral studies investigating the immune responses elicited upon viral infection [91].

Inbred Mice for Pathogenesis and Therapeutic Response Studies

Mouse strains of inbred nature that are available widely can also be adapted in the experimental designs to understand various parameters associated with the pathogenesis and pathophysiology of COVID-19. For example, age-related mortality can be studied in more detail in mouse models that are infected with SARS-CoV-2 [19]. The pneumonitis and clinical symptoms of SARS have been mimicked in several inbred mouse species, including BALB/c, C57BL/6, and 129S [84, 92 - 94]. The main reason for inbred mice being animals of choice for COVID-19 disease is their cost-effectiveness, smaller size, larger numbers to include a valid statistical output, and ease of manipulation at the genetic level [95]. 129S6 strain of mice is observed to report SARS susceptibility higher than BALB/c or B6 mice because the infection led to mild interstitial pneumonitis 2 days post-infection [84].

Similarly, TNF-alpha, a known pro-inflammatory cytokine, was reported at higher levels in BALB/c mice when recorded 2-9 days post-infection [94]. Age-related severity of SARS has already been demonstrated in aged BALB/c mice, which is observed in previous SARS outbreaks as well [93]. As seen in COVID-19 patients, viral replication is observed in the respiratory tract, and BALB/c also shows the same pattern of viral replication upon infection with viral agents in experimental conditions, leading to respiratory distress. Other clinical signs of weight loss, edema, dehydration, and pneumonitis were also observed in such mice strains when infected with SARS-CoV [96].

Humanized Immune System Mice for Vaccine Approaches

COVID-19 has overwhelmed many healthcare systems and has impacted economies negatively since its spread globally. If a COVID-19 vaccine becomes available for public immunization, life globally can go back to normalcy. Many vaccine candidates for COVID-19 are under investigation, and some are in clinical trials [74, 97]. Preclinical studies to develop an approach against SARS-CoV-2 require animal models corresponding to the immune responses as elicited in humans against the viral agent [98]. The antigens presented to the Major Histocompatibility Complex (MHC), however, vary between different species. Therefore, the mice models that can carry human leukocyte antigen genes can mimic the human response to the epitope-based vaccines and assist in developing or discovering the vaccines for COVID-19 in animal models [99].

Moreover, the vaccine discovery process can become rapid if the humanized immune system containing mice model is used for this purpose [100]. They can enhance the discovery process by speedily eliciting the response for efficacy studies and the immune response or memory generated upon vaccinated and un-immunized mice [37, 101 - 103]. Human immune cell engrafted mice have also been instrumental in determining the immune response for a vaccine candidate and include a promising approach in combating COVID-19 [104, 105]. Immuno-deficient mice, when engrafted with peripheral blood mononuclear cells, exhibit another vaccine modeling approach [106].

CONCLUSION AND FUTURE PERSPECTIVES

Although there are many mice strains available that have assisted in understanding the pathogenesis of SARS and SARS-CoV previously, COVID-19 caused by SARS-CoV-2 presents a new challenge to the scientific community. Although mice and humans have shared genes, mice as *in vivo* replicas of COVID-19 or disease models require overcoming the challenges that are unique to the virus. The challenges include the model not possessing the receptor for the virus as human cells have mouse protein expression not being similar to human proteins. The binding affinity is different among viral and animal proteins. It also has a slightly distinct immune system among different species. Due to the aforementioned challenges, certain approaches have been utilized to overcome certain challenges, including transgenic mice representing the human version of certain aspects of the pathogenesis, knockout mice revealing the functions of intracellular programs required for the disease patterns, and inbred mice as age-related mortality models for disease, *etc*. In the end, mice models can also provide a great tool in discovering the therapeutic targets for the disease, which are not obvious at first but can be unearthed upon functional studies. Moreover, the information obtained through studies conducted in various types of mouse models consequently leads to the development phases of the vaccine or a drug target. Therefore, recently used immunized or immuno-deficient mice for investigating vaccine candidates or drug targets will ultimately lead to our understanding of rapidly concluding the different phases of discovery, therefore providing a gateway to quick response in times like COVID-19.

CONSENT FOR PUBLICATION

Not applicable.

CONFLICT OF INTEREST

The author confirms that this chapter contents have no conflict of interest.

ACKNOWLEDGEMENT

Declared none.

REFERENCES

[1] Huang C, Wang Y, Li X, *et al.* Clinical features of patients infected with 2019 novel coronavirus in Wuhan, China. Lancet 2020; 395(10223): 497-506. [http://dx.doi.org/10.1016/S0140-6736(20)30183-5] [PMID: 31986264]

[2] Li Q, Guan X, Wu P, *et al.* Early transmission dynamics in Wuhan, China, of novel coronavirus-infected pneumonia. N Engl J Med 2020; 382(13): 1199-207.
[http://dx.doi.org/10.1056/NEJMoa2001316] [PMID: 31995857]

[3] Saadat S, Rawtani D, Hussain CM. Environmental perspective of COVID-19. Sci Total Environ 2020; 728: 138870.
[http://dx.doi.org/10.1016/j.scitotenv.2020.138870] [PMID: 32335408]

[4] Ross J. The exacerbation of burnout during COVID19: A major concern for nurse safety. J PeriAnesthesia Nurs 2020. 35(4): 439–440.
[http://dx.doi.org/10.1016/j.jopan.2020.04.001]

[5] Paraskevis D, Kostaki EG, Magiorkinis G, Panayiotakopoulos G, Sourvinos G, Tsiodras S. Full-genome evolutionary analysis of the novel corona virus (2019-nCoV) rejects the hypothesis of emergence as a result of a recent recombination event. Infect Genet Evol 2020; 79: 104212.
[http://dx.doi.org/10.1016/j.meegid.2020.104212] [PMID: 32004758]

[6] Wu F, Zhao S, Yu B, *et al.* A new coronavirus associated with human respiratory disease in China. Nature 2020; 579(7798): 265-9.
[http://dx.doi.org/10.1038/s41586-020-2008-3] [PMID: 32015508]

[7] World Health Organization. WHO Coronavirus Disease (COVID-19). Dashboard. World Heal Organ 2020.

[8] Verity R, Okell LC, Dorigatti I, *et al.* Estimates of the severity of coronavirus disease 2019: a model-based analysis. Lancet Infect Dis 2020; 20(6): 669-77.
[http://dx.doi.org/10.1016/S1473-3099(20)30243-7] [PMID: 32240634]

[9] Onder G, Rezza G, Brusaferro S. Case-fatality rate and characteristics of patients dying in relation to covid-19 in Italy. JAMA 2020; 323(18): 1775-6.
[http://dx.doi.org/10.1001/jama.2020.4683] [PMID: 32203977]

[10] Rajgor DD, Lee MH, Archuleta S, Bagdasarian N, Quek SC. The many estimates of the COVID-19 case fatality rate. Lancet Infect Dis 2020; 20(7): 776-7.
[http://dx.doi.org/10.1016/S1473-3099(20)30244-9] [PMID: 32224313]

[11] He W, Yi GY, Zhu Y. Estimation of the basic reproduction number, average incubation time, asymptomatic infection rate, and case fatality rate for COVID-19: Meta-analysis and sensitivity analysis. J Med Virol 2020; 92(11): 2543-50.
[http://dx.doi.org/10.1002/jmv.26041] [PMID: 32470164]

[12] He F, Deng Y, Li W. Coronavirus disease 2019: what we know? J Med Virol 2020; 92(7): 719-25.
[http://dx.doi.org/10.1002/jmv.25766] [PMID: 32170865]

[13] Wang Y, Wang Y, Chen Y, Qin Q. Unique epidemiological and clinical features of the emerging 2019 novel coronavirus pneumonia (COVID-19) implicate special control measures. J Med Virol 2020; 92(6): 568-76.
[http://dx.doi.org/10.1002/jmv.25748] [PMID: 32134116]

[14] Gretebeck LM, Subbarao K. Animal models for SARS and MERS coronaviruses. Curr Opin Virol 2015; 13: 123-9.
[http://dx.doi.org/10.1016/j.coviro.2015.06.009] [PMID: 26184451]

[15] Yong CY, Ong HK, Yeap SK, Ho KL, Tan WS. Recent advances in the vaccine development against middle east respiratory syndrome-coronavirus. Front Microbiol 2019; 10: 1781.
[http://dx.doi.org/10.3389/fmicb.2019.01781] [PMID: 31428074]

[16] Bartlett JG. Virology: SARS virus infection of cats and ferrets. Infect Dis Clin Pract 2004.
[http://dx.doi.org/10.1097/01.idc.0000129853.80250.2c]

[17] Roberts A, Wood J, Subbarao K, Ferguson M, Wood D, Cherian T. Animal models and antibody assays for evaluating candidate SARS vaccines: summary of a technical meeting 25-26 August 2005,

London, UK. Vaccine 2006; 24(49-50): 7056-65.
[http://dx.doi.org/10.1016/j.vaccine.2006.07.009] [PMID: 16930781]

[18] Lamirande EW, DeDiego ML, Roberts A, *et al.* A live attenuated severe acute respiratory syndrome coronavirus is immunogenic and efficacious in golden Syrian hamsters. J Virol 2008; 82(15): 7721-4.
[http://dx.doi.org/10.1128/JVI.00304-08] [PMID: 18463152]

[19] Roberts A, Lamirande EW, Vogel L, *et al.* Animal models and vaccines for SARS-CoV infection. Virus Res 2008; 133(1): 20-32.
[http://dx.doi.org/10.1016/j.virusres.2007.03.025] [PMID: 17499378]

[20] Zhao J, Li K, Wohlford-Lenane C, *et al.* Rapid generation of a mouse model for Middle East respiratory syndrome. Proc Natl Acad Sci USA 2014; 111(13): 4970-5.
[http://dx.doi.org/10.1073/pnas.1323279111] [PMID: 24599590]

[21] Yang XH, Deng W, Tong Z, *et al.* Mice transgenic for human angiotensin-converting enzyme 2 provide a model for SARS coronavirus infection. Comp Med 2007; 57(5): 450-9.
[PMID: 17974127]

[22] Munster VJ, de Wit E, Feldmann H. Pneumonia from human coronavirus in a macaque model. N Engl J Med 2013; 368(16): 1560-2.
[http://dx.doi.org/10.1056/NEJMc1215691] [PMID: 23550601]

[23] Menachery VD, Gralinski LE, Mitchell HD, *et al.* Combination attenuation offers strategy for live attenuated coronavirus vaccines. J Virol 2018; 92(17): e00710-18.
[http://dx.doi.org/10.1128/JVI.00710-18] [PMID: 29976657]

[24] Zhou Y, Jiang S, Du L. Prospects for a MERS-CoV spike vaccine. Expert Rev Vaccines 2018; 17(8): 677-86.
[http://dx.doi.org/10.1080/14760584.2018.1506702] [PMID: 30058403]

[25] Cockrell AS, Yount BL, Scobey T, *et al.* A mouse model for MERS coronavirus-induced acute respiratory distress syndrome. Nat Microbiol 2016; 2: 16226.
[http://dx.doi.org/10.1038/nmicrobiol.2016.226] [PMID: 27892925]

[26] Leist SR, Cockrell AS. Genetically engineering a susceptible mouse model for MERS-CoV-induced acute respiratory distress syndrome. Methods Mol Biol 2020; 2099: 137-59.
[http://dx.doi.org/10.1007/978-1-0716-0211-9_12] [PMID: 31883094]

[27] Dhama K, Sharun K, Tiwari R, *et al.* COVID-19, an emerging coronavirus infection: advances and prospects in designing and developing vaccines, immunotherapeutics, and therapeutics. Hum Vaccines Immunother 2020; 16: pp. (6)1232-38.
[http://dx.doi.org/10.1080/21645515.2020.1735227]

[28] Doudna JA, Charpentier E. The new frontier of genome engineering with CRISPR-Cas9. Science 2014. 346(6213).
[http://dx.doi.org/10.1126/science.1258096]

[29] Cong L, Ran FA, Cox D, *et al.* Multiplex genome engineering using CRISPR/Cas systems. Science 2013. 339(6121): 819-23.
[http://dx.doi.org/10.1126/science.1231143]

[30] Pardee K, Green AA, Takahashi MK, *et al.* Rapid, low-cost detection of zika virus using programmable biomolecular components. Cell 2016; 165(5): 1255-66.
[http://dx.doi.org/10.1016/j.cell.2016.04.059] [PMID: 27160350]

[31] Guk K, Keem JO, Hwang SG, *et al.* A facile, rapid and sensitive detection of MRSA using a CRISPR-mediated DNA FISH method, antibody-like dCas9/sgRNA complex. Biosens Bioelectron 2017; 95: 67-71.
[http://dx.doi.org/10.1016/j.bios.2017.04.016] [PMID: 28412663]

[32] Myhrvold C, Freije CA, Gootenberg JS, *et al.* Field-deployable viral diagnostics using CRISPR-Cas13. Science 2018. 360(6387): 444-448.

[http://dx.doi.org/10.1126/science.aas8836]

[33] Kellner MJ, Koob JG, Gootenberg JS, Abudayyeh OO, Zhang F. SHERLOCK: nucleic acid detection with CRISPR nucleases. Nat Protoc 2019; 14(10): 2986-3012. [http://dx.doi.org/10.1038/s41596-019-0210-2] [PMID: 31548639]

[34] Xiang X, Qian K, Zhang Z, *et al.* CRISPR-cas systems based molecular diagnostic tool for infectious diseases and emerging 2019 novel coronavirus (COVID-19) pneumonia. J Drug Target 2020; 28(7-8): 727-31. [http://dx.doi.org/10.1080/1061186X.2020.1769637] [PMID: 32401064]

[35] Broughton JP, Deng X, Yu G, *et al.* CRISPR-Cas12-based detection of SARS-CoV-2. Nat Biotechnol 2020; 38(7): 870-4. [http://dx.doi.org/10.1038/s41587-020-0513-4] [PMID: 32300245]

[36] Wei J, Alfajaro M, Hanna R, *et al.* Genome-wide CRISPR screen reveals host genes that regulate SARS-CoV-2 infection BioRxiv 2020. [http://dx.doi.org/10.1101/2020.06.16.155101]

[37] Soldatov VO, Kubekina MV, Silaeva YY, Bruter AV, Deykin AV. On the way from SARS-Co--sensitive mice to murine COVID-19 model. Res Results Pharmacol 2020. 6(2): 1-7 [http://dx.doi.org/10.3897/rrpharmacology.6.53633]

[38] Tipnis SR, Hooper NM, Hyde R, Karran E, Christie G, Turner AJ. A human homolog of angiotensin-converting enzyme. Cloning and functional expression as a captopril-insensitive carboxypeptidase. J Biol Chem 2000; 275(43): 33238-43. [http://dx.doi.org/10.1074/jbc.M002615200] [PMID: 10924499]

[39] Lambert DW, Yarski M, Warner FJ, *et al.* Tumor necrosis factor-α convertase (ADAM17) mediates regulated ectodomain shedding of the severe-acute respiratory syndrome-coronavirus (SARS-CoV) receptor, angiotensin-converting enzyme-2 (ACE2). J Biol Chem 2005; 280(34): 30113-9. [http://dx.doi.org/10.1074/jbc.M505111200] [PMID: 15983030]

[40] Li W, Zhang C, Sui J, *et al.* Receptor and viral determinants of SARS-coronavirus adaptation to human ACE2. EMBO J 2005; 24(8): 1634-43. [http://dx.doi.org/10.1038/sj.emboj.7600640] [PMID: 15791205]

[41] To KF, Lo AWI. Exploring the pathogenesis of severe acute respiratory syndrome (SARS): the tissue distribution of the coronavirus (SARS-CoV) and its putative receptor, angiotensin-converting enzyme 2 (ACE2). J Pathol 2004; 203(3): 740-3. [http://dx.doi.org/10.1002/path.1597] [PMID: 15221932]

[42] Crackower MA, Sarao R, Oudit GY, *et al.* Angiotensin-converting enzyme 2 is an essential regulator of heart function. Nature 2002; 417(6891): 822-8. [http://dx.doi.org/10.1038/nature00786] [PMID: 12075344]

[43] Hamming I, Timens W, Bulthuis MLC, Lely AT, Navis G, van Goor H. Tissue distribution of ACE2 protein, the functional receptor for SARS coronavirus. A first step in understanding SARS pathogenesis. J Pathol 2004; 203(2): 631-7. [http://dx.doi.org/10.1002/path.1570] [PMID: 15141377]

[44] Jia HP, Look DC, Shi L, *et al.* ACE2 receptor expression and severe acute respiratory syndrome coronavirus infection depend on differentiation of human airway epithelia. J Virol 2005; 79(23): 14614-21. [http://dx.doi.org/10.1128/JVI.79.23.14614-14621.2005] [PMID: 16282461]

[45] Lu R, Zhao X, Li J, *et al.* Genomic characterisation and epidemiology of 2019 novel coronavirus: implications for virus origins and receptor binding. Lancet 2020; 395(10224): 565-74. [http://dx.doi.org/10.1016/S0140-6736(20)30251-8] [PMID: 32007145]

[46] Hofmann H, Geier M, Marzi A, *et al.* Susceptibility to SARS coronavirus S protein-driven infection correlates with expression of angiotensin converting enzyme 2 and infection can be blocked by soluble

receptor. Biochem Biophys Res Commun 2004; 319(4): 1216-21.
[http://dx.doi.org/10.1016/j.bbrc.2004.05.114] [PMID: 15194496]

[47] Zhao Y, Zhao Z, Wang Y, Zhou Y, Ma Y, Zuo W. Single-Cell RNA expression profiling of ACE2, the receptor of SARS-CoV-2. Am J Respir Crit Care Med 2020; 202(5): 756-9.
[http://dx.doi.org/10.1164/rccm.202001-0179LE] [PMID: 32663409]

[48] Rothe C, Schunk M, Sothmann P, *et al.* Transmission of 2019-NCOV infection from an asymptomatic contact in Germany. N Engl J Med 2020; 382(10): 970-1.
[http://dx.doi.org/10.1056/NEJMc2001468] [PMID: 32003551]

[49] Cao Y, Li L, Feng Z, *et al.* Comparative genetic analysis of the novel coronavirus (2019-nCoV/SAR--CoV-2) receptor ACE2 in different populations. Cell Discov 2020; 6: 11.
[http://dx.doi.org/10.1038/s41421-020-0147-1] [PMID: 32133153]

[50] Kuba K, Imai Y, Rao S, *et al.* A crucial role of angiotensin converting enzyme 2 (ACE2) in SARS coronavirus-induced lung injury. Nat Med 2005; 11(8): 875-9.
[http://dx.doi.org/10.1038/nm1267] [PMID: 16007097]

[51] Imai Y, Kuba K, Rao S, *et al.* Angiotensin-converting enzyme 2 protects from severe acute lung failure. Nature 2005; 436(7047): 112-6.
[http://dx.doi.org/10.1038/nature03712] [PMID: 16001071]

[52] Rey-Parra GJ, Vadivel A, Coltan L, *et al.* Angiotensin converting enzyme 2 abrogates bleomycin-induced lung injury. J Mol Med (Berl) 2012; 90(6): 637-47.
[http://dx.doi.org/10.1007/s00109-012-0859-2] [PMID: 22246130]

[53] Treml B, Neu N, Kleinsasser A, *et al.* Recombinant angiotensin-converting enzyme 2 improves pulmonary blood flow and oxygenation in lipopolysaccharide-induced lung injury in piglets. Crit Care Med 2010; 38(2): 596-601.
[http://dx.doi.org/10.1097/CCM.0b013e3181c03009] [PMID: 19851091]

[54] Khan A, Benthin C, Zeno B, *et al.* A pilot clinical trial of recombinant human angiotensin-converting enzyme 2 in acute respiratory distress syndrome. Crit Care 2017; 21(1): 234.
[http://dx.doi.org/10.1186/s13054-017-1823-x] [PMID: 28877748]

[55] Subbarao K, Roberts A. Is there an ideal animal model for SARS? Trends Microbiol 2006; 14(7): 299-303.
[http://dx.doi.org/10.1016/j.tim.2006.05.007] [PMID: 16759866]

[56] Li W, Greenough TC, Moore MJ, *et al.* Efficient replication of severe acute respiratory syndrome coronavirus in mouse cells is limited by murine angiotensin-converting enzyme 2. J Virol 2004; 78(20): 11429-33.
[http://dx.doi.org/10.1128/JVI.78.20.11429-11433.2004] [PMID: 15452268]

[57] McCray PB Jr, Pewe L, Wohlford-Lenane C, *et al.* Lethal infection of K18-hACE2 mice infected with severe acute respiratory syndrome coronavirus. J Virol 2007; 81(2): 813-21.
[http://dx.doi.org/10.1128/JVI.02012-06] [PMID: 17079315]

[58] Koehler DR, Chow YH, Plumb J, *et al.* A human epithelium-specific vector optimized in rat pneumocytes for lung gene therapy. Pediatr Res 2000; 48(2): 184-90.
[http://dx.doi.org/10.1203/00006450-200008000-00011] [PMID: 10926293]

[59] Bao L, Deng W, Huang B, *et al.* The pathogenicity of SARS-CoV-2 in hACE2 transgenic mice. Nature 2020; 583(7818): 830-3.
[http://dx.doi.org/10.1038/s41586-020-2312-y] [PMID: 32380511]

[60] Peeri NC, Shrestha N, Rahman MS, *et al.* The SARS, MERS and novel coronavirus (COVID-19) epidemics, the newest and biggest global health threats: what lessons have we learned? Int J Epidemiol 2020; 49(3): 717-26.
[http://dx.doi.org/10.1093/ije/dyaa033] [PMID: 32086938]

[61] Iwata-Yoshikawa N, Okamura T, Shimizu Y, Hasegawa H, Takeda M, Nagata N. TMPRSS2

contributes to virus spread and immunopathology in the airways of murine models after coronavirus infection. J Virol 2019; 93(6): e01815-18.
[http://dx.doi.org/10.1128/JVI.01815-18] [PMID: 30626688]

[62] Matsuyama S, Nagata N, Shirato K, Kawase M, Takeda M, Taguchi F. Efficient activation of the severe acute respiratory syndrome coronavirus spike protein by the transmembrane protease TMPRSS2. J Virol 2010; 84(24): 12658-64.
[http://dx.doi.org/10.1128/JVI.01542-10] [PMID: 20926566]

[63] Glowacka I, Bertram S, Müller MA, *et al.* Evidence that TMPRSS2 activates the severe acute respiratory syndrome coronavirus spike protein for membrane fusion and reduces viral control by the humoral immune response. J Virol 2011; 85(9): 4122-34.
[http://dx.doi.org/10.1128/JVI.02232-10] [PMID: 21325420]

[64] Tarnow C, Engels G, Arendt A, *et al.* TMPRSS2 is a host factor that is essential for pneumotropism and pathogenicity of H7N9 influenza A virus in mice. J Virol 2014; 88(9): 4744-51.
[http://dx.doi.org/10.1128/JVI.03799-13] [PMID: 24522916]

[65] Cheng Z, Zhou J, To KKW, *et al.* Identification of TMPRSS2 as a susceptibility gene for severe 2009 pandemic A(H1N1) influenza and A(H7N9) influenza. J Infect Dis 2015; 212(8): 1214-21.
[http://dx.doi.org/10.1093/infdis/jiv246] [PMID: 25904605]

[66] Böttcher E, Matrosovich T, Beyerle M, Klenk H-D, Garten W, Matrosovich M. Proteolytic activation of influenza viruses by serine proteases TMPRSS2 and HAT from human airway epithelium. J Virol 2006; 80(19): 9896-8.
[http://dx.doi.org/10.1128/JVI.01118-06] [PMID: 16973594]

[67] Chaipan C, Kobasa D, Bertram S, *et al.* Proteolytic activation of the 1918 influenza virus hemagglutinin. J Virol 2009; 83(7): 3200-11.
[http://dx.doi.org/10.1128/JVI.02205-08] [PMID: 19158246]

[68] Hoffmann M, Kleine-Weber H, Schroeder S, *et al.* SARS-CoV-2 Cell entry depends on ACE2 and TMPRSS2 and is blocked by a clinically proven protease inhibitor. Cell 2020; 181(2): 271-280.e8.
[http://dx.doi.org/10.1016/j.cell.2020.02.052] [PMID: 32142651]

[69] Stopsack KH, Mucci LA, Antonarakis ES, Nelson PS, Kantoff PW. TMPRSS2 and COVID-19: serendipity or opportunity for intervention? Cancer Discov 2020; 10(6): 779-82.
[http://dx.doi.org/10.1158/2159-8290.CD-20-0451] [PMID: 32276929]

[70] Xiao L, Sakagami H, Miwa N. ACE2: the key molecule for understanding the pathophysiology of severe and critical conditions of COVID-19: Demon or angel? Viruses 2020; 12(5): E491.
[http://dx.doi.org/10.3390/v12050491] [PMID: 32354022]

[71] Djomkam ALZ, Olwal CO, Sala TB, Paemka L. Commentary: SARS-CoV-2 cell entry depends on ace2 and tmprss2 and is blocked by a clinically proven protease inhibitor. Front Oncol 2020; 10: 1448.
[http://dx.doi.org/10.3389/fonc.2020.01448] [PMID: 32974166]

[72] University Y. Camostat mesylate in COVID-19 outpatients. Clin Trials 2020.

[73] Hoffmann M, Schroeder S, Kleine-Weber H, Müller MA, Drosten C, Pöhlmann S. Nafamostat mesylate blocks activation of SARS-CoV-2: New treatment option for COVID-19. Antimicrob Agents Chemother 2020; 64(6): e00754-20.
[http://dx.doi.org/10.1128/AAC.00754-20] [PMID: 32312781]

[74] Stahlmann R, Lode H. Medication for COVID-19-an overview of approaches currently under study. Dtsch Arztebl Int 2020; 117(13): 213-9.
[http://dx.doi.org/10.3238/arztebl.2020.0213] [PMID: 32343658]

[75] Sakai K, Ami Y, Tahara M, *et al.* The host protease TMPRSS2 plays a major role in *in vivo* replication of emerging H7N9 and seasonal influenza viruses. J Virol 2014; 88(10): 5608-16.
[http://dx.doi.org/10.1128/JVI.03677-13] [PMID: 24600012]

[76] Schneider WM, Chevillotte MD, Rice CM. Interferon-stimulated genes: a complex web of host

defenses. Annu Rev Immunol 2014; 32: 513-45.
[http://dx.doi.org/10.1146/annurev-immunol-032713-120231] [PMID: 24555472]

[77] Claverie JM. A putative role of de-mono-ADP-ribosylation of STAT1 by the SARS-CoV-2 Nsp3 protein in the cytokine storm syndrome of COVID-19. Viruses 2020; 12(6): E646.
[http://dx.doi.org/10.3390/v12060646] [PMID: 32549200]

[78] Liu YJ. IPC: professional type 1 interferon-producing cells and plasmacytoid dendritic cell precursors. Annu Rev Immunol 2005; 23: 275-306.
[http://dx.doi.org/10.1146/annurev.immunol.23.021704.115633] [PMID: 15771572]

[79] Ivashkiv LB, Donlin LT. Regulation of type I interferon responses. Nat Rev Immunol 2014; 14(1): 36-49.
[http://dx.doi.org/10.1038/nri3581] [PMID: 24362405]

[80] Schoggins JW, Rice CM. Interferon-stimulated genes and their antiviral effector functions. Curr Opin Virol 2011; 1(6): 519-25.
[http://dx.doi.org/10.1016/j.coviro.2011.10.008] [PMID: 22328912]

[81] Frieman M, Yount B, Heise M, Kopecky-Bromberg SA, Palese P, Baric RS. Severe acute respiratory syndrome coronavirus ORF6 antagonizes STAT1 function by sequestering nuclear import factors on the rough endoplasmic reticulum/Golgi membrane. J Virol 2007; 81(18): 9812-24.
[http://dx.doi.org/10.1128/JVI.01012-07] [PMID: 17596301]

[82] Kopecky-Bromberg SA, Martínez-Sobrido L, Frieman M, Baric RA, Palese P. Severe acute respiratory syndrome coronavirus open reading frame (ORF) 3b, ORF 6, and nucleocapsid proteins function as interferon antagonists. J Virol 2007; 81(2): 548-57.
[http://dx.doi.org/10.1128/JVI.01782-06] [PMID: 17108024]

[83] Sallard E, Lescure FX, Yazdanpanah Y, Mentre F, Peiffer-Smadja N. Type 1 interferons as a potential treatment against COVID-19. Antiviral Res 2020; 178: 104791.
[http://dx.doi.org/10.1016/j.antiviral.2020.104791] [PMID: 32275914]

[84] Hogan RJ, Gao G, Rowe T, *et al.* Resolution of primary severe acute respiratory syndrome-associated coronavirus infection requires Stat1. J Virol 2004; 78(20): 11416-21.
[http://dx.doi.org/10.1128/JVI.78.20.11416-11421.2004] [PMID: 15452265]

[85] Frieman MB, Chen J, Morrison TE, *et al.* SARS-CoV pathogenesis is regulated by a STAT1 dependent but a type I, II and III interferon receptor independent mechanism. PLoS Pathog 2010; 6(4): e1000849.
[http://dx.doi.org/10.1371/journal.ppat.1000849] [PMID: 20386712]

[86] Zornetzer GA, Frieman MB, Rosenzweig E, *et al.* Transcriptomic analysis reveals a mechanism for a prefibrotic phenotype in STAT1 knockout mice during severe acute respiratory syndrome coronavirus infection. J Virol 2010; 84(21): 11297-309.
[http://dx.doi.org/10.1128/JVI.01130-10] [PMID: 20702617]

[87] Fung SY, Yuen KS, Ye ZW, Chan CP, Jin DY. A tug-of-war between severe acute respiratory syndrome coronavirus 2 and host antiviral defence: lessons from other pathogenic viruses. Emerg Microbes Infect 2020; 9(1): 558-70.
[http://dx.doi.org/10.1080/22221751.2020.1736644] [PMID: 32172672]

[88] Gu H, Chen Q, Yang G, *et al.* Rapid adaptation of SARS-CoV-2 in BALB/c mice: Novel mouse model for vaccine efficacy BioRxiv 2020.
[http://dx.doi.org/10.1101/2020.05.02.073411]

[89] Dinnon KH, Leist SR, Schäfer A, Edwards CE, Martinez DR, Montgomery SA, *et al.* A mouse-adapted SARS-CoV-2 model for the evaluation of COVID-19 medical countermeasures. BioRxiv 2020.
[http://dx.doi.org/10.1101/2020.05.06.081497]

[90] Van den Steen PE, Geurts N, Deroost K, *et al.* Immunopathology and dexamethasone therapy in a new

model for malaria-associated acute respiratory distress syndrome. Am J Respir Crit Care Med 2010; 181(9): 957-68.
[http://dx.doi.org/10.1164/rccm.200905-0786OC] [PMID: 20093644]

[91] Lundberg P, Ramakrishna C, Brown J, *et al.* The immune response to herpes simplex virus type 1 infection in susceptible mice is a major cause of central nervous system pathology resulting in fatal encephalitis. J Virol 2008; 82(14): 7078-88.
[http://dx.doi.org/10.1128/JVI.00619-08] [PMID: 18480436]

[92] Glass WG, Subbarao K, Murphy B, Murphy PM. Mechanisms of host defense following severe acute respiratory syndrome-coronavirus (SARS-CoV) pulmonary infection of mice. J Immunol 2004; 173(6): 4030-9.
[http://dx.doi.org/10.4049/jimmunol.173.6.4030] [PMID: 15356152]

[93] Roberts A, Deming D, Paddock CD, *et al.* A mouse-adapted SARS-coronavirus causes disease and mortality in BALB/c mice. PLoS Pathog 2007; 3(1): e5.
[http://dx.doi.org/10.1371/journal.ppat.0030005] [PMID: 17222058]

[94] Subbarao K, McAuliffe J, Vogel L, *et al.* Prior infection and passive transfer of neutralizing antibody prevent replication of severe acute respiratory syndrome coronavirus in the respiratory tract of mice. J Virol 2004; 78(7): 3572-7.
[http://dx.doi.org/10.1128/JVI.78.7.3572-3577.2004] [PMID: 15016880]

[95] Tuttle AH, Philip VM, Chesler EJ, Mogil JS. Comparing phenotypic variation between inbred and outbred mice. Nat Methods 2018; 15(12): 994-6.
[http://dx.doi.org/10.1038/s41592-018-0224-7] [PMID: 30504873]

[96] Cleary SJ, Pitchford SC, Amison RT, *et al.* Animal models of mechanisms of SARS-CoV-2 infection and COVID-19 pathology. Br J Pharmacol 2020; 177(21): 4851-65.
[http://dx.doi.org/10.1111/bph.15143] [PMID: 32462701]

[97] Corey L, Mascola JR, Fauci AS, Collins FS. A strategic approach to COVID-19 vaccine R & D. Science 2020; 368(6494): 948-50.
[http://dx.doi.org/10.1126/science.abc5312]

[98] Li H, Zhou Y, Zhang M, Wang H, Zhao Q, Liu J. Updated approaches against SARS-CoV-2. Antimicrob Agents Chemother 2020; 64(6): e00483-20.
[http://dx.doi.org/10.1128/AAC.00483-20] [PMID: 32205349]

[99] Deb B, Shah H, Goel S. Current global vaccine and drug efforts against COVID-19: Pros and cons of bypassing animal trials. J Biosci 2020; 45: 82.
[http://dx.doi.org/10.1007/s12038-020-00053-2] [PMID: 32554907]

[100] Wang H, Zhang Y, Huang B, *et al.* Development of an inactivated vaccine candidate, BBIBP-CorV, with potent protection against SARS-CoV-2. Cell 2020; 182(3): 713-721.e9.
[http://dx.doi.org/10.1016/j.cell.2020.06.008] [PMID: 32778225]

[101] Lakdawala SS, Menachery VD. The search for a COVID-19 animal model. Science (80-) 2020.
[http://dx.doi.org/10.1126/science.abc6141]

[102] Cimolai N. Defining protective epitopes for COVID-19 vaccination models. J Med Virol 2020; 92(10): 1772-3.
[http://dx.doi.org/10.1002/jmv.25876] [PMID: 32285942]

[103] Padron-Regalado E. Vaccines for SARS-CoV-2: Lessons from Other Coronavirus Strains. Infect Dis Ther 2020; 1-20.
[http://dx.doi.org/10.1007/s40121-020-00300-x] [PMID: 32328406]

[104] Janice Oh HL, Ken-En Gan S, Bertoletti A, Tan YJ. Understanding the T cell immune response in SARS coronavirus infection. Emerg Microbes Infect 2012; 1(9): e23.
[http://dx.doi.org/10.1038/emi.2012.26] [PMID: 26038429]

[105] Florindo HF, Kleiner R, Vaskovich-Koubi D, *et al.* Immune-mediated approaches against COVID-19.

Nat Nanotechnol 2020; 15(8): 630-45.
[http://dx.doi.org/10.1038/s41565-020-0732-3] [PMID: 32661375]

[106] Brehm MA, Wiles MV, Greiner DL, Shultz LD. Generation of improved humanized mouse models for human infectious diseases. J Immunol Methods 2014; 410: 3-17.
[http://dx.doi.org/10.1016/j.jim.2014.02.011] [PMID: 24607601]

CHAPTER 2

Different Cell Lines for SARS-CoV-2

Sonali Bajaj[1], Neha Sharma[1], Abhinav Anand[1,2], Devesh Tewari[1] and Navneet Khurana[1,*]

[1] *School of Pharmaceutical Sciences, Lovely Professional University, Phagwara, Punjab, PIN- 144 411, India*

[2] *CT Institute of Pharmaceutical Sciences, CT Group of Institutions, Shahpur, Jalandhar, Punjab, PIN- 144 020, India*

Abstract: The recent emergence of the novel *betacoronavirus*, pathogenic severe acute respiratory syndrome-coronavirus-2 (SARS-CoV-2) with high nucleotide identity to SARS-CoV represents the causative agent of a potentially deadly disease coronavirus disease-19 (COVID-19) in Wuhan, China, and spreading across several countries globally pose a great global public health concern. Until a vaccine is available, effective therapy must be identified, and many clinical trialshave been executed worldwide. Various *in vitro* investigations are ongoing using different cell cultures to find alternative treatment options, allowing SARS-CoV-2 replications. Various cell lines are susceptible to the SARS-CoV-2 infection. In this chapter, literature regarding SARS-CoV-2 isolated in several cell lines commonly used for diagnostic or research purposes has been summarized. It also shows that SARS-CoV-2 can achieve high titers in various cell cultures derived from different species. In addition, these cell lines are extensively used in the diagnosis, to study pathophysiology, genome studies, and the finding of new targets for drug development and provide new ideas for the discovery of lead compounds with potential therapeutic agents against novel COVID-19.

Keywords: Anti-viral, Betacoronavirus, Cell lines, Clinical trials, Lead compounds, SARS-CoV-2.

INTRODUCTION

The first outbreak of the novel coronavirus occurred in Wuhan on December 12, 2019, in China, and abruptly spread to several other nations. The World Health Organization (WHO) declared a name for 2019-nCoV infectious disease coronavirus disease-19 (COVID-19) on February 11, 2020. The virus name was renamed Severe Acute Respiratory Syndrome-coronavirus-2 (SARS-CoV-2) by the International Committee of Taxonomy of Viruses, earlier called 2019-nCoV [1].

[*] **Corresponding author Navneet Khurana:** School of Pharmaceutical Sciences, Lovely Professional University, Phagwara, Punjab, PIN- 144 411, India; E-mail: navi.pharmacist@gmail.com

During the last 20 years, three infectious diseases, such as SARS and the Middle East Respiratory Syndrome (MERS), have been triggered by coronaviruses.

This suggests that COVID-19 is not the first infection caused by coronavirus [2]. According to the classification of the CoVs, it belongs to the Coronaviridae family having Coronavirinae subfamily of the Nidovirales order, which their subfamily comprises of 4 genera coronavirus, namely α, β, γ and δ [3]. The nucleotide arrangements of the SARS-CoV-2 were associated with SARS-CoV and MERS-CoV that demonstrated greater homology to SARS-CoV, although they were comparably weak with the MERS-CoV [4]. It is not surprising that many researchers have newly verified the genomic similarities associated with the SARS-CoV-2 and bat *betacoronavirus,* which belongs to the sub-genus *Sarbecovirus* [5]. The researchers have also found that the SARS-CoV-2 utilizes the identical receptor known as the Angiotensin-Converting Enzyme 2 (ACE2), similarly to the SARS-CoV [6]. Tyrell and Bynoe first identified the coronaviruses in 1966 and grown the viruses by taking samples of the patients suffering from the common cold [7]. The enclosed, positive single-stranded giant RNA viruses of about 30 kb in size are the characteristics of coronaviruses that infect individuals and the wide-ranging of creatures. Genomic sequencing of the SARS-CoV-2 has already been done. It has been found that the SARS-CoV-2 has originated from the bat that emerged from a photogenetic study [8]. Entry of this virus into the host organism is facilitated with the transmembrane S-glycoprotein (spike), which makes homotrimers protruding from the virus's surface.

Currently, no approved treatment is available for managing COVID-19. There are no specific drugs for the treatment, so there are many supporting measures that are usually given to the patients, including oxygen treatment, antimicrobial agents, antifungal drugs, and Extracorporeal Membrane Oxygenation (ECMO), *etc.*, [9]. This chapter aims to comprehensively gather all the medical literature highlighting the various cell lines that are useful in replicating SARS-CoV-2 that can be fruitful for *in vitro* studies of an anti-viral drug effective in managing COVID-19 disease. Also, not only for evaluating the anti-viral drugs but also for these cell lines are useful for various purposes. For instance, to study the pathogenesis, study the genome of this virus, and find the new targets for drug development is important to highlight.

Role of Cell Lines in Scientific Research

Instead of individual cells, immortal cell lines are also used to explore the plethora of biological processes. The benefits include cost-effectiveness, easy-t--use, limitless availability of products, and it avoids the ethical questioning involved with human and animal tissues [10]. In vaccine development, monitoring of the drug metabolism and cytotoxicity, antibody development, the analysis of genetic material regulation, and artificial tissue creation, in addition to the development of biological substances such as therapeutic proteins and cell lines, have revolutionized medical science [11]. Traditionally, the diagnosis of the viral disease has focused on viral pathogens in cell culture isolation. Even though this technique is always sluggish and needs significant scientific skill. The laboratory diagnosis for the viral disease has been recognized as a "gold standard" for decades. Cell lines are extracted from cells separated from the original tissues after broken down through various methods, including enzymatic, mechanical, or chemical. It has been given a huge quantity of cells appropriate for isolation, allowed the monitoring that helps reduction in the use of laboratory animals, and has contributed to antibiotic and clean air pollution [12]. However, in confirming the causative agent of the disease during high prevalence, the culture of cells has always been essential [13]. In current years, however, technical advances, from monoclonal antibody production to molecular diagnosis, have created powerful methods useful in detecting the various forms of viruses. Molecular identification of viral deoxyribonucleic acid (DNA) and ribonucleic acid (RNAs), molecular multiplication using Polymerase Chain Reaction (PCR), and additional methods in diagnostic laboratories have become increasingly usable. Using an RT-PCR multiplex for SARS-CoV detection, scientists evaluated several human and animal cell lines [14]. The goals of the RT-PCR (real time-PCR) technique are:

1. Glyceraldehyde 3-phosphate dehydrogenase, as an internal RNA integrity regulation and help in the development of cDNA.
2. For the input virus identification process, SARS-CoV genomic RNA is targeted.
3. It also showed the 3' co-terminal specific sub genomic RNAs representative of viral ingestion and appropriate for the viral replication initiation process.

As the SARS-CoV is extremely pathogenic, most laboratories are unwilling to separate this virus in culture. Because of the high pathogenic nature of these viruses, co-cultured cell lines serve as the best alternatives, for instance, R-Mix (Diagnostic Hybrids, Inc.). R-Mix is a blend of the mink pulmonary cells and human adenocarcinoma cells, consisting of the strains Mv1Lu and A549, respectively [15].

Table 1. Summary of the different cell cultures with their species of origin and cell type.

Cell Line	Species of Origin	Cell Type
Caco–2	*Homo sapiens*	Colon carcinoma
Huh-7	*Homo sapiens*	Liver hepatocellular carcinoma

(Table 1) cont.....

Cell Line	Species of Origin	Cell Type
A549	*Homo sapiens*	Lung carcinoma epithelium
Intestinal organoids	*Homo sapiens*	Intestinal epithelium
HAE	*Homo sapiens*	Airway epithelium
HEK-293	*Homo sapiens*	Fetal kidney
Calu-3	*Homo sapiens*	Bronchial epithelium
Vero	*Chlorocebus aethiops*	Kidney epithelium
Vero E6	*Chlorocebus aethiops*	Kidney epithelium

There are nine different types of cell lines used in the culturing of SARS-CoV-2, which include Caco–2, Huh-7, A549, intestinal organoids, HAE, HEK-293, Calu-3, Vero, and Vero E6 as shown in Fig. (**1**) and Table **1**. All cell lines originate from the human cell cultures except Vero cell lines obtained from kidney epithelium cells of African green monkeys. Human cell cultures include; colon carcinoma, hepatocellular carcinoma, lung carcinoma epithelium, intestinal epithelium, airway epithelium, fetal kidney cultures, and bronchial epithelium.

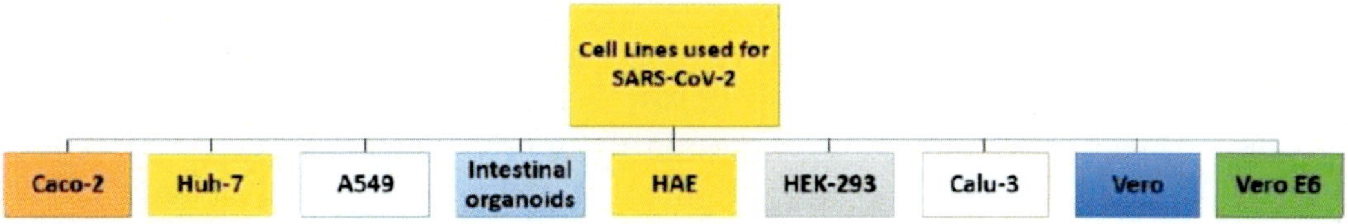

Fig. (1). Various cell lines used for the SARS-CoV-2 replication.

Caco-2 cells

In 1977, Fogh and his colleagues developed the cell culture Caco-2 from a human colon adenocarcinoma to assess anticancer medications' cytotoxic effects and evaluate the various pathways of drug resistance [16]. Across several scientific fields like pharmaceutical science, intestinal epithelial cell lines, including Caco-2, have increased significantly in recent years. The initial experiments on the Caco-2 lines indicate that the cells display a wide range of morphological and biochemical features of small intestine enterocytes after differentiation. This model has become a standard way of predicting human absorption of intestinal drugs and mechanisms underlying the drug transport experiments [17]. The cell's surface confronting the top medium forms a brush border similar to the intestinal epithelium's luminal membrane. The cell surface that binds to the permeable membrane and faces the lowermost medium is transformed into the basolateral membrane [18]. These Caco-2 cell cultures are usually grown in monolayers, display a cylindrical polarized structure, microvilli on the apical surface, tight junctions among neighboring cells, and exhibit hydrolase enzyme activities on the surface of the apical membrane. However, these activities of the hydrolase enzymes in the human fetal colon are identified to be transiently expressed in the 15th week of their pregnancy. It was observed that in the adult human colon, such hydrolase enzymes are absent. Further research on the features of the Caca-2 differentiated cells in the enzyme indicated that they are more similar to the fetal than to adult ilea intestinal absorptive cells [19]. Numerous transporters as well as receptors and enzymes that are involved in the metabolism namely, sulfotransferases (SULTs), UDP glucuronosyltransferases (UGTs) and glutatathione- S- transfers (GSTs), and cytochrome P450 1A (CYP1A) are involved in the Caco-2 cell lines [20].

These cell lines support various types of viral replications. Recently, Caco-2 cell cultures are utilized in the culturing of the SARS-CoV-2 collected from human samples. The efficacy of the Darunavir, which is an oral nonpeptidic HIV-1 protease inhibitor for the treatment of COVID-19, was assessed. But, it was found by the researchers that Darunavir fails to show anti-viral activity in the SARS-CoV-2 infection [21].

Huh-7 cells

The related cell cultures used in *in vitro* research are varied in their genetic and phenotypic profiles, as are human hepatocellular carcinoma (HCC) [22]. For instance, differential proliferative response to Src /Abl blocker in HCC cell cultures, *i.e.*, dasatinib [23], and growth factor-β such as transforming growth factor-beta (TGF-β) stimulation are known [24]. A permanent cancer cell line from the hepatoma tissue, which was operatively removed from a Japanese patient of 57 age in 1985, is Hereafter Huh7 (HuH-7) [25]. It is worth mentioning that Huh-7 cell lines were the long-sought-out cellular system that is permitted full molecular research related to the Hepatitis C Virus (HCV). In several investigations, including research related to iron metabolism, Huh-7 cells have been extensively used and support various viral replications [26].

As a conventional Chinese drug, Lianhuaqingwen (LH) has been used to manage influenza and had a wide-spectrum anti-viral activity on several influenza viruses. It is also used in the regulation of the immune system of the body [27]. The recent *in vitro* investigation of LH has been done to find effectiveness in treating the novel SARS-CoV-2 virus and possible effects on the regulation of the human immune system. In the cell culture of Huh-7, pro-inflammatory cytokine expression levels were assessed by real-time quantitative PCR screening against SARS-CoV-2 infection. In contrast, its anti-viral effects were determined by the Vero E6 cells. These findings suggest that LH shows an anti-inflammatory effect due to decreases the release of the cytokine from the host cells and halts the virus replication [28]. Besides, Huh-7 cells are used in the culturing of SARS-CoV-2 in the plethora. For instance, Huh-7 is used to evaluate the susceptibility of T-lymphocytes in SARS-CoV-2 infection [29] and the examination of the viral architecture of SARS-CoV-2 with the help of electron microscopy [30].

A549 cells

Different forms of cells, including alveolar type I and type II, lead to the pulmonary barrier. Type I cells occupy about 96% of the pulmonary epithelium surface and therefore cannot be segregated. Type II cells have several different roles, even as they occupy a much smaller surface region of the alveolus [31]. In parts of the lung tissue, alveolar cells of type II may be recognized by their characteristic morphological features, the typical pattern of staining using histochemical dyes, and a distinct cytoplasmic organelle. It has multilamellar bodies, a single membrane, and electron-rich materials are the two characteristics features of the suicidal bags, *i.e.*, lysosomes [32]. These type II cells are susceptible to the numerous microbes. These can enter the air sacs of the lungs and be infected by multiple viruses and bacteria, namely influenza virus, SARS coronavirus, *Legionella pneumophelia*, *Bacillus anthracis,* or *Mycobacterium tuberculosis*, which has a capability of replication and survival within type II alveolar epithelial cells [33].

Moreover, most human tumor cell line A549 were done, which is known as the human model of type II alveolar epithelial cells. The cell cultures A549, which was developed in 1972, were taken from the cancerous human alveolar cell and had pulmonary epithelial Type II cells, like lamellar bodies [34]. The ultrastructure of A549 cells has reported various morphological features including, the diameter of the cells were 4.93 μm and 10.59 μm. It was estimated with the help of inverted microscopy and transmission electron microscopy, respectively, and the total volume and surface area of suicidal bags, *i.e.*, lysosomes, were 21.69 μm^3 and 212.04 $\mu m^{2,}$ respectively [35]. The A549 cell line is an excellent model in many aspects since the endocytic role and localization of cytochrome P450 systems primarily depend on the alveoli's surface epithelial type II cells. A549 cell cultures do not exhibit any functional tight junctions between neighboring cells [32].

Comparative study of host transcriptional response by the SARS-CoV-2 with the seasonal Influenza A Virus (IAV) along with human orthopneumovirus (usually called human Respiratory Syncytial Virus (RSV), which is achieved by infecting A549 cells with these three viruses. Data showed a unique transcriptional response, as it does not contain Type I and III interferons (IFN). Also, secreted peptides involved in respiratory disease are the only genes that seem to be distinctive to the SARS-CoV-2 infection [36].

Atazanavir is the first once-daily protease inhibitor (PI) that is licensed in several nations marketed as a therapeutic agent in the Antiretroviral Therapy (ART) regimens in the management of adults, and in certain nations in pediatric, also for patients who are suffering from the HIV-1 infection [37]. SARS-CoV-2 infection was managed *via* atazanavir as a therapeutic agent. *In vitro* research was performed in which A549 cell lines are infected with the SARS-CoV-2 virus. Findings revealed that reduced interleukin-6 (IL-6) levels in SARS-CoV-2 human primary monocyte and cellular mortality and cytokine storm-linked mediators decreased. Mortality of the patients with SARS-CoV-2 infection linked with the increased levels of IL-6 and apoptosis. Research points atazanavir as a new alternative among commercially approved medicines to be considered for successfully managing SARS-CoV-2 infection in ongoing clinical trials [38].

Human Intestinal Organoids

In adult mammals, epithelial cells of the intestine are the quickest in dividing and regenerating various tissues. Intestinal epithelium regeneration is strictly regulated with the help of intestinal stem cells (ISC) and self-renewal [39]. Histologically, epithelial cells of the small intestine are partitioned into two sections:

1. The crypts

2. The villi

Crypts are predominantly made of the proliferative compartment and contain undifferentiated cells, including transit amplification cells and ISCs. Within this area, the epithelium ensures a significant cell turnover and protects the stem cell's niche [40]. On the other hand, villi are a functioning compartment in the epithelial cells that include differentiated cells that lose the power of multiplication and have the characteristics of the developing epithelium. These segregated epithelial cells comprise the villi and can be classified depending on their role such as enterocytes that act to absorb nutrients, goblet cells involved in a defensive mucus layer, and cells of enteroendocrine that produce gastrointestinal hormones [41]. The ISCs regularly regenerate themselves throughout the individual's life cycle and contribute to all sorts of distinct tissue lines. Experiments including genetic lineage tracing systems have presented that the columnar cells present in the crypt region, recognized by the expression of Leucine-rich repeat-containing the G protein-coupled receptor 5 (Lgr5), act as ISCs [42].

Researchers have developed stem cells *in vitro* for many years, driven both by fundamental scientific research and therapeutic goals. Ten years ago, Sasai showed that apart from leading the pluripotent stem cells into a certain lineage, they obtain distinct cell populations. Their stem cells and progeny may follow and organize themselves into similar structures representing several histological and functional aspects of actual organs [43]. The advancement of organoid technology has been scientifically transforming with vast applications in the different research areas, including epithelial and cell biology and clinical applications like organoid biobanks derived from the patients [44]. Such *in vitro* organ mimetic is labeled as organoids. The source of the extracted tissue often determines the structure and characteristics features of the subsequent organoid when it refers to intestinal organoids [45]. Organoids are extensively used in studying various host-bacterial pathologies and used in studies associated with the commonly occurring and problematic pathogens so that new drug targets can be found. In the U.S, for the management of diarrhea which is caused by *Clostridium difficile*, at an annual expense to healthcare approaching 1 billion US$ per year was estimated [46]. The illness caused by *Clostridium difficile* and also to study the various pathologies associated with it, numerous immortalized cell lines are widely used. However, organoid production has made it possible to validate existing theories and further helps in the improvement in the cellular mechanisms related to cytotoxicity [47].

While the clinical manifestation of COVID-19 comprises majorly respiratory symptoms, a minority of patients report gastrointestinal symptoms [48]. In addition, the diagnosis of the COVID-19 rectal swab can be used as it showed the presence of viral RNA [49], even after the nasopharyngeal screening is showing negative results. So, it suggests a pathway of transmission of gastrointestinal and fecal-oral infection [48].

The first *in vitro* culturing of Norovirus was done with the help of the Human Small Intestinal Organoids (hSIOs) [50]. To discover the pathway of SARS-Co--2 that is followed during the transmission of gastrointestinal and fecal-oral infection, researchers cultured ileal hSIOs in four distinct culture mediums. These include 'High Expansion Medium (EXP)', 'Differentiation Medium (DIF)', 'Differentiation Medium-Basic Metabolic Panel (DIF-BMP)' and 'Enteroendocrine Cells (EEC)' which help in the amplification of the virus. hSIOs cultured with a significant proportion of stem cells and enterocyte progenitors in the WNT- EXP. DIF is used to culture organoids, including enterocytes, goblet cells, and a very small number of EECs. BMP2/4 incorporation to the DIF (DIF-BMP) further helps in differentiation and the growth of the cells [51]. It was reported that the SARS-CoV-2 virus utilized the identical receptor, which SARS-CoV already uses, *i.e.*, ACE2, and this receptor is found in the differentiated enterocytes. The study found that enterocytes were readily infected by these two viruses, *i.e.*, SARS-CoV and SARS-CoV-2 which was displayed by the help of the confocal and electron-microscopy in the hSIOs. As a result, significant titers have been identified as infectious viral particles. The mRNA expression screening indicates that the available viral response system has been highly induced. It is stated that hSIOs serve as *in vitro* models for coronavirus infection. These organoids support multiplications of the SARS-CoV-2 and may be utilized in the findings of the pathogenesis of the COVID-19 disease [52].

HAE cells

The nasal cavity, trachea, and bronchi are lined by the epithelium, which acts as a prominent part in defending the host from several harmful substances such as chemical and particulate contaminants and infections [53]. Foreign particles are stuck in mucus on the surface of the mucus membrane and expelled *via* coordinated beating of cilia and/or coughing. Airway inherent host protection involves physical trapping and elimination of toxic compounds associated with baseline or inducible release of antimicrobial agents, antioxidants, and protease blockers and the mobilization of non-specific immune cells that includes neutrophils and monocytes [54]. Epithelial cells of the air sacs have thin and wider surface area which is guarded *via* alveolar macrophages, and this epithelium composed of has a pseudo-stratified surface consisting of a total of six different forms of epithelial cells [55]: a) Ciliated, b) Mucous, c) Clara, d) Serous, e) Basal and f) Dense core- granulated.

Cancer and cystic fibrosis (CF) study are the two key factors behind the production of human airway epithelial cell cultures (HAE) [56], which is stimulated by the shortage of tissue. Scientists have now established a range of specified systems for cell culture, which involves the biochemical and genetic factorsaffecting these and many other airway diseases [57]. Retroviral and lentiviral vectors are the main components of the HAE study toolbox, and many researchers can access their development through individual laboratories. Through collaborating surgeons and pathologists with the appropriate institutional, local and national guidelines, airway epithelial cells may be removed from trachea or bronchi, nasal turbinate, or polyp specimens [54].

In HAE models, airway architectural design and cellular complexity are easy to infect with various human and Zoonotic CoV, such as SARS-CoV and MERS-CoV [58]. In recent investigations, HAE models were used to assess the potential of the various anti-viral drugs in managing the SARS-CoV virus. One of the broad actions as an anti-viral agent ribonucleoside analog β-D-N4-deoxycytidine (NHC, and EIDD-1931) is used to treat the distinct RNA viruses, namely influenza, Ebola virus, CoV, and the Venezuelan Equine Encephalitis Virus (VEEV). Cell lines and preclinical research have revealed that NHC is a successful anti-SARS-CoV-2, MERS-CoV, SARS-CoV, and bat-CoVs in related zoonotic classes 2b or 2c. It also effective against resistance due to the mutations to other nucleoside analog blockers in the treatment of a coronavirus [59].

Remdesivir is a nucleotide analog agent that has board spectrum anti-viral activity [60]. It belongs to the class of antihypertensive agents. Diltiazem is a marketed drug that acts by inhibiting voltage-gated Ca^{2+} channel commonly prescribed to manage angina pectoris and cardiac arrhythmia. The researchers used repurposing of diltiazem as a potential host-directed influenza antagonist due to its so far unknown potential of inducing the IFN anti-viral response, especially type III IFNs [61]. Another *in vitro* study concluded that remdesivir and a combination with diltiazem could be used as an alternative in the management of the COVID-19 with the help of HAE models [62].

HEK 293T cells

In the year 1977, the human embryonic kidney 293 (HEK 293) cell lines were produced by the transformation of the DNA of the human embryonic kidney cell derived from the sheared Adenovirus5 (Ad5) [63]. For the production of the adenovirus or its related viral vectors, there has been a rise in the importance of 293 cells from the last 20 years. This employs various types of uses in gene therapy. For the recombinant adenoviral vector generation, the HEK 293 cell line and associated cell lines were used as the most prominent host [64]. In addition, these HEK 293 cell cultures can also be used in the cancer cells model for transformation *in cellulo* and preclinical experiments. HEK-293 cell lines have the following benefits.

(1) An easily transfected human cell line

(2) Readily available

(3) No deposition of collagen is seen

HEK 293T cells are used in various *in vitro* studies. These cell lines can infect and culturing the SARS-CoV-2 and are used in various types of research work. One of the *in vitro* studies reported that the human 47D11 monoclonal antibody effective against the SARS-CoV-2 and SARS-CoV in the HEK 293T cells. This antibody targets the communal epitope on both viruses and can serve as therapeutic approaches for treating the SARS-CoV-2 infection [65].

In another study, 26 out of the 29 viral proteins were cloned, labeled, and expressed in HEK 293T cell lines. These were detected physically aligned with the human proteins using affinity-purification mass spectrometry that reported 332 high confidence SARS-CoV-2-human protein-protein interactions (PPI). They found that only 67 druggable human protein and host factors can be targeted by the 69 FDA-licensed medications, pharmaceutical products in clinical trials, and *in vivo* studies. Identification of various host dependence factors responsible for the viral infections can provide a valuable understanding of the effective molecular targets that can be beneficial in synthesizing wide-spectrum anti-viral drugs in the management of the COVID-19 and other fatal strains of the coronavirus [66].

Calu-3 cells

A Calu-3 2B4 cell culture is among the few human bronchial epithelial cell cultures that form tight junctions *in vitro* , ideal for modeling the epithelial barrier of the airways used in the pulmonary research work [67]. These cell lines are becoming highly popular in drug delivery and toxicological study. Before spending significant resources on these investigations, the characterization of the epithelium produced in distinct cultural environments is necessary [68]. In the year 1975, Calu-3 cell lines taken from adenocarcinoma epithelium and have serious origin from the proximal bronchial airways of Caucasians at the age of 25 were developed by Fogh [69]. Immuno-staining of desmoplakin shows desmosomes, and E-cadherin shows zonulae adherents in the Calu-3 cell lines. These cell cultures exhibit an mRNA and protein profile belong to the pulmonary epithelial cells [70]. These cell cultures consist of a diverse phenotype that includes secretory and ciliated cells. These differentiates having "tight" junctions, shown with the help of the high Transepithelial Electrical Resistance (TEER) >1000 ohm-cm^2. It also has less permeability to paracellular transport markers [71].

The most commonly used Calu-3 has the following benefits:

(a) It is comparable to other cell lines well distinguished, characterized, and derived from sub-mucosal bronchial glands.

(b) At an Air-Liquid Interface (ALI), these cell lines can be cultured easily to form polarized cells compared to other respiratory cell lines. These cells form a pseudo-stratified layer of columnar cells, exhibit an improved ciliogenesis process. It produces a thick mucus gel layer on the surface of epithelial cells and hold superior barrier integrity, typically in the upper airway epithelium.

These cells exhibit the CF transmembrane conductance regulator (cAMP)-

dependent chloride secretion. In addition, these cells also have the lung surfactant-specific protein proSP-C and comprise mucin granules [72]. These cell cultures have a system where we can evaluate organic cation transporters-inhaled drug-drug interactions. These all are physiologically appropriate, reproducible, inexpensive, and convenient to work with these cell lines [73]. Specifically, these cells cultured under the ALI medium exhibit a more *in vivo* like apical surface compared to those cultured in the submerged medium. Therefore, they are more secure from various xenobiotic challenges [74].

Nafamostat Mesylate (NM) is a wide-spectrum serine protease antagonist [75]. Generally, this drug is prescribed in the management of pancreatitis [76], disseminated intravascular coagulation (DIC) [77], and systemic inflammatory response syndrome by inhibition of several factors including thrombin, plasmin, kallikrein, trypsin, and Cl-esterase in the supplementary system [75]. It is also used in the coagulation cascade as it suppresses the factors such as VIIa, Xa, and XIIa [78].

The earlier investigations found that NM antagonized the MERS-CoV protein-initiated membrane fusion *via* inhibiting transmembrane protease serine2 (TMPRSS2) priming activity. Based on the earlier work, NM was chosen to be the best drug candidate for the COVID-19. Calu-3 cells easily infect SARS-Co--2. It was found that NM antagonized membrane fusion step at the entry of the virus and inhibited SARS-CoV-2 virus [79].

Another drug candidate for the treatment of COVID-19 was tested in the *in vitro* study with the help of Calu-3 cell cultures. Suramin is an anti-parasitic drug [80]. This medication is used to manage sleeping sickness in humans due to infection of trypanosomes and onchocerciasis [81]. Further, it is an effective blocker of the reverse transcriptase enzyme (RNA-directed DNA polymerase) found in retroviruses. Scientists revealed that multiplication of SARS-CoV-2 was blocked at the earlier stages, and also drop in the viral load was found in the Calu-3 cell lines treated with the suramin. Also, this drug slows the progression of the disease [82].

Vero Cells

Being a crucial tool for the life sciences, cell cultures that are derived from mammalian tissues are often significant substrates of animal cells for the development of different forms for biological purposes. Vero cell lines are established from the parent source, *i.e.*, from an African green monkey (*Cercopithecus aethiops*) kidney. Vero cells are one of the utmost frequently utilized mammalian cell cultures [83]. The primary culturing of this tissue was begun on March 27, 1962, by the two scientists Yasumura and Kawikata in Japan.

Numerous continuous cell sub-lines were collected afterward passages of a lot of time, and sub-lines were then selected as the standard known as Vero cell line. After their worldwide spread, usage of these cells broadened from virology in research laboratories to medical procedures that include diagnostic procedures of particular diseases in clinics and bacterial toxin testing.

These cell lines are most susceptible to different forms of viruses: a) SV-40 (Simian polyomavirus), b) SARS-CoV and SARS-CoV-2, c) Influenza A and B viruses, d) Arboviruses, e) Adenoviruses, and f). MERS.

It also reported that these cell lines are also susceptible to various toxins of bacteria such as diphtheria toxin and Vero toxins [84]. These cells possess pseudo-diploid karyotype, and they do not form tumors until the cell passage number was not high [85]. The use of animal substrates for the production of the vaccine is needed to be moved from animals and eggs to certain immortal cell cultures, as animal substrates have various concerns that include quality control, stability, and animal ethics. Thus, these cell lines are widely utilized in the cell substrate to produce human vaccines at a large scale [86]. Genetic variations may occur and develop the tumorigenic phenotype of the Vero cells based on the passage number. For instance, high passage numbers (passage 162) indicate genomic instability and tumorigenic potential. Therefore, only a lower passage number of Vero cells has the non-tumorigenic potential that can be used for vaccine development, which might increase concerns as the seed stocks are now declining due to the extensive usage of this cell substrate [87]. These cell lines are the only immortal cell lines approved by the WHO that serve as the cell's substrate for the production of vaccines and other biological purposes to use in humans against different forms of viruses or bacterial toxins. At the beginning of the 1980s, the first use of these Vero cell lines was made by Montagnon and colleagues at the Institute Merieux to develop Inactivated Poliovirus Vaccine (IPV) for human use. For several years, these cells are widely used for oral poliovirus live vaccine production [88]. Subsequently, inactivated rabies vaccine was also manufactured with the usage of Vero cells [89]. An additional key benefit of these cultures for the manufacturing of vaccines is that it is used in the cultivation and infection on micro-carrier beads and cultured in fermenters to facilitate vaccines production. Anton Van Wezel developed this technology, and this can be used for manufacturing polio and rabies virus vaccines [90]. Several vaccines that are effective for chikungunya, dengue fever, Ross River fever, SARS, smallpox, West Nile encephalitis, and influenza have been produced with the help of these cell lines [86]. These cell lines possessed extensive cytopathic effects and plaque formation, which made them an efficient and reproducible direct technique for the demonstration of several viruses and particular neutralizing antibodies [91]. Vero-cells cannot develop type I IFN in response to the virus, the principal reason behind the highly susceptible behavior of these cell lines towards several types of microorganisms [92]. A classical DNA hybridization analysis was already carried out in which researchers found that homozygous deletion of α- and β1-IFN genes were observed in cell lines [93]. There are a variety of commercial cell lines of Vero cells (namely Vero, Vero 76 and Vero E6), but basically all cell lines obtained from the same parent source *i.e.* African Green Monkey [83].

Literature reported that SARS-CoV-2 infection is highly susceptible to IFN-I pretreatment, although SARS-CoV-2 exhibits almost identical viral replication kinetics in Vero cell culture compared to SARS-CoV. SARS-CoV-2, with type 1 IFN, induces STAT1 phosphorylation and enhances IFN-stimulated genes (ISG) while analyzing the activation of the transcriptional factors and the induction of ISG. On the other side, the original SARS-CoV has no proof of the rise in phosphorylation of STAT1 or ISG protein even though IFN pretreatment is used. The findings together describe significant variations in IFN-I pretreatment responses of SARS-CoV in contrast to SARS-CoV-2. These results can benefit in finding the novel 'therapeutics' for the COVID-19 and help develop the *in vivo* models [94].

Therapeutic Agents Using *in vitro* Models Especially Vero and Vero Derived Cell Lines

Remdesivir

American pharmaceutical industry Gilead Sciences launched a drug Remdesivir that is a prodrug of a 1'-cyano-substituted nucleotide derivative shown potential effect during Ebola virus spread owing to its low 50% effective concentrations (EC_{50}) along with its selectivity to host polymerase in the treatment of the Ebola virus [95]. The compound has shown a wide-spectrum anti-viral potential. It is widely used in the management of the members of several virus families, namely filoviruses (*e.g.,* Ebola virus), paramyxoviruses (*e.g.,* Nipah virus), and coronaviruses (*e.g.,* SARS-CoV and MERS-CoV). For RNA viruses such as SARS-CoV-2, multiplication depends on the viral RNA-dependent RNA polymerase (RdRp), which presents an optimal target due to its important role in RNA synthesis [96]. A recent cell line study showed that remdesivir has potency and has very few adverse effects in the SARS-CoV-2 infection in Vero E6 cell lines. The reported EC_{50} value of this drug was 23.15 μM against this infection [97]. Remdesivir is an adenosine analog that is resistant to exonuclease. It is intracellularly changed into active metabolite nucleoside triphosphates. It helps to efficiently inhibit the RNA chain elongation by terminating the enzyme RNA polymerase. However, this drug cannot be absorbed by viral exonuclease (nsp14) having proofreading activity [98]. So, this is a promising drug amongst all drugs to manage the SARS-CoV-2 virus [96].

Lopinavir

Lopinavir is a potent protease blocker and is prescribed to manage HIV type 1 (HIV-1), a crucial enzyme used to produce mature infectious viruses. It works by preventing HIV-1 maturation, thus blocking infectivity [99]. Therefore, the mechanism behind the anti-viral activity of lopinavir is to prevent consequent susceptible cell infections. It also does not show an effect on cells that have integrated viral DNA. Lopinavir has a higher *in vitro* activity against both wild-type and mutant HIV-1 proteases than ritonavir (an inhibitor of the cytochrome P450 3A isoenzyme). But, its efficacy is critically reduced due to the poor bioavailability of the pre-systemic metabolism *in vivo* model. Lopinavir is used in combination with a reduced dosage of ritonavir that considerably improves plasma concentrations of the drug and helps achieve high and consistent levels of lopinavir [100]. Both protease inhibitors prevent viral nucleic acid multiplication by blocking 3CLpro [101]. In the cell line, investigations of lopinavir as an anti-SARS-CoV-2 in the Vero E6 cell lines were found to be effective.

In addition, co-administration of lopinavir with the other effective drugs against the treatment of COVID-19. It enhances synergism and decreases the inhibitory concentration of lopinavir [97]. Therefore, lopinavir warrants further study for possible benefits in the treatment of COVID-19 shown in Table **2**.

Homorringtonine

Homoharringtonine (HHT) is an alkaloid obtained from *Cephalotoxus fortunei* with anti-leukemic activity and had been the drug of choice for treating patients suffering from acute and chronic myeloid leukemia. The main mechanism by which HHT works is the interruption of the translation process, which is dependent on dose and time as it binds to the ribosome and prevents polypeptide chain elongation [102]. In 2012, Omacetaxine, a semisynthetic derivative of HHT, was licensed by the FDA to manage chronic myeloid leukemias. According to past investigations, HHT has shown anti-viral action and can be used to manage herpesviruses, coronaviruses, and rhabdoviruses [103]. HHT binds to the 80S ribosome and blocked viral protein translation machinery *via* interrupting chain elongation [104]. In a recent investigation, it was observed that HHT is effective against SARS-CoV-2 infection with EC_{50} 2.10 μM in the cell cultures of Vero E6 [97]. Altogether, as a phytoconstituents, HHT is extensively distributed however, its potent anti-viral action in a plethora of viruses requires more exploration.

Emetine hydrochloride

Emetine is an alkaloid obtained from the *Psychotria ipecacuanha* Stokes (Rubiaceae). This herbal plant is called *Cephaelis ipecacuanha.* It is among the major active constituents in ipecac syrup marketed as an emetic and has been widely utilized in herbal medication as an anti-protozoan agent. The mode of action by which it works is that it blocked both ribosomal and mitochondrial protein translation machinery synthesis and hinders the synthesis and functions of nucleic acids. Emetine is used in the management of both intestinal and extraintestinal amoebiasis. It helps in amebic dysentery caused by the infection of *Entamoeba histolytica,* an anaerobic parasitic protozoan [105]. Emetine works as an anti-viral action. According to the past findings, emetine interferes with the viral protein synthesis by inhibiting the 40S ribosomal protein S14 in cells of the host. It has been reported that emetine inhibits HIV reverse transcriptase enzyme, block viral polymerases [106]. In the studies related to the COVID-19 treatment, emetine has shown positive results. In the cell line study, emetine inhibits the SARS-CoV-2 viral multiplication in the Vero E6 cells [97]. Overall, emetine has an anti-viral action, which indicated that emetine is a potential remedy in managing the SARS-CoV-2.

Ivermectin

Ivermectin is a macrocyclic lactone structurally similar to its naturally occurring fermentation product, avermectin B_1, obtained from an actinomycete, *Streptomyces avermitilis*. Ivermectin is an anti-parasitic agent and mainly active against two main phyla of the animal kingdom- a) the Nemathelminthes or nematodes (roundworms) and b) the arthropod (insects, ticks, and mites). The mode of action of ivermectin is the same as avermectin B_1 [107]. They paralyze body-wall muscle in nematodes and arthropods *via* disrupting gamma-aminobutyric acid (GABA)-mediated chloride ion conductance of nerve signals. It has been extensively prescribed to manage the patients having the infection caused by nematode *Onchocerca volvulus,* which is the main reason for blindness in natives of some tropical regions [108]. Subsequently, the latest research showed that ivermectin has an effective role in the SARS-CoV-2 infection in the Vero/hSLAM cell lines, and half inhibitory concentration (IC_{50}) was found to be ~2 μM [109]. The possible anti-viral mechanism of ivermectin acts by inhibition of IMPα/β1 responsible for the nuclear import proteins of the virus [110] shown in Table **2**. Overall, this drug requires further investigation for its efficacy in human to manage the SARS-CoV-2 virus.

Chloroquine/Hydroxychloroquine

Chloroquine and its less toxic derivative hydroxychloroquine are two inexpensive drugs that have been used traditionally as a wide-spectrum therapy for malaria and autoimmune disease [111]. The underlying mechanism of chloroquine and hydroxychloroquine as an anti-viral agent against coronavirus is still unclear. Earlier investigations have suggested that both these drugs block virus infection from entering into the host *via* inhibition of glycosylation of host cell receptors and proteolytic processing by increasing endosomal pH. Moreover, they improve immunity *via* reducing the number of cytokines that inhibit the autophagy and lysosomal action in the cells [112, 113]. The latest investigation suggested that chloroquine worked at entry and post-entry stages of the SARS-CoV-2 virus in Vero E6 cell lines, and EC_{50} was 1.13 μM and half-cytotoxic concentration (CC_{50}) was less than 100 μM [114]. Hydroxychloroquine also showed its potential in the management of COVID-19 in Vero E6 cells [115]. Therefore, it can be reasonably speculated that these are potential drugs for SARS-CoV-2 infection. So, its effective against COVID-19 deserves further study for its efficacy in the human.

Nelfinavir

Nelfinavir is a nonpeptidic, specific, and HIV protease competitive antagonist. It is the main enzyme required for post-translational modifications of HIV propeptides [116]. Nelfinavir has a good safety profile and potent drug in the management of HIV-1 and HIV-2 viruses. Nelfinavir was developed by the private pharmaceutical industry and gained popularity for the management of AIDS in combination with other antiretroviral agents [117]. This drug has been investigated due to its off-target anticancer mechanism [118]. Nelfinavir is also tested for the treatment of COVID-19 in Vero E6 cell cultures in recent investigations. Findings suggested that this protease inhibitor significantly inhibits cell fusion of the viral envelope caused by spike (S) glycoprotein, a key factor in virus infectivity [119 - 121]. *in vitro* studies, nelfinavir has shown high potency against SARS-CoV-2 infection, requiring further exploration for managing COVID-19.

Indomethacin

Indomethacin categorizes in the class as a non-steroidal anti-inflammatory drug (NSAIDs) are extensively prescribed painkillers in the treatment of headache and many of the primary headache disorders [122]. It has a potent inhibitory action on the synthesis of prostaglandins that has a crucial role in the anti-inflammatory response. The production of prostaglandins is blocked as it inhibits cyclooxygenases (COX) 1 and 2 enzymes and is important for most NSAIDs. Indomethacin is prescribed to manage arthritis, fever, several headache syndromes, and dysmenorrhea [123]. Past investigations showed that indomethacin has potency in treating the SARS-CoV virus. In the latest experiments where indomethacin has shown its potency in treating the SARS-CoV-2 virus in the Vero E6 cells. The molecular mechanism underlying the anti-viral activity of indomethacin in the management of the SARS-CoV-2 virus is not fully known and requires further investigation. Results suggested that the possible mechanism of indomethacin as an anti-viral agent may be due to the reduction in the IL-6 and inhibit RNA synthesis [124 - 126] mentioned in Table **2**. Overall, indomethacin is a potent inhibitor of SARS-CoV-2 infection and warrants further exploration.

Merimepodib

Merimepodib is an orally bioavailable, potent, selective, reversible, and uncompetitive antagonist of inosine-5'-monophosphate dehydrogenase (IMPDH) [127]. A crucial component catalyzes the rate-limiting step in the de novo synthesis of the purine nucleotides biosynthesis pathway. Thus, blocking IMPDH could reduce the intracellular guanosine triphosphate (GTP) that is mandatory for the transcription process at the time of viral replication. Merimepodib was marketed for the managing of the hepatitis C virus (HCV) [128]. Literature reveals that merimepodib has *in vitro* anti-viral activity against Ebola, Lassa, and Zika virus [129]. The *in vitro* investigations suggested that merimepodib work as an anti-coronavirus agent against SARS-CoV-2 virus in the Vero E6 cell lines found to be effective and 50% tissue culture, infectious dose ($TCID_{50}$) was 3.3 μM. It is probably due to its IMPDH suppression, which is responsible for guanosine depletion when replication by viral polymerase [130]. Consequently, merimepodib may be a promising COVID-19 therapy alternative that should be further explored for efficacy in humans.

Scutellaria baicalensis

Scutellaria baicalensis (S. baicalensis), also known as Chinese skullcap or Huangqin, is amongst the utmost important medicinal herb prescribed in Chinese herbal medicine and is formally mentioned in the Chinese Pharmacopoeia. This herb possesses a plethora of biological and pharmacological actions, including anti-inflammatory, anticancer, anti-viral, anti-bacterial, anti-hypertensive, and sedative effects. This herb comprises several flavonoids [131]. Baicalin, baicalein, wogonin, and oroxylin A are the major active constituents found in *S. baicalensis* (Georgi), are flavone derivatives containing a phenylbenzopyrone moiety [132]. Various studies are ongoing to find the treatment options for the COVID-19. One of the study ethanolic extracts of *S. baicalensis* (Georgi) and baicalein, one of the flavonoids of this herbal drug, exhibits anti-coronavirus activity as they inhibit the multiplication of SARS-CoV-2 virus in Vero E6 cell cultures. The proposed mechanism behind its anti-viral activity is due to the inhibition of 3CLpro and prevents viral nucleic acid multiplication [133]. Taken together, the results of this investigation provide evidence that *S. baicalensis* Georgi and baicalein may serve as a viable treatment alternative for COVID-19.

Gemcitabine

Gemcitabine is a novel pyrimidine nucleoside derivative of cytarabine (cytosine arabinoside) in which two fluorine atoms have been introduced into deoxyribofuranosyl ring widely used as a standard chemotherapeutic agent [134]. Gemcitabine is different from other anticancer drugs due to its comparatively few adverse effects (typically mild fatigue and modest bone-marrow suppression). Its wide range of activity against different cancers and potency inhibit deoxynucleotide metabolism at clinically effective doses [135]. This drug also possesses anti-viral action in managing various RNA viruses, including enterovirus 71, human rhinoviruses (HRVs), MERS-CoV, SARS-CoV, and coxsackievirus B3. The anti-viral mechanism of gemcitabine hinders the salvage pathway of pyrimidine synthesis and improves innate immunity [136]. Recently, the study reported that gemcitabine has anti-viral action against SARS-CoV-2 infection (EC_{50}= 1.24 μM) in Vero E6 cell cultures [137]. These results demonstrated that gemcitabine may be the alternative option in the COVID-19 therapy but requires preclinical and clinical studies to evaluate the efficacy.

Carmofur

Carmofur (HCFU; 1-Hexylcarbamoyl-5-fluorouracil, Mifurol) is a fluorinated pyrimidine derivate of 5-fluorouracil (5-FU) has an anticancer action, is one of the key drug prescribed to manage individuals suffering from a variety of malignancies [138]. Carmofur is orally bioavailable, used as a solo compound. It is used as adjuvant therapy in cervical carcinoma, breast, colorectal cancer, and gastrointestinal carcinomas. Carmofur is an orally administered prodrug that metabolized intracellularly to active form 5-FU. It helps to inhibits thymidylate synthetase, which is responsible for catalyzing the deoxyuridine monophosphate (dUMP) into deoxythymidine monophosphate (dTMP). Thus, it will inhibit tumor proliferation [139]. HCFU drug is also a potent acid human ceramidase inhibitor marketed as an adjuvant chemotherapeutic agent in Japan since 1981 [140]. In numerous RNA and DNA viruses, proteases have a crucial role in the viral multiplication process. Thus, proteases are frequently used as therapeutic targets during the development of anti-coronavirus drugs [141]. A recent *in silico* study showed with the help of the X-ray crystallography structure of SARS-CoV-2 main protease (M^{pro}) forms a complex with HCFU. Moreover, *in vitro* evaluation of carmofur reveals that this drug inhibits viral replication in Vero E6 cell culture (EC_{50} = 24.30 μM) [142]. Therefore, carmofur serves as a potential lead molecule that can be utilized to manage COVID-19.

Arbidol

The anti-viral medicine arbidol (ARB) is a derivative of indole used in Russia and China in 1993 and 2006, respectively to prevent and manage influenza A, B, and C viruses [143]. In preclinical *in cellulo* studies, ARB has potential anti-viral action against several numbers of RNA or DNA viruses [144]. The mechanism behind the anti-viral action of this molecule acts on important steps of host-virus interactions. It may directly act on the interaction of membrane fusion with the chief players of the primary steps of virus entry and prevents multiplication. Consequently, ARB may also have the potential role to serve as a host-targeting agent (HTA) [145]. Recently, ARB also tested for the SARS-CoV-2 virus treatment, and positive results were seen in Vero E6 cells. ARB inhibits the SARS-CoV-2 virus as it interferes with attachment and intracellular vesicle trafficking [146]. Therefore, results suggested that ARB may be a promising COVID-19 therapy alternative that should be further explored for efficacy in clinical trials.

Table 2. Summary of the possible drugs against SARS-CoV-2 infection.

S. No.	Drug Candidate	Pharmacological Activity	Subjects	EC_{50} (μM)	IC_{50}	CC_{50} (μM)	Mechanism of Action	References
1.	Remdesivir	Adenosine analog	Vero E6 cells	23.15	-	> 100	Inhibits RdRp	[96, 97]
2.	Lopinavir	Protease inhibitor	Vero E6 cells	26.63	-	49.75	Inhibits 3CLpro	[97, 101]
3.	Homorringtonine	Anticancer	Vero E6 cells	2.55	-	59.75	Inhibits protein synthesis	[97, 104]
4.	Emetine hydrochloride	Anti- protozoal	Vero E6 cells	0.46	-	56.46	Inhibits protein synthesis	[97, 105]
5.	Ivermectin	Anti-parasitic	Vero/hSLAM cells	-	2	-	Inhibits IMPα/β1 responsible for nuclear import of proteins of the virus	[109, 110]

(Table 2) cont.....

S. No.	Drug Candidate	Pharmacological Activity	Subjects	EC_{50} (μM)	IC_{50}	CC_{50} (μM)	Mechanism of Action	References
6.	Chloroquine/ Hydroxychloroquine	Anti-malarial	Vero E6 cells	1.13 / 5.47	-	> 100	Inhibits endosomal acidification fusion and improves immunity	[114, 115],
7.	Nelfinavir	Protease antagonist	VeroE6/ TMPRSS2 cells	1.13	-	24.32	Inhibits cell fusion mediated by SARS-CoV□2 spike (S) glycoprotein	[120, 121]
8.	Indomethacin	Cyclooxygenases inhibitor	Vero E6 cells	1	-	-	Inhibits RNA synthesis, reduces IL-6 production	[125, 126]
9.	Merimepodib	IMPDH inhibitor	Vero cells	-	-	-	Reduction in the GTP involved in the viral replication	[130]
10.	*Scutellaria baicalensis*	Anti-viral, anti-hypertensive, anti-bacterial, anticancer.	Vero cells	-	8.5 μg/ml (extract) 0.39 μM (baicalein)	-	Inhibits 3CLpro	[133]
11.	Gemcitabine	Anticancer	Vero E6 cells	1.24	-	>40	Inhibits pyrimidine biosynthesis and improves innate immunity	[136, 137]
12.	Carmofur	Anti-cancer	Vero E6 cells	24.30	-	133.4	Inhibits SARS-CoV-2 main protease (M^{pro})	[142]
13.	Arbidol	Anti-influenza	Vero E6 cells	4.11	-	31.79	Interferes viral binding	[146]

CONCLUDING REMARKS

In conclusion, these cell lines such as Vero, Calu-3, A549, Huh-7, and Caco-2 make accessible to the national and international public health, academia, and pharmaceutical industries for fundamental studies, diagnostic purposes, evaluation of anti-viral agents, and manufacturing of vaccine. We look forward to the collaboration of all researchers worldwide to expedite countermeasure development and testing for SARS-CoV-2. It could assist a good understanding of the pathophysiology of this novel SARS-CoV-2 infection. Moreover, these cell lines can be used as effective drug development candidates to manage the recent and upcoming potential of the SARS-CoV-2 virus. It is also used to control the further spread of this pandemic. However, preclinical and clinical studies are equivalently crucial for effective drug development in managing the COVID-19.

CONSENT FOR PUBLICATION

Not applicable.

CONFLICT OF INTEREST

The author confirms that this chapter contents have no conflict of interest.

ACKNOWLEDGEMENT

Declared none.

REFERENCES

[1] Lai CC, Shih TP, Ko WC, Tang HJ, Hsueh PR. Severe acute respiratory syndrome coronavirus 2 (SARS-CoV-2) and coronavirus disease-2019 (COVID-19): the epidemic and the challenges. Intern. J Antimicrobial Agents. Elsevier B.V. 2020; Vol. 55: p. 105924.

[2] Li X, Geng M, Peng Y, Meng L, Lu S. Molecular immune pathogenesis and diagnosis of COVID-19 J Pharmaceut Analysis. Xi'an Jiaotong University 2020.

[3] Chen Y, Liu Q, Guo D. Emerging coronaviruses: genome structure, replication, and pathogenesis. J Med Virol 2020; 92(4): 418-23.
[http://dx.doi.org/10.1002/jmv.25681] [PMID: 31967327]

[4] Tortorici MA, Veesler D. Structural insights into coronavirus entry. Advances in Virus Research. Academic Press Inc. 2019; pp. 93-116.

[5] Wu A, Peng Y, Huang B, *et al.* Genome composition and divergence of the novel coronavirus (2019-ncov) originating in China. Cell Host Microbe 2020; 27(3): 325-8.
[http://dx.doi.org/10.1016/j.chom.2020.02.001] [PMID: 32035028]

[6] Zhou P, Yang X-L, Wang X-G, Hu B, Zhang L, Zhang W, *et al.* Discovery of a novel coronavirus associated with the recent pneumonia outbreak in humans and its potential bat origin. Nature 2020; 579(7798): 270-3.
[http://dx.doi.org/10.1038/s41586-020-2012-7]

[7] Velavan TP, Meyer CG. The COVID-19 epidemic. Tropical Medicine & International Health 2020; 25(3): 278.
[http://dx.doi.org/10.1101/2020]

[8] Lu R, Zhao X, Li J, *et al.* Genomic characterisation and epidemiology of 2019 novel coronavirus: implications for virus origins and receptor binding. Lancet 2020; 395(10224): 565-74.
[http://dx.doi.org/10.1016/S0140-6736(20)30251-8] [PMID: 32007145]

[9] Chen N, Zhou M, Dong X, *et al.* Epidemiological and clinical characteristics of 99 cases of 2019 novel coronavirus pneumonia in Wuhan, China: a descriptive study. Lancet 2020; 395(10223): 507-13.
[http://dx.doi.org/10.1016/S0140-6736(20)30211-7] [PMID: 32007143]

[10] Gómez-Lechón MJ, Donato MT, Castell JV, Jover R. Human hepatocytes as a tool for studying toxicity and drug metabolism. Curr Drug Metab 2003; 4(4): 292-312. [http://dx.doi.org/10.2174/1389200033489424] [PMID: 12871046]

[11] MacDonald C. Development of new cell lines for animal cell biotechnology. Crit Rev Biotechnol 1990; 10(2): 155-78.http://www.ncbi.nlm.nih.gov/pubmed/2202521 [http://dx.doi.org/10.3109/07388559009068265] [PMID: 2202521]

[12] Birch JR. Culture of animal cells: A manual of basic technique: By R. I. Freshney. J Chem Technol Biotechnol. New York: Alan R. Liss, Inc. 2007; 45: p. (4)330. [http://dx.doi.org/10.1002/jctb.280450414]

[13] Hudu SA, Alshrari AS, Syahida A, Sekawi Z. Cell Culture, Technology: Enhancing the Culture of Diagnosing Human Diseases. J Clin Diagn Res 2016; 10(3): DE01-5. [http://dx.doi.org/10.7860/JCDR/2016/15837.7460] [PMID: 27134874]

[14] Gillim-Ross L, Taylor J, Scholl DR, Ridenour J, Masters PS, Wentworth DE. Discovery of novel human and animal cells infected by the severe acute respiratory syndrome coronavirus by replication-specific multiplex reverse transcription-PCR. J Clin Microbiol 2004; 42(7): 3196-206. http://www.ncbi.nlm.nih.gov/pubmed/15243082 [http://dx.doi.org/10.1128/JCM.42.7.3196-3206.2004] [PMID: 15243082]

[15] Barenfanger J, Drake C, Mueller T, Troutt T, O'Brien J, Guttman K. R-Mix cells are faster, at least as sensitive and marginally more costly than conventional cell lines for the detection of respiratory viruses. J Clin Virol 2001; 22(1): 101-10. https://linkinghub.elsevier.com/retrieve/pii/S1386653201001718 [Internet]. [http://dx.doi.org/10.1016/S1386-6532(01)00171-8] [PMID: 11418357]

[16] Zucco F, Batto A, Bises G, *et al.* An inter-laboratory study to evaluate the effects of medium composition on the differentiation and barrier function of Caco-2 cell lines. JC-A 2005. Available from: journals.sagepub.com journals.sagepub.com [Internet]. [cited 2020 Apr 29]. [http://dx.doi.org/10.1177/026119290503300618]

[17] Artursson P. Epithelial transport of drugs in cell culture. I: A model for studying the passive diffusion of drugs over intestinal absorptive (Caco-2) cells. J Pharm Sci 1990; 79(6): 476-82. [http://dx.doi.org/10.1002/jps.2600790604] [PMID: 1975619]

[18] Yi W, Akoh CC, Fischer J, Krewer G. Absorption of anthocyanins from blueberry extracts by caco-2 human intestinal cell monolayers. J Agric Food Chem 2006; 54(15): 5651-8. [http://dx.doi.org/10.1021/jf0531959] [PMID: 16848559]

[19] Chantret I, Rodolosse A, Barbat A, Dussaulx E, Brot-Laroche É, Zweibaum A, *et al.* Differential expression of sucrase-isomaltase in clones isolated from early and late passages of the cell line Caco-2: evidence for glucose-dependent negative regulation. J Cell Sci 1994; 107(Pt 1): 213-5.

[20] Chiu E, Chow Y, Sun H, Chow EC, Liu S, Du Y, *et al.* The Caco-2 cell monolayer: Usefulness and limitations. Artic Expert Opin Drug Metab Toxicol [Internet] 2008; 4(4): 395-411. [cited 2020 Apr 29] Available from: https://www.researchgate.net/publication/5420246 [http://dx.doi.org/] [PMID:]

[21] De Meyer S, Bojkova D, Cinatl J, Van Damme E, Meng CB, Van Loock M, *et al.* Lack of anti-viral activity of darunavir against SARS-CoV-2. Int J Infect Dis 2020; 97: 7-10. [http://dx.doi.org/10.1101/2020.04.03.20052548]

[22] Nault JC, Galle PR, Marquardt JU. The role of molecular enrichment on future therapies in hepatocellular carcinoma. J Hepatol 2018; 69(1): 237-47. [http://dx.doi.org/10.1016/j.jhep.2018.02.016]

[23] Finn RS, Aleshin A, Dering J, *et al.* Molecular subtype and response to dasatinib, an Src/Abl small molecule kinase inhibitor, in hepatocellular carcinoma cell lines *in vitro* . Hepatology 2013; 57(5): 1838-46. [Internet].

[http://dx.doi.org/10.1002/hep.26223] [PMID: 23299860]

[24] Dzieran J, Fabian J, Feng T, Coulouarn C, Ilkavets I, Kyselova A, *et al.* Comparative Analysis of TGF-β/Smad Signaling Dependent Cytostasis in Human Hepatocellular Carcinoma Cell Lines. PLoS One [Internet] 2013; 8(8): e72252.
[http://dx.doi.org/10.1371/journal.pone.0072252]

[25] Nakabayashi H, Taketa K, Miyano K, Yamane T, Sato J. Growth of human hepatoma cells lines with differentiated functions in chemically defined medium. Cancer Res 1982; 42(9): 3858-63.
[PMID: 6286115]

[26] Lohmann V, Körner F, Koch JO, Herian U, Theilmann L, Bartenschlager R. Replication of subgenomic hepatitis C virus RNAs in a hepatoma cell line. Science 1999; 285(5424): 110-3.
[http://dx.doi.org/10.1126/science.285.5424.110]

[27] Ding Y, Zeng L, Li R, *et al.* The Chinese prescription lianhuaqingwen capsule exerts anti-influenza activity through the inhibition of viral propagation and impacts immune function. BMC Complement Altern Med 2017; 17(1): 130.
[http://dx.doi.org/10.1186/s12906-017-1585-7] [PMID: 28235408]

[28] Runfeng L, Yunlong H, Jicheng H, *et al.* Lianhuaqingwen exerts anti-viral and anti-inflammatory activity against novel coronavirus (SARS-CoV-2). Pharmacol Res 2020; 156: 104761.
[http://dx.doi.org/10.1016/j.phrs.2020.104761] [PMID: 32205232]

[29] Wang X, Xu W, Hu G, Xia S, Sun Z, Liu Z, *et al.* SARS-CoV-2 infects T lymphocytes through its spike protein-mediated membrane fusion. Cellular and Molecular Immunology. Springer Nature 2020; pp. 1-3.

[30] Liu C, Yang Y, Gao Y, Shen C, Ju B, Liu C, *et al.* Viral architecture of SARS-CoV-2 with post-fusion spike revealed by Cryo-EM. Structure 2020; 28(11): 1218-1224.e4.
[http://dx.doi.org/10.1016/j.str.2020.10.001]

[31] Ryan RM, Mineo-Kuhn MM, Kramer CM, Finkelstein JN. Growth factors alter neonatal type II alveolar epithelial cell proliferation. Am J Physiol 1994; 266(1 Pt 1): L17-22. http://www.ncbi.nlm.nih.gov/pubmed/8304465 [Internet].
[PMID: 8304465]

[32] Foster KA, Oster CG, Mayer MM, Avery ML, Audus KL. Characterization of the A549 cell line as a type II pulmonary epithelial cell model for drug metabolism. Exp Cell Res 1998; 243(2): 359-66.
[http://dx.doi.org/10.1006/excr.1998.4172] [PMID: 9743595]

[33] Corbière V, Dirix V, Norrenberg S, Cappello M, Remmelink M, Mascart F. Phenotypic characteristics of human type II alveolar epithelial cells suitable for antigen presentation to T lymphocytes. Respir Res 2011; 12(1): 15.http://respiratory-research.biomedcentral.com/articles/10.1186/1465-9921-12-15 [Internet].
[http://dx.doi.org/10.1186/1465-9921-12-15] [PMID: 21261956]

[34] Lieber M, Smith B, Szakal A, Nelson-Rees W, Todaro G. A continuous tumor-cell line from a human lung carcinoma with properties of type II alveolar epithelial cells. Int J Cancer 1976; 17(1): 62-70.
[http://dx.doi.org/10.1002/ijc.2910170110] [PMID: 175022]

[35] Jiang RD, Shen H, Piao YJ. The morphometrical analysis on the ultrastructure of A549 cells. Rom J Morphol Embryol 2010; 51(4): 663-7.
[PMID: 21103623]

[36] Blanco-Melo D, Nilsson-Payant BE, Liu W-C, Møller R, Panis M, Sachs D, *et al.* SARS-CoV-2 launches a unique transcriptional signature from *in vitro*, *ex vivo*, and *in vivo* systems. bioRxiv 2020.
[http://dx.doi.org/10.1101/2020.03.24.004655]

[37] Busti AJ, Hall RG, Margolis DM. Atazanavir for the treatment of human immunodeficiency virus infection. Pharmacotherapy 2004; 24(12): 1732-47. http://doi.wiley.com/10.1592/phco.24.17.1732.52347

[http://dx.doi.org/10.1592/phco.24.17.1732.52347] [PMID: 15585441]

[38] Fintelman-Rodrigues N, Sacramento CQ, Ribeiro Lima C, Souza da Silva F, Ferreira AC, Mattos M, *et al.* Atazanavir inhibits SARS-CoV-2 replication and pro-inflammatory cytokine production. Antimicrob Agents Chemother 2020; 64(10): e00825-20. [http://dx.doi.org/10.1101/2020.04.04.020925]

[39] Barker N, van Es JH, Kuipers J, *et al.* Identification of stem cells in small intestine and colon by marker gene Lgr5. Nature 2007; 449(7165): 1003-7. [http://dx.doi.org/10.1038/nature06196] [PMID: 17934449]

[40] Wright NA. Epithelial stem cell repertoire in the gut: clues to the origin of cell lineages, proliferative units and cancer. Int J Exp Pathol 2000; 81(2): 117-43. [http://dx.doi.org/10.1046/j.1365-2613.2000.00146.x] [PMID: 10762441]

[41] Cheng H, Leblond CP. Origin, differentiation and renewal of the four main epithelial cell types in the mouse small intestine. V. Unitarian Theory of the origin of the four epithelial cell types. Am J Anat 1974; 141(4): 537-61.http://doi.wiley.com/10.1002/aja.1001410407 [Internet]. [http://dx.doi.org/10.1002/aja.1001410407] [PMID: 4440635]

[42] Sato T, Vries RG, Snippert HJ, *et al.* Single Lgr5 stem cells build crypt-villus structures *in vitro* without a mesenchymal niche. Nature 2009; 459(7244): 262-5. [http://dx.doi.org/10.1038/nature07935] [PMID: 19329995]

[43] Y Sasai. Next-generation regenerative medicine: organogenesis from stem cells in 3D culture. Cell stem cell 2013; 12(5): 520-30. [http://dx.doi.org/10.1016/j.stem.2013.04.009]

[44] van de Wetering M, Francies HE, Francis JM, *et al.* Prospective derivation of a living organoid biobank of colorectal cancer patients. Cell 2015; 161(4): 933-45. [http://dx.doi.org/10.1016/j.cell.2015.03.053] [PMID: 25957691]

[45] Okita K, Ichisaka T, Yamanaka S. Generation of germline-competent induced pluripotent stem cells. Nature 2007; 448(7151): 313-7. http://www.jwildlifedis.org/doi/10.7589/0090-3558-37.4.755 [Internet]. [http://dx.doi.org/10.1038/nature05934] [PMID: 17554338]

[46] O'Brien JA, Lahue BJ, Caro JJ, Davidson DM. The emerging infectious challenge of *clostridium difficile*-associated disease in Massachusetts hospitals: clinical and economic consequences. Infect Control Hosp Epidemiol 2007; 28(11): 1219-27. [http://dx.doi.org/10.1017/S0195941700026072] [PMID: 17926270]

[47] Engevik MA, Engevik KA, Yacyshyn MB, *et al.* Human *Clostridium difficile* infection: inhibition of NHE3 and microbiota profile. Am J Physiol Gastrointest Liver Physiol 2015; 308(6): G497-509. [http://dx.doi.org/10.1152/ajpgi.00090.2014] [PMID: 25552580]

[48] Gu J, Han B, Wang J. COVID-19: gastrointestinal manifestations and potential fecal–oral transmission. Gastroenterology 2020; 158(6): 1518-9.

[49] Wang W, Xu Y, Gao R, Lu R, Han K, Wu G, *et al.* Detection of SARS-CoV-2 in different types of clinical specimens. Jama 323(18): 1843-4.

[50] Ettayebi K, Crawford S, *et al.* Replication of human noroviruses in stem cell–derived human enteroids. 2016. [cited 2020 May 6]; Available from: https://science.sciencemag.org/content/353/6306/1387.short

[51] Beumer J, Artegiani B, Post Y, Reimann F, *et al.* Enteroendocrine cells switch hormone expression along the crypt-to-villus BMP signalling gradient. [cited 2020 May 6]; Available from: https://www.nature.com/articles/s41556-018-0143-y

[52] Lamers MM, Beumer J, van der Vaart J, Knoops K, Puschhof J, Breugem TI, *et al.* SARS-CoV-2 productively infects human gut enterocytes. Science 2020. [http://dx.doi.org/doi/10.1126/science.abc1669]

[53] Fulcher ML, Randell SH. Human nasal and tracheo-bronchial respiratory epithelial cell culture. Methods Mol Biol 2013; 945: 109-21.
[http://dx.doi.org/10.1007/978-1-62703-125-7_8] [PMID: 23097104]

[54] Fulcher ML, Gabriel S, Burns KA, Yankaskas JR, Randell SH. Well-differentiated human airway epithelial cell cultures. Methods Mol Med 2005; 107: 183-206.
[http://dx.doi.org/10.1385/1-59259-861-7:183] [PMID: 15492373]

[55] Gruenert DC, Finkbeiner WE, Widdicombe JH. Culture and transformation of human airway epithelial cells. Am J Physiol 1995; 268(3 Pt 1): L347-60.
[http://dx.doi.org/10.1152/ajplung.1995.268.3.L347] [PMID: 7900815]

[56] Forbes I. Human airway epithelial cell lines for *in vitro* drug transport and metabolism studies. Pharm Sci Technol Today 2000; 3(1): 18-27. https://linkinghub.elsevier.com/retrieve/pii/S146153479900231X
[http://dx.doi.org/10.1016/S1461-5347(99)00231-X] [PMID: 10637597]

[57] Yankaskas JR, Cotton CU, Knowles MR, Gatzy JT, Boucher RC. Culture of human nasal epithelial cells on collagen matrix supports. A comparison of bioelectric properties of normal and cystic fibrosis epithelia. Am Rev Respir Dis 1985; 132(6): 1281-7.
[PMID: 4073668]

[58] Sheahan T, Sims A, *et al.* Broad-spectrum anti-viral GS-5734 inhibits both epidemic and zoonotic coronaviruses. RG-S translational, 2017 undefined RG-S translational, 2017 undefined. Broad-spectrum anti-viral GS-5734 inhibits both epidemic and zoonotic coronaviruses. stm.sciencemag.org [Internet]. [cited 2020 May 13]; Available from: https://stm.sciencemag.org

[59] Sheahan TP, Sims AC, Zhou S, Hill C, Leist SR, Schaefer A, *et al.* An orally bioavailable broadspectrum anti-viral inhibits SARS-CoV-2 and multiple endemic, epidemic and bat coronavirus. Science (80-) 2020.https://www.biorxiv.org/content/10.1101/2020.03.19.997890v1

[60] PubChem [Internet]. [cited 2020 May 13]. Available from: https://pubchem.ncbi.nlm.nih.gov/#query=remdesivir

[61] Diltiazem | C22H26N2O4S - PubChem [Internet]. [cited 2020 May 13]. Available from: https://pubchem.ncbi.nlm.nih.gov/compound/39186

[62] Pizzorno A, Padey B, Julien T, Trouillet-Assant S, Traversier A, Errazuriz-Cerda E, *et al.* Characterization and treatment of SARS-CoV-2 in nasal and bronchial human airwayepithelia bioRxiv 2020.http://biorxiv.org/content/early/2020/04/02/2020.03.31.01788

[63] Graham FL, Smiley J, Russell WC, Nairn R. Characteristics of a human cell line transformed by DNA from human adenovirus type 5. J Gen Virol 1977; 36(1): 59-74. https://www.microbiologyresearch.org/content/journal/jgv/10.1099/0022-1317-36-1-59 [Internet].
[http://dx.doi.org/10.1099/0022-1317-36-1-59] [PMID: 886304]

[64] Berkner KL. Development of adenovirus vectors for the expression of heterologous genes. Biotechniques 2020; 6(7): 29-616.
[PMID: 3078719]

[65] Wang C, Li W, Drabek D, *et al.* A human monoclonal antibody blocking SARS-CoV-2 infection. Nat Commun 2020; 11(1): 2251.http://www.nature.com/articles/s41467-020-16256-y [Internet].
[http://dx.doi.org/10.1038/s41467-020-16256-y] [PMID: 32366817]

[66] Gordon DE, Jang GM, Bouhaddou M, Xu J, Obernier K. O Meara MJ, *et al.* A SARS-CoV-2-Human Protein-Protein Interaction Map Reveals Drug Targets and Potential Drug-Repurposing bioRxiv http://biorxiv.org/content/early/2020/03/27/2020.03.22.002386

[67] Florea BI, Cassara ML, Junginger HE, Borchard G. Drug transport and metabolism characteristics of the human airway epithelial cell line Calu-3. J Control Release. Elsevier 2003; pp. 131-8.
[http://dx.doi.org/10.1016/S0168-3659(02)00356-5]

[68] Forbes B, and CE-E journal of pharmaceutics, 2005 undefined. Human respiratory epithelial cell culture for drug delivery applications. Elsevier [Internet]. [cited 2020 May 19]; Available from: https://www.sciencedirect.com

[69] WE F. SD C, CE T. Reverse transcription-polymerase chain reaction (RT-PCR) phenotypic analysis of cell cultures of human tracheal epithelium, tracheobronchial glands, and lung carcinomas. Am J Respir Cell Mol Biol 1993; 9(5)

[70] Wan H, Winton H, Soeller C, Stewart G, Thompson P, Gruenert D, *et al.* Tight junction properties of the immortalized human bronchial epithelial cell lines Calu-3 and 16HBE14o-Tight junction properties of the immortalized human bronchial epithelial cell lines Calu-3 and 16HBE14o. Eur Respir J 2000; 15(6): 1058-68.

[71] Shen BQ, Finkbeiner WE, Wine JJ, Mrsny RJ, Widdicombe JH. Calu-3: A human airway epithelial cell line that shows cAMP-dependent Cl- secretion. Eur Respir J 2000; 16(6): 1058-68.

[72] Kreft ME, Jerman UD, Lasič E, *et al.* The characterization of the human cell line Calu-3 under different culture conditions and its use as an optimized *in vitro* model to investigate bronchial epithelial function. Eur J Pharm Sci 2015; 69: 1-9. https://linkinghub.elsevier.com/retrieve/pii/S0928098714004758 [Internet].
[http://dx.doi.org/10.1016/j.ejps.2014.12.017] [PMID: 25555374]

[73] Mukherjee M, Pritchard DI, Bosquillon C. Evaluation of air-interfaced Calu-3 cell layers for investigation of inhaled drug interactions with organic cation transporters *in vitro* . Int J Pharm 2012; 426(1-2): 7-14.https://linkinghub.elsevier.com/retrieve/pii/S0378517311011628 [Internet].
[http://dx.doi.org/10.1016/j.ijpharm.2011.12.036] [PMID: 22265910]

[74] Jeong MH, Kim HR, Bang IJ, *et al. in vitro* model for predicting acute inhalation toxicity by using a Calu-3 epithelium cytotoxicity assay. J Pharmacol Toxicol Methods 2019; 98: 106576.https://linkinghub.elsevier.com/retrieve/pii/S1056871918307019 [Internet].
[http://dx.doi.org/10.1016/j.vascn.2019.04.002] [PMID: 31026561]

[75] Fujii S. (BBA)-Enzymology YH-B et BA, 1981 undefined. New synthetic inhibitors of C1r, C1 esterase, thrombin, plasmin, kallikrein and trypsin. Elsevier [Internet]. [cited 2020 May 21]; Available from: https://www.sciencedirect.com/science/article/pii/0005274481900231

[76] Iwaki M, Ino Y, Motoyoshi A, Ozeki M, Sato T, Kurumi M, *et al.* Pharmacological studies of FUT-175, nafamostat mesilate v. Effects on the Pancreatic Enzymes and Experimental Acute Pancreatitis in Rats [Internet] https://jstage.jst.go.jp.

[77] Minakata D, Fujiwara SI, Ikeda T, *et al.* Comparison of gabexate mesilate and nafamostat mesilate for disseminated intravascular coagulation associated with hematological malignancies. Int J Hematol 2019; 109(2): 141-6.
[http://dx.doi.org/10.1007/s12185-018-02567-w] [PMID: 30536180]

[78] Ohtake Y, Hirasawa H, Sugai T, *et al.* SO-C, 1991 undefined. Nafamostat mesylate as anticoagulant in continuous hemofiltration and continuous hemodiafiltration. karger.com [Internet]. [cited 2020 May 21]; Available from: https://www.karger.com

[79] Yamamoto M, Kiso M, Sakai-Tagawa Y, Iwatsuki-Horimoto K, Imai M, Takeda M, *et al.* The anticoagulant nafamostat potently inhibits SARS-CoV-2 infection *in vitro* : an existing drug with multiple possible therapeutic effects. Viruses 2020; 12(6): 629.
[http://dx.doi.org/10.1101/2020.04.22.054981]

[80] De Clercq E. Suramin: a potent inhibitor of the reverse transcriptase of RNA tumor viruses. Cancer Lett 1979; 8(1): 9-22.
[http://dx.doi.org/10.1016/0304-3835(79)90017-X] [PMID: 92362]

[81] McGeary R, Bennett A, *et al.* QT-M reviews in, 2008 undefined. Suramin: clinical uses and structure-activity relationships. europepmc.org [Internet]. [cited 2020 May 22]; Available from: https://europepmc.org/abstract/med/18991754

[82] da Silva CSB, Thaler M, Tas A, Ogando NS, Bredenbeek PJ, Ninaber DK, *et al.* Suramin inhibits SARS-CoV-2 infection in cell culture by interfering with early steps of the replication cycle bioRxiv 2020.

[83] Ammerman NC, Beier-Sexton M, Azad AF. Growth and maintenance of vero cell lines. Curr Protoc Microbiol 2008.
[http://dx.doi.org/10.1002/9780471729259.mca04es11]

[84] Osada N, Kohara A, Yamaji T, Hirayama N, Kasai F, Sekizuka T, *et al.* The Genome Landscape of the African Green Monkey Kidney-Derived Vero Cell Line [cited 2020 May 23]; Available from: http://picard.sourceforge.net
[http://dx.doi.org/10.1093/dnares/dsu029]

[85] Levenbook IS, Petricciani JC, Elisberg BL. Tumorigenicity of vero cells. J Biol Stand 1984; 12(4): 391-8.
[http://dx.doi.org/10.1016/S0092-1157(84)80063-3] [PMID: 6526826]

[86] Barrett PN, Mundt W, Kistner O, Howard MK. Vero cell platform in vaccine production: moving towards cell culture-based viral vaccines. Expert Rev Vaccines 2009; 8(5): 607-18.
[http://dx.doi.org/10.1586/erv.09.19] [PMID: 19397417]

[87] Aubrit F, Perugi F, Léon A, *et al.* Cell substrates for the production of viral vaccines. Vaccine 2015; 33(44): 5905-12.https://linkinghub.elsevier.com/retrieve/pii/S0264410X15009329 [Internet].
[http://dx.doi.org/10.1016/j.vaccine.2015.06.110] [PMID: 26187258]

[88] Montagnon B, Fanget B. biological AN-D in, 1981 undefined. The large-scale cultivation of VERO cells in micro-carrier culture for virus vaccine production. Preliminary results for killed poliovirus vaccine. europepmc.org [Internet]. [cited 2020 May 23]; Available from: https://europepmc.org/abstract/med/6785126

[89] Van Wezel A, Van Steenis G, *et al.* CH-D in, 1978 undefined. New approach to the production of concentrated and purified inactivated polio and rabies tissue culture vaccines. europepmc.org [Internet]. [cited 2020 May 23]; Available from: https://europepmc.org/article/med/223908

[90] Vidor E, Meschievitz C. disease SP-TP infectious, 1997 undefined. Fifteen years of experience with Vero-produced enhanced potency inactivated poliovirus vaccine. [Internet] [cited 2020 May 23]; Available from: https://journals.lww.com

[91] Rhim JS, Schell K, Creasy B, Case W. Biological characteristics and viral susceptibility of an African green monkey kidney cell line (Vero). Proc Soc Exp Biol Med 1969; 132(2): 670-8.
[http://dx.doi.org/10.3181/00379727-132-34285] [PMID: 4982209]

[92] Desmyter J, Melnick JL, Rawls WE. Defectiveness of interferon production and of rubella virus interference in a line of African green monkey kidney cells (Vero). J Virol 1968; 2(10): 955-61.
[http://dx.doi.org/10.1128/jvi.2.10.955-961.1968] [PMID: 4302013]

[93] Diaz MO, Ziemin S, Le Beau MM, *et al.* Homozygous deletion of the α- and β 1-interferon genes in human leukemia and derived cell lines. Proc Natl Acad Sci USA 1988; 85(14): 5259-63.
[http://dx.doi.org/10.1073/pnas.85.14.5259] [PMID: 3134658]

[94] Lokugamage KG, Hage A, Schindewolf C, Rajsbaum R, Menachery VD. SARS-CoV-2 is sensitive to type I interferon pretreatment bioRxiv 2020.
[http://dx.doi.org/10.1101/2020.03.07.982264]

[95] Mulangu S, Dodd LE, Davey RT Jr, *et al.* PALM Writing Group; PALM Consortium Study Team. A randomized, controlled trial of ebola virus disease therapeutics. N Engl J Med 2019; 381(24): 2293-303.
[http://dx.doi.org/10.1056/NEJMoa1910993] [PMID: 31774950]

[96] Gordon CJ, Tchesnokov EP, Woolner E, Perry JK, Feng JY, Porter DP, *et al.* Remdesivir is a direct-acting anti-viral that inhibits RNA-dependent RNA polymerase from severe acute respiratory syndrome coronavirus 2 with high potency. J Biol Chem 2020 Apr 13; jbc.RA120.013679.

[97] Choy KT, Wong AYL, Kaewpreedee P, Sia SF, Chen D, Hui KPY, *et al.* Remdesivir, lopinavir, emetine, and homoharringtonine inhibit SARS-CoV-2 replication *in vitro*. Antiviral Res. 2020 June 1; 178: 104786.

[98] Agostini ML, Andres EL, Sims AC, *et al.* Coronavirus susceptibility to the anti-viral remdesivir (GS-5734) is mediated by the viral polymerase and the proofreading exoribonuclease. MBio 2018; 9(2): e00221-18.
[http://dx.doi.org/10.1128/mBio.00221-18] [PMID: 29511076]

[99] Hurst M, Faulds D. Lopinavir. Drugs 2000; 60(6): 1371-9.
[http://dx.doi.org/10.2165/00003495-200060060-00009] [PMID: 11152017]

[100] Cvetkovic RS, Goa KL. Lopinavir/ritonavir: A review of its use in the management of HIV infection. Drugs. Springer 2003; Vol. 63: pp. 769-802.

[101] Mangum EM, Graham KK. Lopinavir-Ritonavir: a new protease inhibitor. Pharmacotherapy 2001; 21(11): 1352-63.http://doi.wiley.com/10.1592/phco.21.17.1352.34419 [Internet].
[http://dx.doi.org/10.1592/phco.21.17.1352.34419] [PMID: 11714208]

[102] Xiu-jin Ye, Mao-fang Lin. Homoharringtonine induces apoptosis of endothelium and down-regulates vegf expression of K562 cells. J Zhejiang Univ Sci 2004; 5(2): 230-4.

[103] Dong HJ, Wang ZH, Meng W, *et al.* The natural compound homoharringtonine presents broad anti-viral activity *in vitro* and *in vivo* . Viruses 2018; 10(11): 601.
[http://dx.doi.org/10.3390/v10110601] [PMID: 30388805]

[104] Ianevski A, Yao R, Fenstad MH, Biza S, Zusinaite E, Lysvand H, *et al.* Potential anti-viral options against SARS-CoV-2 infection bioRxiv 2020.

[105] Akinboye ES, Bakare O. Biological activities of emetine. The Open Natural Products Journal 2011; 4: 8-15.
[http://dx.doi.org/10.2174/1874848101104010008]

[106] Yang S, Xu M, Lee EM, *et al.* Emetine inhibits Zika and Ebola virus infections through two molecular mechanisms: inhibiting viral replication and decreasing viral entry. Cell Discov 2018; 4(1): 31.
[http://dx.doi.org/10.1038/s41421-018-0034-1] [PMID: 29872540]

[107] Campbell WC. Ivermectin: an update. Parasitol Today 1985; 1(1): 10-6.
[http://dx.doi.org/10.1016/0169-4758(85)90100-0] [PMID: 15275618]

[108] Campbell WC, Fisher MH, Stapley EO, Albers-Schönberg G, Jacob TA. Ivermectin: A potent new antiparasitic agent. Science (80-) [Internet] 1983; 221(4613): 8-823.
[http://dx.doi.org/10.1126/science.6308762]

[109] Caly L, Druce JD, Catton MG, Jans DA, Wagstaff KM. The FDA-approved drug ivermectin inhibits the replication of SARS-CoV-2 *in vitro* . Antiviral Res 2020; 178: 104787.
[http://dx.doi.org/10.1016/j.antiviral.2020.104787] [PMID: 32251768]

[110] Yang SNY, Atkinson SC, Wang C, *et al.* The broad spectrum antiviral ivermectin targets the host nuclear transport importin α/β1 heterodimer. Antiviral Res 2020; 177: 104760. https://linkinghub.elsevier.com/retri eve/pii/S0166354219307211 [Internet].
[http://dx.doi.org/10.1016/j.antiviral.2020.104760] [PMID: 32135219]

[111] Liu J, Cao R, Xu M, Wang X, Zhang H, Hu H, *et al.* Hydroxychloroquine, a less toxic derivative of chloroquine, is effective in inhibiting SARS-CoV-2 infection *in vitro.* naturecom [Internet] [cited 2020 May 29]; Available from: https://www.nature.com

[112] Al-Bari MAA. Targeting endosomal acidification by chloroquine analogs as a promising strategy for the treatment of emerging viral diseases. Pharmacol Res Perspect 2017; 5(1): e00293.
[http://dx.doi.org/10.1002/prp2.293] [PMID: 28596841]

[113] Zhou D, Dai S. Antimicrobial QT-J of, 2020 undefined. COVID-19: a recommendation to examine the effect of hydroxychloroquine in preventing infection and progression. academic.oup.com [Internet].

[cited 2020 May 29]; Available from: https://academic.oup.com

[114] Wang M, Cao R, Zhang L, Yang X, Liu J, Xu M, *et al.* Remdesivir and chloroquine effectively inhibit the recently emerged novel coronavirus. Cell Res 2020; 30(3): 269-71.

[115] Liu J, Cao R, Xu M, Wang X, Zhang H, Hu H, *et al.* Hydroxychloroquine, a less toxic derivative of chloroquine, is effective in inhibiting SARS-CoV-2 infection *in vitro*. Cell Discovery Springer Nature 2020; 6: 1-4.

[116] Bardsley-Elliot A, Plosker CL. Nelfinavir: An update on its use in HIV infection. Drugs. Adis International Ltd 2000; 59: pp. 581-620.

[117] Jarvis B, Faulds D. A review of its therapeutic efficacy in HIV infection. Drugs. Springer 1998; Vol. 56: pp. 67-147.

[118] Koltai T. Nelfinavir and other protease inhibitors in cancer: Mechanisms involved in anticancer activity. F1000Research. Faculty of 1000 Ltd 2015; Vol. 4.

[119] Xu Z, Yao H, Shen J, Wu N, Xu Y, Lu X, *et al.* Nelfinavir Is Active Against SARS-CoV-2 in Vero E6 Cells. ChemRxiv 2020.https://chemrxiv.org/articles/Nelfinavir_Is_Active_Against_SARS-Co--2_in_Vero_E6_Cells/12039888/1

[120] Musarrat F, Chouljenko V, Dahal A, Nabi R, Chouljenko T, Jois SD, *et al.* The anti HIV drug nelfinavir mesylate (Viracept) is a potent inhibitor of cell fusion caused by the SARSCoV 2 spike (S) glycoprotein warranting further evaluation as an anti viral against COVID-19 infections. J Med Virol [Internet] 2020 May 17 [cited 2020 May 30]; jmv.25985. Available from: https://onlinelibrary.wiley.com

[121] Yamamoto N, Matsuyama S, Hoshino T, Yamamoto N. Nelfinavir inhibits replication of severe acute respiratory syndrome coronavirus 2 *in vitro*. bioRxiv 2020.

[122] Summ O, Andreou AP, Akerman S, Goadsby PJ. A potential nitrergic mechanism of action for indomethacin, but not of other COX inhibitors: relevance to indomethacin-sensitive headaches. J Headache Pain 2010; 11(6): 477-83. https://thejournalofheadacheandpain.biomedcentral.com /articles/10.1007/s10194-010-0263-7 [Internet]. [http://dx.doi.org/10.1007/s10194-010-0263-7] [PMID: 20978816]

[123] Summ O, Evers S. Mechanism of action of indomethacin in indomethacin-responsive headaches. Curr Pain Headache Rep 2013; 17(4): 327. [http://dx.doi.org/10.1007/s11916-013-0327-x] [PMID: 23423598]

[124] Martella V, Decaro N. Indomethacin has a potent anti-viral activity against SARS coronavirus [Internet]. 2006 [cited 2020 May 30]. Available from: https://www.researchgate.net /publication/6503810

[125] Xu T, Gao X, Wu Z, Selinger DW, Zhou Z. Indomethacin has a potent anti-viral activity against SARS CoV-2 *in vitro* and canine coronavirus *in vivo*. bioRxiv 2019. https://www.biorxiv.org/content/10.1101 /2020.04.01.017624v1

[126] Gomeni R, Xu T, Gao X. Françoise Bressolle-Gomeni. Model based approach for estimating the dosage regimen of indomethacin a potential anti-viral treatment of patients infected with SARS CoV-2. J Pharmacokinet Pharmacodyn 2020; 43(3): 189-98. [http://dx.doi.org/10.1007/s10928-020-09690-4] [PMID: 32435882]

[127] Rustgi VK, Lee WM, Lawitz E, *et al.* MErimepodib TRiple cOmbination Study Group. Merimepodib, pegylated interferon, and ribavirin in genotype 1 chronic hepatitis C pegylated interferon and ribavirin nonresponders. Hepatology 2009; 50(6): 1719-26. [http://dx.doi.org/10.1002/hep.23204] [PMID: 19852040]

[128] Li S fang, Gong M jiao, Shao J jun, Sun Y feng, Zhang Y guang, Chang H yun. Anti-viral activity of merimepodib against foot and mouth disease virus *in vitro* and *in vivo*. Mol Immunol 2019; 114: 226-32.https://linkinghub.elsevier.com/retrieve/pii/S0161589019301774 [Internet]. [http://dx.doi.org/10.1016/j.molimm.2019.07.021]

[129] Tong X, Smith J, Bukreyeva N, *et al.* Merimepodib, an IMPDH inhibitor, suppresses replication of Zika virus and other emerging viral pathogens. Antiviral Res 2018; 149: 34-40.https://linkinghub.elsevier.com/retrieve/pii/S0166354217302371 [Internet]. [http://dx.doi.org/10.1016/j.antiviral.2017.11.004] [PMID: 29126899]

[130] Bukreyeva N, Mantlo EK, Sattler RA, Huang C, Paessler S, Zeldis J. The IMPDH inhibitor merimepodib suppresses SARS-CoV-2 replication *in vitro* bioRxiv.

[131] Gao Z, Huang K, Xu H. Protective effects of flavonoids in the roots of *Scutellaria baicalensis* Georgi against hydrogen peroxide-induced oxidative stress in HS-SY5Y cells. Pharmacol Res 2001; 43(2): 173-8.
[http://dx.doi.org/10.1006/phrs.2000.0761] [PMID: 11243719]

[132] H Bin Li, Y Jiang, F Chen. Separation methods used for *Scutellaria baicalensis* active components. Journal of Chromatography B: Analytical Technologies in the Biomedical and Life Sciences 2004; 812: 90-277.
[http://dx.doi.org/] [PMID:]

[133] Liu H, Ye F, Sun Q, Liang H, Li C, Lu R, *et al. Scutellaria baicalensis* extract and baicalein inhibit replication of SARS-CoV-2 and its 3C-like protease *in vitro* J Enzyme Inhib Med Chem 2021; 36(1): 497-503.
[http://dx.doi.org/10.1101/2020.04.10.035824]

[134] S Noble, KL Goa. Gemcitabine A review of its pharmacology and clinical potential in non-small cell lung cancer and pancreatic cancer. International Publishing: Springer 1997; pp. 72-447.

[135] Lawrence TS, Eisbruch A, Mcginn CJ, Fields MT, Shewach DS. Radiosensitization by gemcitabine published on physicians practice. 1999 [cited 2020 Jun 1]. Available from: http://www.physicianspractice.com

[136] Lee K, Kim D eun, Jang KS, Kim SJ, Cho S, Kim C. Gemcitabine, a broad-spectrum anti-viral drug, suppresses enterovirus infections through innate immunity induced by the inhibition of pyrimidine biosynthesis and nucleotide depletion. Oncotarget 2017; 8(70): 115315-25.
[http://dx.doi.org/10.18632/oncotarget.23258] [PMID: 29383162]

[137] Gemcitabine, lycorine and oxysophoridine inhibit novel coronavirus (SARS-CoV-2) in cell culture. Emerg Microbes Infect [Internet] 2020 May 20 [cited 2020 June 1];1–10. Available from: https://www.tandfonline.com/doi/full/10.1080/22221751.2020.1772676

[138] Zhang P, Liu S. Solvent Effects on the UV Absorption Spectrum of Carmofur. Detection [Internet]. 2016 [cited 2020 June 1];4:25–31. Available from: http://www.scirp.org

[139] Domraceva I, Petrova M, Duburs G. 2-Dimyristoyl-sn-glycero-3-phosphocholine (DMPC) increases Carmofur stability and *in vitro* antiproliferative effect Cardiovascular drugs View project Inhibitors of multidrug resistance View project. [cited 2020 June 1] :http://dx.doi.org/doi:10.1016/j.toxrep.2015.01.009

[140] Govindarajah N, Clifford R, Bowden D, Sutton PA, Parsons JL, Vimalachandran D. Sphingolipids and acid ceramidase as therapeutic targets in cancer therapy. Critical Reviews in Oncology/Hematology. Elsevier Ireland Ltd 2019; Vol. 138: pp. 104-11. https://linkinghub.elsevier.com/retrieve/pii/S1040842818305079 Internet

[141] Khaerunnisa S, Kurniawan H, Awaluddin R, Suhartati S. Potential Inhibitor of COVID-19 Main Protease (M pro) from Several Medicinal Plant Compounds by Molecular Docking Study Preprints 2020. https://www.preprints.org/manuscript/202003.0226/v1

[142] Jin Z, Zhao Y, Sun Y, *et al.* Structural basis for the inhibition of SARS-CoV-2 main protease by antineoplastic drug carmofur. Nat Struct Mol Biol 2020; 27(6): 529-32.
[http://dx.doi.org/10.1038/s41594-020-0440-6] [PMID: 32382072]

[143] Leneva IA, Russell RJ, Boriskin YS, Hay AJ. Characteristics of arbidol-resistant mutants of influenza virus: implications for the mechanism of anti-influenza action of arbidol. Antiviral Res 2009; 81(2):

132-40. https://linkinghub.elsevier.com/retri eve/pii/S0166354208004312 [Internet]. [http://dx.doi.org/10.1016/j.antiviral.2008.10.009] [PMID: 19028526]

[144] Blaising J, Polyak SJ, Pécheur EI. Arbidol as a broad-spectrum anti-viral: An update. Antiviral Research. Elsevier 2014; Vol. 107: pp. 84-94.

[145] Boriskin YS, Leneva IA, Pécheur E-I, Polyak SJ. Arbidol: a broad-spectrum antiviral compound that blocks viral fusion. Curr Med Chem 2008; 15(10): 997-1005. [http://dx.doi.org/10.2174/092986708784049658] [PMID: 18393857]

[146] Wang X, Cao R, Zhang H, Liu J, Xu M, Hu H, *et al.* The anti-influenza virus drug, arbidol is an efficient inhibitor of SARS-CoV-2 in vitro . Cell Discovery. Springer Nature 2020; Vol. 6: pp. 1-5.

CHAPTER 3

Histopathologic Evaluation and Scoring of SARS-CoV-2 Infection

Muhammad Mazhar Ayaz[1,*], **Ihtisham Ulhaq**[2] and **Kashif Rahim**[3]

[1] *Department of Parasitology, Faculty of Veterinary Science, Cholistan University of Veterinary and Animal Sciences, Bahawalpur, Pakistan*

[2] *Department of Biosciences, COMSATS University Islamabad (CUI)45550, Pakistan*

[3] *Department of Microbiology, Faculty of Veterinary Science, Cholistan University of Veterinary and Animal Sciences (CUVAS), Punjab, Bahawalpur 63100, Pakistan*

Abstract: The recent emergent coronaviruses in the 21st century, such as Severe Acute Respiratory Syndrome-Coronavirus (SARS-CoV), Middle East Respiratory Syndrome-Coronavirus (MERS-CoV), and severe acute respiratory syndrome-coronavirus-2 (SARS-CoV-2), has caused significant morbidity and mortality around the world. The lung is the most affected organ in the infection of human pathogenic coronaviruses. There is always a scarcity of human signs, symptoms, and modes of transmission. So to study the viral pathogenesis and evaluated interventions of therapies and vaccines, animals need to be used as models, especially at early epidemics. Lesions scoring can be identified from histopathological studies, and it can be helpful to understand the viral pathogenesis and damages to the cells to design effective therapies or vaccines. Histopathology uses the cells to determine viral host receptors and viral host tropism to relate with disease severity and lesions. Moreover, histopathology also plays a role in the qualitative description of affected organs to determine the micro-anatomic location of cells, type of cells, and cellular consequences during and post-infection. Comparatively, this approach has various limitations, but still, it is significant in comparing treatment groups. In comparing various groups, semi-quantitative and quantitative tissue scores are used for statistical analysis to increase the reproducibility of the study. This chapter refers to different features, including the importance of histopathology, principles, technique, scoring methods, and pathological characteristics of COVID-19, which can be valuable to assess the lung infection caused by SARS-CoV-2 and animal models and real situations.

Keywords: COVID-19, Infection, Lung, Pathology, RNA, Scoring.

* **Corresponding author Dr. Muhammad Mazhar Ayaz:** Department of Parasitology, Faculty of Veterinary Science, Cholistan University of Veterinary and Animal Sciences, Bahawalpur, Pakistan. E-mail: mmazharayaz@cuvas.edu.pk

Kamal Niaz & Muhammad Farrukh Nisar (Eds.)

INTRODUCTION

Severe Acute Respiratory Syndrome-Coronavirus-2 (SARS-CoV-2) belongs to the group of *betacoronaviruses*, enveloped, and genetic material is present in the form of single-stranded RNA which size is approximate ~30 kb. A single-stranded RNA genome codes a variety of structural and non-structural proteins. The non-structural proteins are comprised of various vital enzymes, including protease, helicase, and RNA-dependent RNA polymerase, which play a key role in the pathogenesis and survival of the virus inside the cell. The sequence analysis of pair-wise non-structural proteins indicated that the pathogen belongs to the Severe Acute Respiratory Syndrome-Coronavirus (SARS) coronaviruses group [1]. However, structural proteins comprised of glycoproteins of spikes and other accessory proteins role in the virus binding to the host receptor and its entry into the cell [2]. The structural proteins reported in the outbreak of SARS and the Middle East Respiratory Syndrome-Coronavirus (MERS) can help develop antiviral drugs as a potential target. Therefore, these proteins are documented as potential targets to develop antiviral drugs against SARS and MERS [3], and possibly representing in coronavirus disease-19 (COVID-19) case, according to the genetic analysis of recent SARS-COV-2 isolated from Wuhan [4]. However, new antiviral drugs or vaccines can be developed by using structural proteins as recommended. The phylogenetic analysis of the full-length genome is suggested that SARS-CoV-2 shares 79.5% sequence similarity with SARS-CoV [5 - 7], which indicated that SARS-CoV-2 belongs to subgenus Sarbecovirus [5 - 8]. Various novel coronaviruses have been identified from animals and humans after the emergence of SARS and MERS coronaviruses. It delivers track for the evolutionary origin of incipient coronaviruses from bats source only. Though, camels were also recognized as immediate hosts for the MERS-CoV outbreak. The emergence of SARS-CoV and MERS-CoV from zoonotic source indicate zoonosis in the case of COVID-19 as well [9, 10]. The sputum sample of a patient who suffered from acute pneumonia and kidney failure was found with MERS-CoV. It was isolated for the first time and genetically closed to PiBatCoV HKU5 (*Pipistrellus* bat CoV HKU5) of japan and Ty-BatCoV HKU4 (*Tylonycteris* bat CoV HKU4) in Hong Kong from *Tylonycteris pachypus* (bamboo bat). The lineage C *β*-CoVs associated to MERS-CoV was detected in bats, together with Hypsugo BatCoV HKU25 and BtVsβCoV/SC2013 from China bats, and coronavirus Bat CoV PREDICT/PDF-2180, BtCoVNeo5038/KZN/RSA/2015, and Neoromicia/PML-PHE1/RSA/2011 (NeoCoV), from African bats [11 - 15]. Additionally, a lineage C *β*-CoVs, Erinaceus CoV VMC/DEU, afterward well-defined as a novel species, Hedgehog coronavirus 1 was detected in European hedgehogs that are closely related to bats phylogenetically [16]. Likewise, palm civets and raccoon dogs were found with similar coronavirus like the SARS-CoV isolated from China during the early outbreak, which indicated that these animals have the potential of intermediate host between bats and humans [17].

Humans appeared to be susceptible to bat-sourced SARS-CoVs without before variations that indicated the re-emergence of SARS-CoVs or related to it [18, 19]. There is a similarity in the spike proteins of Ty-Bat CoV HKU4 and MERS-CoV, which indicated that the primary host of the ancestor of coronaviruses in bats [20, 21]. Two different highly human pathogenic coronaviruses, such as SARS and MERS emerged in the 21st century in 2002 and 2012 respectively [22, 23]. At the end of December 2019, another coronavirus that was named SARS-CoV-2 has emerged in the Chinese population who had epidemiologically linked to the seafood market in Wuhan, Hubei Province [24]. The SARS-CoV-2 appeared to be transmitted to humans by nasal route, orally and through the membrane of eyes, which indicated that it has broad-scale transmission modes [25]. The recently identified SARS-CoV-2 has 88% sequence similarity with two bat-derived SARS coronaviruses such as bat-SL-CoVZXC21 and bat-SL-CoVZC45 and 79% genetic similarity with SARS-CoV and 50% with MERS-CoV [4]. After phylogenetic analysis, it was revealed that SARS-CoV-2 belongs to the genus of *betacoronavirus*, which comprises SARS/SARS-like-CoV and others isolated from bats and few wild animals [26]. Spikes proteins (also called S proteins) determined the host and tissue tropism of the SARS-CoV-2. S1 and S2 are the two domains of spikes proteins, which have a role in the virus attachment to host cell and membrane fusion, respectively. There is a high sequence similarity found in the S proteins of SARS-CoV-2 and SARS-CoV and both coronaviruses using the same cellular receptor for pathogenesis, which may be due to similarity in the S proteins [27]. Compared with SARS and MERS coronaviruses, the receptor domain of SARS-CoV-2 has a high mutation rate but still uses the ACE2 receptor during pathogenesis. The transmissibility and pathogenesis of SARS-CoV-2 are reported to enhance significantly because of mutation at Furin protease. The lessons learned through experiences result in tremendous advances, and valuable insight near separating the physiognomies of SARS-CoV-2 has been accomplished at an extraordinary speed from coronaviruses' epidemics, occurrence over the last two decades. It is still able to use this binding receptor. Whether mutations in ACE2 affect its binding or change receptor tropism need to explore in detail [4]. This chapter refers to different features, including the importance of histopathology, principles, technique, scoring methods, recent case studies of coronavirus and its types, virological examination, blood cell examination, and counts and pathological characteristic of COVID-19, which can be valuable to assess the lung infection caused by SARS-CoV-2 and animal models and real situation.

Importance of Histopathology Technique

Some years ago, the technique of histopathology was developed to study the abnormal activities happening inside the cell. The pioneer of the very first published book on histopathology is Johannes Miller, who published the book "On Nature and Structure Characteristics of Cancer" in 1938. In 1591, the compound microscope was constructed for the first time but writhed from various problems, including optical problems [28]. The simple microscopes were upgraded by Anton van Leeuwenhoek in 1673 with single lenses by improving the resolution and magnification [29]. Popular manufacturers such as Cambridge Rocker, Minot, and Sledge microtomes solved the issues of sectioning with the first microtome, which is ideal for animal tissues sectioning [28]. During the mid of 19th century, embedding Paraffin wax for infiltration and maintenance throughout sectioning was introduced [30]. From time to time, various chemicals in the laboratory have been investigated to be used as preservatives [31], including formalin introduced in 1893 for the first time. In 1945, hand processing was replaced by automatic tissue processors through the industrial revolution. In 1951, the cryostat was manufactured for the first time [32]. From the past 50 years, histochemistry, electron, and polarizing microscopy have been used as diagnostic tools [28]. In 1980, a cancer diagnosis was revolutionized with the beginning of frequent use of immune-histochemistry but still under progress (Michael Titford, 2006). The human pathogenic coronaviruses, including SARS-CoV, MERS-CoV, and SARS-CoV-2, are associated with high morbidity and mortality rates. However, WHO did not permit the postmortem of dead body organs infected with SARS-CoV-2 to observe pathologic changes among them due to transmission to healthy individuals [33].

Principles

The principles for histopathology were based on the differential coloring of the cells present in the tissue(s). The coloring ability of many dyes resides in either their acid or basic radical [34]. The acid components of a cell nucleus chromatin or chromosomes stain with basic dyes (mostly by hematoxylin). These components are referred to as basophilic or hematoxylin-ophilic dye (blue). The characteristics of cells and tissues fluctuated when they were examined by microscope due to inappropriate techniques. Vigilant fixation can kill the cells due to the reduction of adjustments *in vivo* morphology. The most reliable method to directly observe the living cells' interior is to separate them for the organism, make a smear, staining and observes them by dark-field or phase-contrast microscopy. Following dispensation ends with tissues implanted in a material that simplifies thin sectioning through microtome; for light microscopy, this is usually done with the help of paraffin [35].

Techniques and Types

For non-invasive tissue collection and slight harm, numerous methods have been evaluated and for the depth study of cellular activities earlier, throughout, and at the end of the pathological process, which is either created intentionally or during the study of any infection [36, 37]. Here in the pathological study, few are discussed, like histopathology and immune-histopathology, to study the COVID-19 model. The point to point procedures of histology processes are as follows:

1. *Elimination or Biopsy taking of the tissue:* The first work for histopathology starts from tissue removal [38]. The tissues can be removed for cellular histopathology by various methods, including (a) Living cell biopsy (b) Autopsy samples for this COVID-19 issue.
2. *Fixation of sample:* The sample, preferably a small piece of tissue, is employed in a chemical or reagent, most commonly formalin, a 10% aqueous solution of 40% formaldehyde that preserves substances structures in the cells and tissues. It also prevents autolytic changes. Depending on the size and nature of the tissue, it should be fixed from 4 to 24 hours [39].
3. *Dehydration and Washing:* Washing is done before the fixation of the specimen, and this is done to remove excess water prior [31]. The tissue is then placed in increasing strengths of alcohol or other dehydrating agents. So to remove the original water in the tissue.
4. *Clearing:* The process of removing the dehydrating agent with some fluid that is miscible both with the dehydrating and embedding medium [31]. Usually, it is an oil-based chemical (paraffin) that is clearing agents frequently substitute oils that are not advanced by formalin, including triglycerides in fat cells.
5. *Embedding and Infiltration:* In this process, the clearing agent is usually replaced with the embedding medium, paraffin [31].
6. *Slicing or Cutting:* Slicing is usually done with 3 μ and 10 μ (micrometers, microns) thick sections of the tissues with the help of a microtome [31].
7. *Section Growing:* Section growing is accomplished by transferring sections to a clean glass microscope slide [31].
8. *Removal of Embedding Material or Decoration:* This is the removal of the embedding agent is very much important. After these eight exhausting steps then we start the process of staining [31].
9. *Staining:* A process for increasing the visibility of cells by the application of dyes or by their reaction(s) with chemical or staining agent(s) to form visual substances or real happenings at the cellular level [31].
10. *Mounting:* This is done after clearing to cover the thin tissue section with a bit of drop of mounting medium like DPX and with the help of a thin glass cover-slip, thus making the preparation permanent [31].

Technique for Immuno-histopathology, RNA scope, or immunofluorescent staining

This technique is a colorimetric immune-alkaline phosphatase immune-histochemistry method that requires certain different that requires certain chemicals and specific antibodies (Abs) developed with a mouse anti-SARS-CoV antibody COVID-19 purpose [40 - 42]. In brief, the following steps can be followed which are already established, and the first step starts with:

1. *Tissues and Sections:* 3 μm sections from formalin-fixed.
2. *Deparaffinization and Rehydration:* Paraffin-embedded tissues may be de-paraffinized, rehydrated.
3. *Staining:* Placed in an auto-stainer.
4. *Enzyme Digestion:* The sections may be digested in 0.1 mg of proteinase K per ml and then,
5. *Incubation with hyper-immune Serum:* Incubate for 1 hour with an ascetic fluid of hyper-immune mouse reactive with SARS-CoV antigen at a 1:1,000 dilution.
6. *Dilution:* Optimal dilutions of the antibody and the requirement for predigestion may be determined (already performed by various workers by a series of pilot studies performed on SARS-CoV-infected Vero cells).
7. *Immunoglobulin-associated incubation:* The slides are washed and evaluated for incubation with a biotinylated anti-mouse immunoglobulin antibody.
8. *Visualization:* Streptavidin-alkaline phosphatase complex is used to visualize the attached antigen; subsequently, for colorimetric detection, a naphthol-fast red substrate is used [43].
9. *Counterstaining:* Sections may be counterstained with Mayer's hematoxylin [44].

Scoring Methods

Evaluating the damage(s) caused by any etiology through histopathology is not an easy job. No such method has been developed even several hundreds of thousands of studies based on histopathology here before. It is a mere attempt to enumerate the COVID-19 pathological signs and score the damaging caused, as shown in Table **1**. In the COVID-19 infection, the most important clinical feature is lung-associated symptoms that indicate the severity of the disease [45]. During the emergence of any novel disease that has no treatment option or vaccines, different animals are used as a model to test the newly developed drug or vaccines against the disease. Animal models are often required to study viral infections and therapies, especially during an initial outbreak [46]. Histopathological studies can identify better understanding of viral pathogenesis, replication, and destruction of lesions of affected cells. It can be helpful to develop any efficient therapeutics.

The detection of presumed viral receptors and viral tropism for cells can be evaluated to correlate with lesions using immune-staining [47]. In the lung, lesions and immune-staining can be qualitatively described to define the cell types involved, micro-anatomic location(s), and type of pathological changes seen at the cellular level. There is also acute diffuse alveolar damage (DAD), a common clinical feature of MERS-CoV infection in the form of lung lesions characterized by septal injury in alveoli, inflammation, and edema. SARS-CoV-2 caused different lesions in the lung, such as thrombi congestion, as shown in Fig. (**1**).

Table 1. Lesions recording as seen in COVID-19 or MERS-CoV in lung infection(s).

S.No	Pathological Condition	Mild	Moderate	Severe
1.	Lesions in Necrosis/cell death	---	---	---
2.	Inflammation	---	---	---
3.	Hyaline membranes/fibrin	---	---	---
4.	Edema	---	---	---
5.	Thrombi	---	---	---
6.	Congestion	---	---	---
7.	Hemorrhage	---	---	---
8.	Pneumonia	---	---	---
9.	Type II hyperplasia	---	---	---
10.	Syncytia	---	---	---
11.	Blackening of lung tissues	---	---	---

Notably, the scoring principle(s) can be applied to tissue lesions at a gross or histopathological level (Table **1**). Immune-stained sections can be used to evaluate the severity or pathogenicity of infection(s) for statistical analysis or comparison purposes. Such robust methods are the need for precise calculation of damage at the site of tissue or cell. This is the reason that scientists remained unable to calculate or enumerate the exact loss. The qualitative loss sometimes cannot be quantified for scoring purposes (s). The mostly used semi-quantitative method(s) produce ordinal scores [48]. The progression of disease severity is defined by assigning grades, which define every score by characteristically 4-5 grades or more being optimal such as 0, 1, 2, 3, 4,5… as presented in Table **2**. The uncertainty must be minimum in the assigned samples, which required each grade to be defined well. The reproducibility score is limited with the use of simple descriptive modifiers including usual, infrequent, acute, slight, modest, and severe, thus making less impact on calculations.

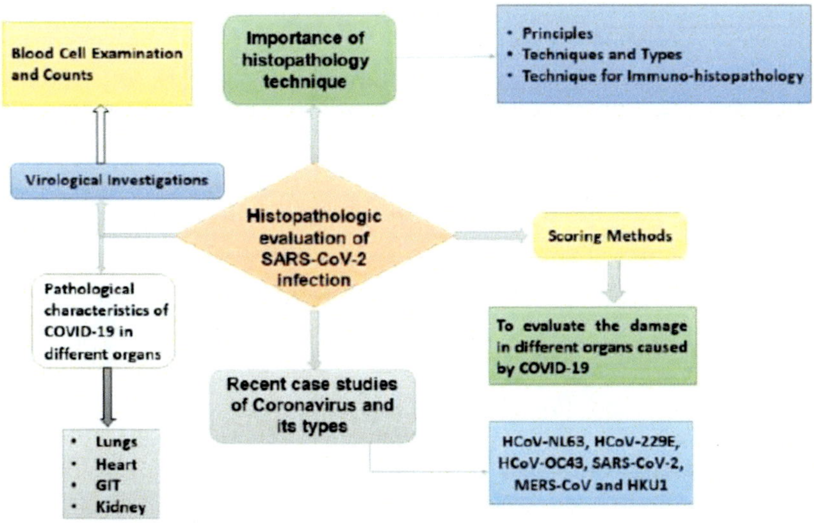

Fig. (1). Some sequences in lung tissues caused by COVID-19.

Quantification of the viral lesion(s) and immune-staining in tissues is an option, though quantification is not commonly performed in tissue sections because of potential confounding factors. Potential confounding factors include random distribution of viral inoculum and difficulty in objectively quantifying lesions. A group of statisticians evaluates the various scoring methods already used in bio-statistics to identify the most applicable tests that help assess differences and benefits in a group [49]. Examples of lung lesions observed in COVID-19 or MERS-CoV infections with quantification that can be numerically analyzed.

Table 2. Scoring of the lesion through the quantitative method.

S.No	Pathological Condition	0	1	2	3
1.	Lesions Necrosis/cell death	---	---	---	---
2.	Edema	---	---	---	---
3.	Hyaline membranes/fibrin	---	---	---	---
4.	Inflammation	---	---	---	---
5.	Thrombi	---	---	---	---
6.	Congestion	---	---	---	---
7.	Hemorrhage	---	---	---	---
8.	Pneumonia	---	---	---	---
9.	Type II hyperplasia	---	---	---	---
10.	Syncytia	---	---	---	---

Recent Case Studies of Coronavirus and its Types

The viruses of coronvirinae have spike protein that given a crown-like appearance under the microscope for the first time, so named coronavirus. All these coronaviruses are classified in Nidovirales order and *Coronaviridae* family [50, 51]. The alpha, beta, gamma, and delta are the subgroups of Coronvirinae that are characterized based on genomic structure. However, these subgroups have different host tropisms. Furthermore, alpha and beta coronaviruses cause respiratory distress, gastroenteritis in humans, and animals, respectively. There were 6 human pathogenic coronaviruses until December 2019. Among 6 viruses, 4 viruses, such as HCoV-NL63, HCoV-229E, HCoV-OC43, and HKU1, cause mild respiratory disease, while others, such as SARS-CoV and MERS-CoV associated with a severe type of respiratory disease [52]. The SARS-CoV emerged in 2002, and the outbreak continues till 2003, causes 10% mortality. The mortality rate was 37% in the case of the MERS-CoV outbreak that was emerged in 2012 [50]. According to the literature, SARS-CoVs and related other coronaviruses related to spikes made of proteins are protruded from the envelope having the receptor-binding domain (RBD). The RBD helps in the binding with the cellular receptor that is angiotensin-converting enzyme-2 (ACE-2), generally present in the respiratory system, kidneys, heart, and gastrointestinal tract (GIT), to which viruses bind and cause infection [53]. The SARS-CoV and SARS-CoV-2 use the same receptor during pathogenesis and having the same biochemical pathways as well. A cascade of inflammation is triggered in the lower respiratory tract when SARS-CoV reaches to lungs and bind with type-II pneumocytes through ACE-2. TMPRSS2 (type-2 trans-membrane protease) is a proteolytic enzyme that cleaves the SARS spike protein and ACE-2 receptor complex. This complex was formed by viral binding to the ACE-2 receptor, and after cleavage spikes, proteins are activated [53]. According to initial studies, in the early outbreak of COVID-19, 41 patients were enrolled in hospital, 98% were having fever, 76% have a cough, and 55% of patients had shortness of breath. During the initial two weeks of infection, the symptoms were mild, and the infection was contagious; however, the shortness of breath symptom increase and dyspnea as well [54]. According to chest CT scan results, 13 out of 41 had developed clinical pneumonia and suffered from hypoxic respiratory failure, and required ventilation. Among them, 2 patients received extracorporeal membrane oxygenation due to refractory hypoxia, 10 patients received mechanical ventilation.

In comparison, 6 patients died due to disease severity. This high CFR triggered alarming situations around the world. Although, most of the patients were having underlying diseases and aged people with an average of 49 age [50,55,56].

Virological Investigations

The flow diagram shows how the spikes get an attachment with receptors on the cell's body (Fig. **2**). It is hypothesized that the mycoplasma-like organisms first paves the way for virus entry at the mucosa level [57]. The mycoplasma-like microorganism removes the villi from the mucous membrane. It denudes where the virus can get entry, and the cell's defense system starts mucous production, especially in the lungs. The whole mechanism of replication has been shown in Fig. (**2**).

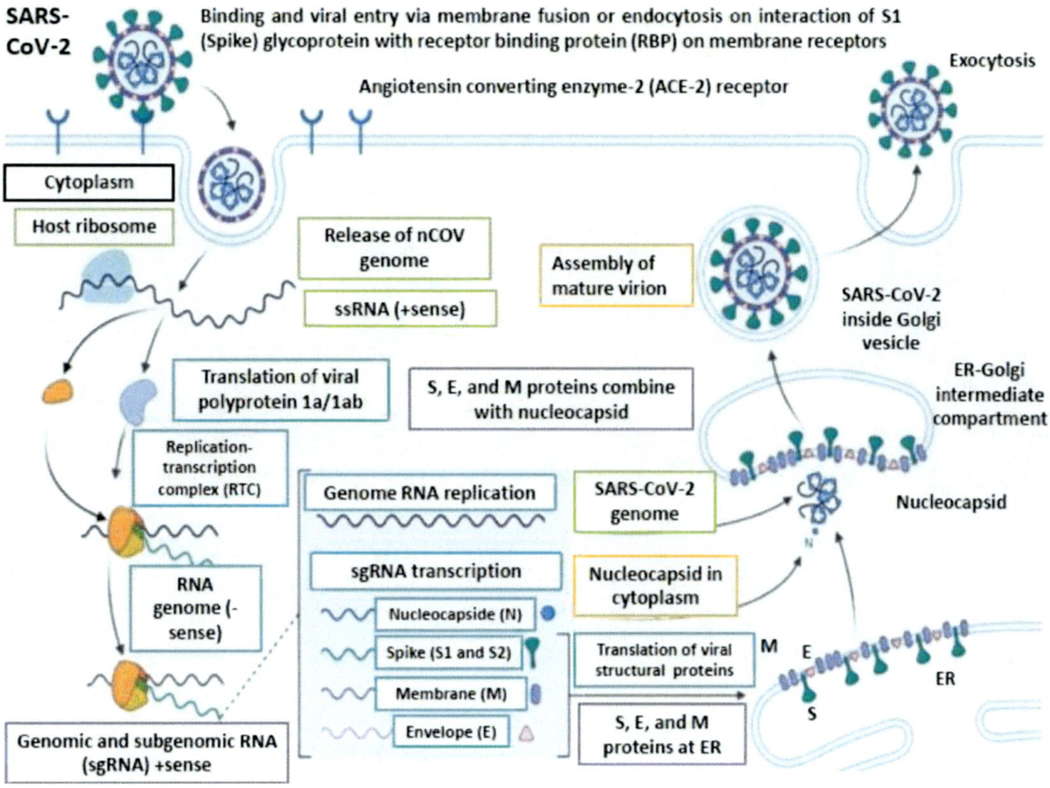

Fig. (2). Replication of SARS-CoV-2 inside the cell.

Blood Cell Examination and Counts

According to the complete blood count of the new hospital admitted patient, the patient has normal white blood cells (WBCs) and platelet counts. Lymphocytes level was reduced, and inadequate normal-sized red blood cells (RBCs). The WBCs and immature neutrophil levels were reported to increase after three days [58, 59], whereas the monocytes level was increased slightly and lymphocytes level reduced. The leuko-erythroblastic showed a reduced level of RBCs but normal in shape and size. Pathologically this is termed normocytic anemia. Moreover, anisocytosis conditions (a mild presence of RBCs with different sizes), nucleated immature RBCs, and dacrocytes (rare tear-drop shaped cells) were observed in the haemogram of the patient. WBCs appeared to be primarily involved in the fight with pathogens as its level was normal when it was analyzed after infection recovery.

Pathological Characteristics of COVID-19

The WHO strictly prohibits the postmortem of dead bodies with COVID-19 infection or die from it [60]. Various organs observed were lung, GIT, heart, liver, kidney, skin, spleen, and blood vessels, and they showed the characteristics of COVID-19.

Lung

Since SARS-CoV-2 is considered respiratory viruses, the lung is one of the well-studied organs in postmortem, autopsies, and biopsies. In postmortem or autopsy of the patient, the visual observation revealed an increasing abundance of gray-white viscous fluid or thick mucus, as discussed earlier. Engagement of vascular, consolidation or thickness, inflammation or edema of pleura developing to pleurisy, mildly erythematous trachea, and evidence of white mucous in lungs along with frothy pink material in airways with aggravation to dark-colored hemorrhage(s) were observed [60]. Moreover, in interstitial regions lymphocytes infiltration, diffused alveolar damage, intra-alveolar fibrin, hyperplasia of pneumocytes, thick exudate formation, and lymphocytic inflammation were also observed. Additionally, in various studies, electron microscopy reported the hyaline membrane formation, presence of fibroblasts around intra-alveolar fibrin, and loose connective tissue [61]. The other changes observed were pulmonary arteries cytoplasmic vacuolization, presence of megakaryocyte in branches of the small vessel, pulmonary microangiopathy, clotting of fibrin in small capillaries around alveoli, congestion of capillary, thrombosis of a small vessel, and alveolar hemorrhage. There was thickening of alveolar capillaries in lungs also.

Gastrointestinal (GI) tract

COVID-19 infection may also affect the GIT due to the presence of ACE2 in the enterocytes. Reports for the presence of SARS-CoV-2 in stool and diarrhea have been reported. No damage has been observed through a histopathology study. The esophagus revealed the lymphocytes intrusion in the squamous epithelium, stomach lamina propria, duodenum, and interstitial edema [62].

Liver

There were high rise in the level of hepatic enzymes, such as aspartate aminotransferase (AST), lactate dehydrogenase (LDH), and alanine aminotransferase (ALT) in COVID 19 patients. It had led to liver function failure. Upon autopsy, it showed a dark red liver with hepatomegaly. Upon histopathological examinations, hepatocyte degeneration, lobular focal necrosis, congested hepatic sinuses, and the microthrombus. It was also noticed that the lung had portal tract fibrosis and mononuclear leukocyte along with neutrophil infiltration [63, 64].

Kidney

Proximal renal tissues have been reported in COVID-19 patients according to histopathological findings of the biopsy. Degeneration in the vacuole, Luminal brush border sloughing, necrosis in tubules, lymphocyte infiltrations in the tubule-interstitial and/or sub-capsular area were also observed. Other kidney-related damages are glomerular epithelial cells hypertrophy, mild focal tubular atrophy, fibrosis in interstitial and cortical parenchyma, and complement membrane attack complex (MAC) deposit in tubules along with glomerular walls [65, 66]. The vascular analysis revealed the infiltration of inflammatory cells in the arcuate artery and glomerulus capillary vessels are dilated. In glomerular capillary loops, fibrin thrombus is shown, which gives a foamy appearance of endothelial cells, and hyperplasia is also observed under the microscope. The reason for kidney failure was collapsing glomerulopathy (CG) in COVID-19 patients.

Skin

Skin tissue alterations have been reported to have clinical features such as petechial rash with thrombocytopenia, widespread urticarial and vesicles on the skin, and erythematous-to-purpuric coalescing macules COVID-19 patients. Moreover, vasculopathy, including peripheral cyanosis leading to bullae and dry gangrene with red papules on fingers resembling chilblains, was also observed. Recently, a study presented skin classification based on lesions that include acral areas of erythema with vesicles or pustules and vesicular eruptions in early cases.

There were common lesions such as urticarial lesions and necrosis and maculopapular eruptions [67, 68]. Other skin-associated histopathological findings are focal acantholytic suprabasal clefts, ballooning herpes-like keratinocytes, mucin deposition in the dermis and hypodermis, and nests of Langerhans cells within the epidermis have been reported frequently. Superficial and deep perivascular dermatitis, lymphocytes around blood vessels, dyskeratotic, thrombus formation, and extravasation of erythrocyte in mid-dermis blood vessels were also reported frequently [69].

Heart

The macroscopic and microscopic features of the heart are also reported to changes with the COVID-19 infection, included cardiomegaly and dilation of right ventricular were prominent. Autopsies showed firm myocardium with a red-brown appearance. Microscopic examination revealed myocyte necrosis in the dispersed area near lymphocytes [70, 71].

Blood

Blood specimens showed coagulation, leukopenia, and lymphocytopenia in infected/suspected live cases in peripheral blood examination [72].

Spleen and lymph nodes

Splenic tissues showed viral nucleocapsid protein (NP) in the red and white pulp. Histopathological examinations showed a reduction of cell composition, atrophied white pulp, neutrophilia, plasma cell infiltration, reduction or absence of lymph follicles, increased red pulp to white pulp proportion, and atrophy of corpuscles in the spleen COVID-19 cases [73]. CD20+B cells were found in abundance.

Brain

Viral particles of SARS-CoV-2/COVID-19 were observed in the frontal lobe and capillary endothelial cells of the brain. There were no recordable findings by histopathologic examination of the brain, despite mild hypoxic changes [74].

Blood vessels and placenta

On postmortem, there was the presence of inflammatory cells and endothelitis. Low-grade fetal vascular malperfusion is reported in the pregnant woman. Other histopathological changes of the pregnant woman were fetal thrombotic vasculopathy, meconium macrophages, intramural nonocclusive thrombi, and intramural fibrin deposition [75].

Animal Models and Real Situation

So far, various animals have been evaluated to study the histopathological changes, but no animal presented similar COVID-19 disease symptoms to a human. Mice were killed by euthanasia to study the effect of COVID-19 on various organs of mice. In the laboratory, access and deal with laboratory animals is easy as they are cheap, but in the case of COVID-19, it is still in infancy. The SARS-CoV-2 replicated potentially in the respiratory tract of young inbred mice and data available in sufficient number(s) for statistical evaluation. Pneumonitis and clinical illness develop in almost 1-year-old mice, but its acquisition is hard, and immune senescence complicates pathogenesis studies [76].

A rat model changed the SARS-CoV (Urbani strain) by serial passage in the respiratory tract of the young virus adopted in BALB/c mice. Later, intranasal inoculation, 15 passages caused in a virus (MA15). The quick and high titer of replicating the virus in the lungs increases disease lethality that causes viremia, lymphopenia, and neutrophilia. Besides, the virus spread to extra-pulmonary sites leads to pathological changes in the lungs. However, focal and mild pneumonitis, airways, and alveoli with debris were also reported due to the extensive distribution of the virus. Bronchial epithelial cells and alveolar pneumocytes were also found with viral antigens. Mice have died from a devastating viral infection, and it was suggested that death occurs due to the destruction of ciliated epithelial cells and pneumocytes [76]. Primate animal models other than humans are required urgently to answer the other critical questions or the questions that have not been answered in clinical patients, such as testing antiviral drugs and vaccine evaluation. In response to this hypothesis, old-world monkeys as primates animal models were inoculated with SARS-CoV-2 experimentally. The monkeys include *Macaca mulatta* (*M. mulatta*) (12), *Macaca fascicularis* (*M. fascicularis*) (6) and 6 were from new world monkeys such as *Callithrix jacchus* (*C. jacchus*). Infection develops after inoculation in the *Macaca mulatta* were found with the symptoms of fever , 2 out of 6 *M. fascicularis* develop fever , and none of the *C. jacchus* found with fever. The abnormality in chest regions included lungs, bronchus, and spleen, was reported in all of the *M. mulatta* and *M. fascicularis*. *C. jacchus* was not found with the genome of the virus. However, severe gross and histopathological changes were seen in the stomach, heart, and lungs [77]. According to another study report, the viral genome in the range of 3.0×10^4 to 1.5×10^7 copies/g was found in the Rhesus monkey till post-infection. In the lower lobes regions of the lungs, the titer of the viral genome identified up to 2.0×10^7 copies/g. The pathologists estimated lung lobes damaged by lesions through necropsy for histopathological analysis. It was identified that the right and left inferior lobe is critically injured and the surroundings of the small bronchus as well. The majority of alveoli had thickened walls due to the proliferation of fibroblasts, formation of pulmonary hyaline-membrane, edema, and hemorrhage also observed in the alveoli [78].

According to the studies of cats and ferrets as animal models, the post-infection consequences were the same as humans. However, they were not observed with hyaline membranes and syncytia. The pathogenesis and consequences of SARS-CoV-2 in cats have primarily been associated with tubercle tracheobronchial lymphadenitis. Lastly, *in vivo* results suggested the ACE2 importance in SARS-CoV-2 infection. In cats, pneumocytes type I and II expressed the ACE2 and facilitated the SARS-CoV-2 infection. In ferrets, ACE2 is expressed only on pneumocytes II [79]. These animal models and techniques like histopathology or immune-histopathology help better understand and develop future strategies for COVID-19 control. Scientists should find the best route to overcome the COVID-19 pandemic and develop vaccines and therapeutics remedies, especially the etiology of innovative origin that happened the first time.

CONCLUSION

Conclusively, the virus induces clinical and histopathological changes that produce vascular harm that caused the failure of multiple organs. Observed the lesions of various organs, including the heart, kidney, brain, lymph nodes, skin, lungs, liver, and GIT simplified the pathophysiology. Our final suggestion is to uphold the speculation that far-reaching endothelial contamination by SARS-CoV-2 could have a function in the pathogenesis of serious type infection and susceptible genes at particular organs. More immune pathological studies are needed to reveal why kids, teenagers, adults, and aged present with restricted skin types of COVID-19, interestingly with the serious multi-organ introductions seen in more aged patients with prior infections.

CONSENT FOR PUBLICATION

Not Applicable.

CONFLICT OF INTEREST

The author confirms that this chapter contents have no conflict of interest.

ACKNOWLEDGEMENT

Declared none.

REFERENCES

[1] Zhou P, Yang X-L, Wang X-G, *et al.* A pneumonia outbreak associated with a new coronavirus of probable bat origin. Nature 2020; 579: 270-3.

[http://dx.doi.org/10.1038/s41586-020-2951-z]

[2] Li G. Erik de clercq, therapeutic options for the. novel coronavirus (2019-Ncov). Nature 2019; 2020.

[3] Zumla A, Chan JF, Azhar EI, Hui DS, Yuen KY. Coronaviruses - drug discovery and therapeutic options. Nat Rev Drug Discov 2016; 15(5): 327-47.
[http://dx.doi.org/10.1038/nrd.2015.37] [PMID: 26868298]

[4] Lu R, Zhao X, Li J, *et al.* Genomic characterisation and epidemiology of 2019 novel coronavirus: implications for virus origins and receptor binding. Lancet 2020; 395(10224): 565-74.
[http://dx.doi.org/10.1016/S0140-6736(20)30251-8] [PMID: 32007145]

[5] Ahmed SF, Quadeer AA, Mckay MR. Preliminary Identification Of Potential Vaccine Targets For The Covid-19 Coronavirus (Sars-Cov-2) Based On Sars-Cov Immunological Studies Biorxiv 2020.

[6] Zhou P, Yang XL, Wang XG, *et al.* A Pneumonia Outbreak Associated With A New Coronavirus Of Probable Bat Origin. Nature 2020.
[http://dx.doi.org/10.1038/s41586-020-2951-z]

[7] Lu R, Zhao X, Li J, *et al.* Genomic Characterisation And Epidemiology Of 2019 Novel Coronavirus: Implications For Virus Origins And Receptor Binding. Lancet (London, England) 2020.

[8] Lu R, Zhao X, Li J, *et al.* Genomic characterisation and epidemiology of 2019 novel coronavirus: implications for virus origins and receptor binding. Lancet 2020; 395(10224): 565-74.
[http://dx.doi.org/10.1016/S0140-6736(20)30251-8] [PMID: 32007145]

[9] Reusken CB, Haagmans BL, Müller MA, *et al.* Middle East respiratory syndrome coronavirus neutralising serum antibodies in dromedary camels: a comparative serological study. Lancet Infect Dis 2013; 13(10): 859-66.
[http://dx.doi.org/10.1016/S1473-3099(13)70164-6] [PMID: 23933067]

[10] Chan JF, Lau SK, To KK, Cheng VC, Woo PC, Yuen K-Y. Middle East respiratory syndrome coronavirus: another zoonotic betacoronavirus causing SARS-like disease. Clin Microbiol Rev 2015; 28(2): 465-522.
[http://dx.doi.org/10.1128/CMR.00102-14] [PMID: 25810418]

[11] Yang L, Wu Z, Ren X, *et al.* MERS-related betacoronavirus in Vespertilio superans bats, China. Emerg Infect Dis 2014; 20(7): 1260-2.
[http://dx.doi.org/10.3201/eid2007.140318] [PMID: 24960574]

[12] Corman VM, Ithete NL, Richards LR, *et al.* Rooting the phylogenetic tree of middle East respiratory syndrome coronavirus by characterization of a conspecific virus from an African bat. J Virol 2014; 88(19): 11297-303.
[http://dx.doi.org/10.1128/JVI.01498-14] [PMID: 25031349]

[13] Anthony SJ, Gilardi K, Menachery VD, *et al.* Further Evidence for Bats as the Evolutionary Source of Middle East Respiratory Syndrome Coronavirus. MBio 2017; 8(2): E00373-17.
[http://dx.doi.org/10.1128/mBio.00373-17] [PMID: 28377531]

[14] Geldenhuys M, Mortlock M, Weyer J, *et al.* A metagenomic viral discovery approach identifies potential zoonotic and novel mammalian viruses in Neoromicia bats within South Africa. PLoS One 2018; 13(3)e0194527
[http://dx.doi.org/10.1371/journal.pone.0194527] [PMID: 29579103]

[15] Lau SKP, Zhang L, Luk HKH, *et al.* Receptor Usage of a Novel Bat Lineage C Betacoronavirus Reveals Evolution of Middle East Respiratory Syndrome-Related Coronavirus Spike Proteins for Human Dipeptidyl Peptidase 4 Binding. J Infect Dis 2018; 218(2): 197-207.
[http://dx.doi.org/10.1093/infdis/jiy018] [PMID: 29346682]

[16] Corman VM, Kallies R, Philipps H, *et al.* Characterization of a novel betacoronavirus related to middle East respiratory syndrome coronavirus in European hedgehogs. J Virol 2014; 88(1): 717-24.
[http://dx.doi.org/10.1128/JVI.01600-13] [PMID: 24131722]

[17] Guan Y, Zheng BJ, He YQ, *et al.* Isolation and characterization of viruses related to the SARS coronavirus from animals in southern China. Science 2003; 302(5643): 276-8. [http://dx.doi.org/10.1126/science.1087139] [PMID: 12958366]

[18] Ksiazek TG, Erdman D, Goldsmith CS, *et al.* A novel coronavirus associated with severe acute respiratory syndrome. N Engl J Med 2003; 348(20): 1953-66. [http://dx.doi.org/10.1056/NEJMoa030781] [PMID: 12690092]

[19] Wu F, Zhao S, Yu B, *et al.* Complete Genome Characterisation Of A Novel Coronavirus Associated With Severe Human Respiratory Disease In Wuhan China. 2020.

[20] Yang Y, Du L, Liu C, *et al.* Receptor usage and cell entry of bat coronavirus HKU4 provide insight into bat-to-human transmission of MERS coronavirus. Proc Natl Acad Sci USA 2014; 111(34): 12516-21. [http://dx.doi.org/10.1073/pnas.1405889111] [PMID: 25114257]

[21] Wang Q, Qi J, Yuan Y, *et al.* Bat origins of MERS-CoV supported by bat coronavirus HKU4 usage of human receptor CD26. Cell Host Microbe 2014; 16(3): 328-37. [http://dx.doi.org/10.1016/j.chom.2014.08.009] [PMID: 25211075]

[22] Zhong NS, Zheng BJ, Li YM, *et al.* Epidemiology and cause of severe acute respiratory syndrome (SARS) in Guangdong, People's Republic of China, in February, 2003. Lancet 2003; 362(9393): 1353-8. [http://dx.doi.org/10.1016/S0140-6736(03)14630-2] [PMID: 14585636]

[23] Rota PA, Oberste MS, Monroe SS, *et al.* Characterization of a novel coronavirus associated with severe acute respiratory syndrome. Science 2003; 300(5624): 1394-9. [http://dx.doi.org/10.1126/science.1085952] [PMID: 12730500]

[24] Wuhan; Commission, M.H., Report Of Clustering Pneumonia Of Unknown Etiology In Wuhan City. Wuhan Municipal Health Commission 2019.

[25] Lu CW, Liu XF, Jia ZF. Ncov transmission through the ocular surface must not be ignored. Lancet 2019; 395(1022): e39. [PMID: 32035510]

[26] Zhu N, Zhang D, Wang W, *et al.* A Novel Coronavirus from Patients with Pneumonia in China, 2019. N Engl J Med 2020; 382(8): 727-33. [http://dx.doi.org/10.1056/NEJMoa2001017] [PMID: 31978945]

[27] Bao L, Deng W, Huang B, *et al.* The Pathogenicity Of Sars-Cov-2 In Hace2 Transgenic Mice Biorxiv 2020. [http://dx.doi.org/10.1101/2020.02.07.939389]

[28] Titford M. A Short History Of Histopathology Technique. J Histotechnol 2006; 29(2): 99-110. [http://dx.doi.org/10.1179/his.2006.29.2.99]

[29] Musumeci G. Past, present and future: overview on histology and histopathology. J Histol Histopathol 2014; 1(1): 5. [http://dx.doi.org/10.7243/2055-091X-1-5]

[30] Ganguly S, Rohlan K, Choudhary S, Kumar V, Shringi N. Chapter-4 embedding techniques in tissue histological process.

[31] Howat WJ, Wilson BA. Tissue fixation and the effect of molecular fixatives on downstream staining procedures. Methods 2014; 70(1): 12-9. [http://dx.doi.org/10.1016/j.ymeth.2014.01.022] [PMID: 24561827]

[32] Kasten FH. In Cell Structure And Function By Microspectrofluorometry. Elsevier 1989; pp. 3-50. [http://dx.doi.org/10.1016/B978-0-12-417760-4.50008-2]

[33] Tian S, Xiong Y, Liu H, *et al.* Novel Coronavirus Disease (Covid-19) Through Postmortem Core Biopsies. Mod Pathol 2019; 2020: 1-8.

[PMID: 32291399]

[34] Zimmermann T, Pepperkok R, Stephens D, Girod A, Rietdorf J. Basic Light Microscopy. *Essential Cell Biology Vol 1*. Cell Structure 2003; 2: 424.

[35] Gautier J-C. Drug Safety Evaluation: Methods And Protocols. Springer 2011. [http://dx.doi.org/10.1007/978-1-60761-849-2]

[36] Comanescu M, Annaratone L, D'Armento G, Cardos G, Sapino A, Bussolati G. Critical steps in tissue processing in histopathology. Recent Pat DNA Gene Seq 2012; 6(1): 22-32. [http://dx.doi.org/10.2174/187221512799303190] [PMID: 22208680]

[37] Feldman AT. Wolfe, D. Histopathology. Springer 2014; pp. 31-43. [http://dx.doi.org/10.1007/978-1-4939-1050-2_3]

[38] Truwit CL, Nelson R. Google Patents 2008.

[39] Cox ML, Schray CL, Luster CN, *et al.* Assessment of fixatives, fixation, and tissue processing on morphology and RNA integrity. Exp Mol Pathol 2006; 80(2): 183-91. [http://dx.doi.org/10.1016/j.yexmp.2005.10.002] [PMID: 16332367]

[40] Taylor CR. Introduction To Immunohistochemistry.Taylor Cr, Lars R. 6th ed., Denmark: Dako 2013.

[41] Duerr JS. In *Wormbook: The Online Review Of C. Elegans Biology*. WormBook 2006. [Internet].

[42] Magaki S. Hojat, S.A.; Wei, B.; So, A.; Yong, W.H.Biobanking. Springer 2019; pp. 289-98. [http://dx.doi.org/10.1007/978-1-4939-8935-5_25]

[43] Ramos-Vara JA. In Drug Safety Evaluation. Springer 2011; pp. 83-96. [http://dx.doi.org/10.1007/978-1-60761-849-2_5]

[44] Garvey W. Modification Of The Mayer Hematoxylin Stain. J Histotechnol 1991; 14(3): 163-5. [http://dx.doi.org/10.1179/his.1991.14.3.163]

[45] Zhao W, Zhong Z, Xie X, Yu Q, Liu J. Relation Between Chest CT Findings and Clinical Conditions of Coronavirus Disease (COVID-19) Pneumonia: A Multicenter Study. AJR Am J Roentgenol 2020; 214(5): 1072-7. [http://dx.doi.org/10.2214/AJR.20.22976] [PMID: 32125873]

[46] Datta PK, Liu F, Fischer T, Rappaport J, Qin X. SARS-CoV-2 pandemic and research gaps: Understanding SARS-CoV-2 interaction with the ACE2 receptor and implications for therapy. Theranostics 2020; 10(16): 7448-64. [http://dx.doi.org/10.7150/thno.48076] [PMID: 32642005]

[47] Sims AC, Burkett SE, Yount B, Pickles RJ. SARS-CoV replication and pathogenesis in an *in vitro* model of the human conducting airway epithelium. Virus Res 2008; 133(1): 33-44. [http://dx.doi.org/10.1016/j.virusres.2007.03.013] [PMID: 17451829]

[48] Soldati G, Smargiassi A, Inchingolo R, *et al.* Proposal for International Standardization of the Use of Lung Ultrasound for Patients With COVID-19: A Simple, Quantitative, Reproducible Method. J Ultrasound Med 2020; 39(7): 1413-9. [http://dx.doi.org/10.1002/jum.15285] [PMID: 32227492]

[49] Meyerholz DK. Beck, A.P.Mers Coronavirus. Springer 2020; pp. 205-20. [http://dx.doi.org/10.1007/978-1-0716-0211-9_16]

[50] Rabi FA, Al Zoubi MS, Kasasbeh GA, Salameh DM, Al-Nasser AD. SARS-CoV-2 and Coronavirus Disease 2019: What We Know So Far. Pathogens 2020; 9(3): 231. [http://dx.doi.org/10.3390/pathogens9030231] [PMID: 32245083]

[51] Dhama K, Sharun K, Tiwari R, *et al.* Coronavirus Disease 2019–Covid-19. 2020.

[52] Dijkman R, Jebbink MF, Gaunt E, *et al.* The dominance of human coronavirus OC43 and NL63 infections in infants. J Clin Virol 2012; 53(2): 135-9. [http://dx.doi.org/10.1016/j.jcv.2011.11.011] [PMID: 22188723]

[53] Nejadi Babadaei MM, Hasan A, Haj Bloukh S, *et al.* The Expression Level Of Angiotensin-Converting Enzyme 2 Determine The Severity Of Covid-19: Lung And Heart Tissue As Targets. Journal Of Biomolecular Structure And Dynamics 2020; (Just-Accepted): 1-13.

[54] Cascella M, Mauro I, De Blasio E, Cascella M. Rapid and impressive response to a combined treatment with single-dose tocilizumab and NIV in a patient with COVID-19 Pneumonia/ARDS. Medicina 2020; 56(8): 377.

[55] Liu K, Chen Y, Lin R, Han K. Clinical features of COVID-19 in elderly patients: A comparison with young and middle-aged patients. J Infect 2020; 80(6): e14-8. [http://dx.doi.org/10.1016/j.jinf.2020.03.005] [PMID: 32171866]

[56] Huang C, Wang Y, Li X, *et al.* Clinical features of patients infected with 2019 novel coronavirus in Wuhan, China. Lancet 2020; 395(10223): 497-506. [http://dx.doi.org/10.1016/S0140-6736(20)30183-5] [PMID: 31986264]

[57] Mirzaei R, Goodarzi P, Asadi M, *et al.* Bacterial co-infections with SARS-CoV-2. IUBMB Life 2020; 72(10): 2097-111. [http://dx.doi.org/10.1002/iub.2356] [PMID: 32770825]

[58] Cao Q, Chen Y-C, Chen C-L, Chiu C-H. SARS-CoV-2 infection in children: Transmission dynamics and clinical characteristics. J Formos Med Assoc 2020; 119(3): 670-3. [http://dx.doi.org/10.1016/j.jfma.2020.02.009] [PMID: 32139299]

[59] Yang P, Wang X, Liu P, *et al.* Clinical characteristics and risk assessment of newborns born to mothers with COVID-19. J Clin Virol 2020; 127104356 [http://dx.doi.org/10.1016/j.jcv.2020.104356] [PMID: 32302955]

[60] Zhang H, Zhou P, Wei Y, *et al.* Histopathologic Changes and SARS-CoV-2 Immunostaining in the Lung of a Patient With COVID-19. Ann Intern Med 2020; 172(9): 629-32. [http://dx.doi.org/10.7326/M20-0533] [PMID: 32163542]

[61] Tian S, Hu W, Niu L, Liu H, Xu H, Xiao S-Y. Pulmonary Pathology of Early-Phase 2019 Novel Coronavirus (COVID-19) Pneumonia in Two Patients With Lung Cancer. J Thorac Oncol 2020; 15(5): 700-4. [http://dx.doi.org/10.1016/j.jtho.2020.02.010] [PMID: 32114094]

[62] Wong SH, Lui RN, Sung JJ. Covid-19 and the digestive system. J Gastroenterol Hepatol 2020; 35(5): 744-8. [http://dx.doi.org/10.1111/jgh.15047] [PMID: 32215956]

[63] Zhang C, Shi L, Wang F-S. Liver injury in COVID-19: management and challenges. Lancet Gastroenterol Hepatol 2020; 5(5): 428-30. [http://dx.doi.org/10.1016/S2468-1253(20)30057-1] [PMID: 32145190]

[64] Sun J, Aghemo A, Forner A, Valenti L. COVID-19 and liver disease. Liver Int 2020; 40(6): 1278-81. [http://dx.doi.org/10.1111/liv.14470] [PMID: 32251539]

[65] Fanelli V, Fiorentino M, Cantaluppi V, *et al.* Acute kidney injury in SARS-CoV-2 infected patients. Crit Care 2020; 24(1): 155. [http://dx.doi.org/10.1186/s13054-020-02872-z] [PMID: 32299479]

[66] Puelles VG, Lütgehetmann M, Lindenmeyer MT, *et al.* Multiorgan and Renal Tropism of SARS-Co--2. N Engl J Med 2020; 383(6): 590-2. [http://dx.doi.org/10.1056/NEJMc2011400] [PMID: 32402155]

[67] Mahé A, Birckel E, Krieger S, Merklen C, Bottlaender L. A distinctive skin rash associated with coronavirus disease 2019? J Eur Acad Dermatol Venereol 2020; 34(6): e246-7. [http://dx.doi.org/10.1111/jdv.16471] [PMID: 32294259]

[68] Diotallevi F, Campanati A, Bianchelli T, *et al.* Skin involvement in SARS-CoV-2 infection: Case series. J Med Virol 2020; 92(11): 2332-4.

[http://dx.doi.org/10.1002/jmv.26012] [PMID: 32410241]

[69] Bataille V, Visconti A, Murray B, *et al.* Diagnostic Value Of Skin Manifestation Of Sars-Cov-2 Infection Medrxiv 2020.

[70] Chen C, Zhou Y, Wang DW. SARS-CoV-2: a potential novel etiology of fulminant myocarditis. Herz 2020; 45(3): 230-2. [http://dx.doi.org/10.1007/s00059-020-04909-z] [PMID: 32140732]

[71] Lindner D, Fitzek A, Bräuninger H, *et al.* Association of Cardiac Infection With SARS-CoV-2 in Confirmed COVID-19 Autopsy Cases. JAMA Cardiol 2020; 5(11): 1281-5. [http://dx.doi.org/10.1001/jamacardio.2020.3551] [PMID: 32730555]

[72] Han H, Yang L, Liu R, *et al.* Prominent Changes In Blood Coagulation Of Patients With Sars-Cov-2 Infection. Clinical Chemistry And Laboratory Medicine (Cclm) 2020; 1(Ahead-Of-Print))

[73] Feng Z, Diao B, Wang R, *et al.* The Novel Severe Acute Respiratory Syndrome Coronavirus 2 (Sars-Cov-2) Directly Decimates Human Spleens And Lymph Nodes. Medrxiv 2020.

[74] Natoli S, Oliveira V, Calabresi P, Maia LF, Pisani A. Does SARS-Cov-2 invade the brain? Translational lessons from animal models. Eur J Neurol 2020; 27(9): 1764-73. [http://dx.doi.org/10.1111/ene.14277] [PMID: 32333487]

[75] Schwartz DA. An Analysis of 38 Pregnant Women With COVID-19, Their Newborn Infants, and Maternal-Fetal Transmission of SARS-CoV-2: Maternal Coronavirus Infections and Pregnancy Outcomes. Arch Pathol Lab Med 2020; 144(7): 799-805. [http://dx.doi.org/10.5858/arpa.2020-0901-SA] [PMID: 32180426]

[76] Jiang R-D, Liu M-Q, Chen Y, *et al.* Pathogenesis Of Sars-Cov-2 In Transgenic Mice Expressing Human Angiotensin-Converting Enzyme 2 Cell 2020; 182(1): 50-58-E58.

[77] Lu S, Zhao Y, Yu W, *et al.* Comparison of Sars-Cov-2 infections among 3 species of non-human primates. Biorxiv 2020.

[78] Shan C, Yao Y-F, Yang X-L, *et al.* Infection with novel coronavirus (SARS-CoV-2) causes pneumonia in Rhesus macaques. Cell Res 2020; 30(8): 670-7. [http://dx.doi.org/10.1038/s41422-020-0364-z] [PMID: 32636454]

[79] van den Brand JM, Haagmans BL, Leijten L, *et al.* Pathology of experimental SARS coronavirus infection in cats and ferrets. Vet Pathol 2008; 45(4): 551-62. [http://dx.doi.org/10.1354/vp.45-4-551] [PMID: 18587105]

CHAPTER 4

Key Proteins and Their Roles in COVID-19

Amjad Islam Aqib[1,*], Iqra Muzammil[2], Qaisar Tanveer[3], Tean Zaheer[4] and Aisha Mahmood[5]

[1] *Department of Medicine, Faculty of Veterinary Science, Cholistan University of Veterinary and Animal Sciences, Bahawalpur-63100, Pakistan*

[2] *Department of Clinical Medicine and Surgery, University of Agriculture, Faisalabad38000, Pakistan*

[3] *Institute of Pharmacy, Physiology and Pharmacology, University of Agriculture, Faisalabad-38000, Pakistan*

[4] *Department of Parasitology, University of Agriculture, Faisalabad-38000, Pakistan*

[5] *Department of Physiology, Faculty of Veterinary and Animal Sciences, The Islamia University of Bahawalpur, Bahawalpur-63100, Pakistan*

Abstract: Severe acute respiratory syndrome-coronavirus-2 (SARS-CoV-2) is a novel member of the *Coronaviridae* family that is the causative agent of coronavirus disease-19 (COVID-19), which is now pandemic in the world. Various proteins characteristically responsible for pathogenesis are categorized as structural proteins (S, M, E, and N), non-structural proteins, and accessory proteins (ORF3a, ORF6, ORF7a, ORF7b, ORF8, and ORF10). Substitution of 380 amino acids and mutations in SARS-CoV-2 compared to other SARS-like coronaviruses characteristically plays a key role in entering the development of infection. S1/S2 of S protein has a specific differential role in SARS-CoV-2 stabilization and resultant infection. In addition to these key proteins, the host and virus-related proteins play risk factors in the spread of this disease. The current chapter will describe the structure of key proteins, their role in pathogenesis, starting from viral attachment leading to the infection in the host compared to the viruses belonging to *Betacoronaviruses*.

Keywords: Coronavirus, Open reading frames, Pathogenesis, Proteins, Risk factors.

INTRODUCTION

Severe acute respiratory syndrome-coronavirus-2 (SARS-CoV-2) is the cause of an outbreak at the world level with the expression of uncommon viral pneumonia

* **Corresponding author Dr. Amjad Islam Aqib:** Department of Medicine, Faculty of Veterinary Science, Cholistan University of Veterinary and Animal Sciences, Bahawalpur-63100, Pakistan; Tel.: +92 343 7474 583; E-mail: amjadwaseer@cuvas.edu.pk

Kamal Niaz & Muhammad Farrukh Nisar (Eds.)

that firstly occurred in Wuhan, China. The virus belongs to genera *Betacoronavirus,* keeping in view genomic structures and phylogeny interactions with other viruses responsible for severe acute respiratory syndrome (SARS) and the Middle East respiratory syndrome (MERS). They all have notable differences in their genomic and phenotypic structures [1]. All *Coronaviridae* family viruses are pleomorphic, having RNA as an essential genetic material. The striking feature is the possession of crown-shaped (thus named corona) peplomers or spikes that surround the genetic material. These spike proteins have facilitated the pathways leading to membrane fusion of the virus with the host cells [2]. These peplomers have a special affinity for binding angiotensin-converting enzyme 2 (ACE2), receptors located abundantly on lungs and the heart tissues. S proteins possess highly variant amino acid sequences than those of Open reading frames (ORFs) [3].

SARS-CoV-2 has been identified as a single standard +RNA comprising 2.9kb nucleotides in length encoding 26 proteins and one RNA-dependent RNA polymerase (RdRp). The proteins of this virus contain large polyproteins, *i.e.,* ORF1a and ORF1ab, which proteolytically slash to form 16 non-structural proteins. Besides these, there are 04 structural proteins, sixteen proteins categorized as non-structural, while 06 of those proteins called accessory proteins (Fig. **1**). Though these proteins are not necessary for *in vitro* replicating viruses, it is important for *in vivo* virus-host interactions [4].

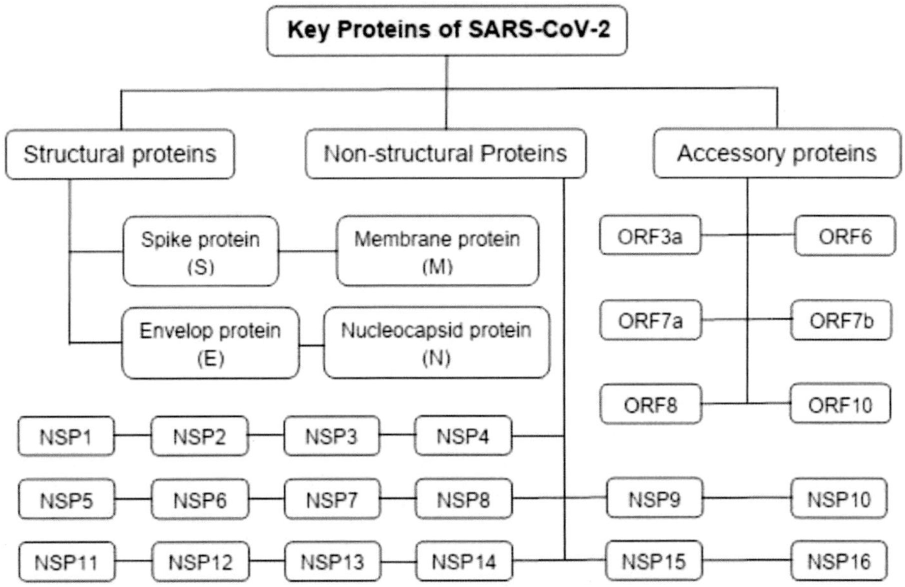

Fig. (1). Structural summary of the proteins expressed by SARS-CoV-2.

Hemagglutinin esterase lacks gene in SARS-CoV-2. Although it is present in a lineage A of *Betacoronavirus* named human coronavirus (hCoV) HKU1 [5]. Spike protein plays a role in binding with receptors and attachment to the membrane, which indicates host tropism and disease spread [6]. In SARS-CoV-2, the S gene is different, having <75% nucleotide sequence resemblance compared to all formerly reported SARS-related coronaviruses [4]. However, the other 03 proteins of the structural category are fairly maintained compared to spike protein and are essential for overall coronavirus function.

The glycosylated spike protein is considered responsible for the induction of an immune response in the host. This spike (S) protein facilitates attack on the host cell by attaching to ACE2 protein receptors found on the host cell membrane. Envelope (E) protein is responsible for performing many functions in the viral replication cycle involving viral assembly, the release of the virion, and viral pathogenesis [7]. Membrane (M) protein is an essential membrane protein of the coronavirus that plays a significant role in viral assembly and induction of apoptosis [5]. The nucleocapsid (N) protein of coronaviruses binds directly to viral RNA, making stability. So it is found to provoke antiviral RNAi in SARS-CoV-2 [8]. These proteins provide a coating to the RNA in protein assemblage (Fig. **2**) responsible for budding, forming an envelope, and pathogenicity of the COVID-19 virus [9].

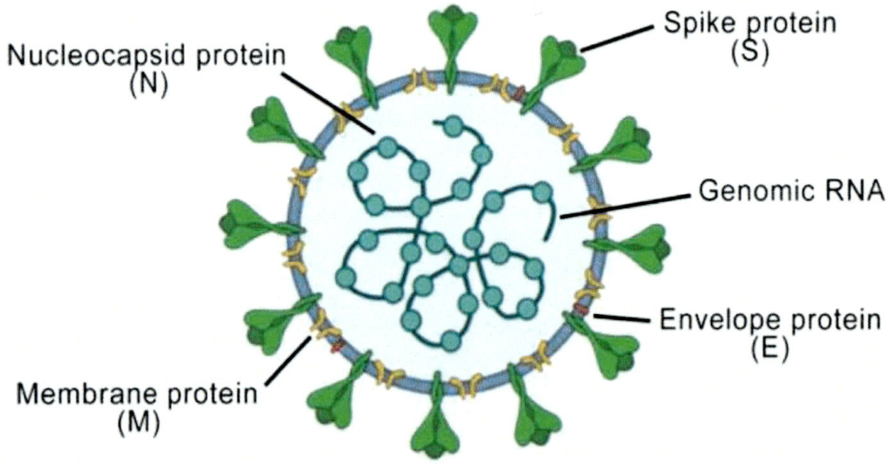

Fig. (2). Structural diagram of the SARS-CoV-2.

Besides these, some non-structural proteins (NSP1-NSP16) in SARS-CoV-2 play an essential role in COVID-19 pathogenesis. Receptor recognition is one of the major differential factors among coronaviruses as a basic primary step of pathogenesis. RdRp acts in combination with non-structural proteins to keep up genome reliability [4]. It is reported that the single guide RNAs of CoVs help in the translation of all structural and accessory proteins. Hence, the genetic and phylogeny of the COVID-19 virus is important to understand its role in the pathogenesis of the disease. The current chapter will significantly focus on the structure of these proteins and their role in pathogenesis, starting from viral attachment leading to the infection in the host compared to other *Betacoronaviruses*.

Classification Track of the SARS-CoV-2

SARS-CoV-2 finds its place in "order" Nidovirales, "family" *Coronaviridae*, and "subfamily" *Orthocoronaviridae*, and "genus" *Coronavirus*. They are 4 genera in their classification, *i.e., Alphacoronaviruses*, *Betacoronaviruses*, *Gammacorona viruses*, and *Deltacoronaviruses*. Former 02 coronaviruses serve as the etiology of infection in mammals. *Gammacoronaviruses* and *Deltacoronavirus* infect avian species and both avian and mammalian species, respectively. *Alphacoronaviruses* own human coronavirus NL63, porcine transmissible gastroenteritis coronavirus, and porcine respiratory coronavirus. On the other hand, *Betacoronaviruses* have a virus SARS-CoV-2 that causes COVID-19. SARS-CoV and MERS-CoV caused SARS, and MERS, bat coronavirus HKU4, bovine coronavirus (BCoV), and mouse hepatitis coronavirus (MHV), respectively. *Gamma* and *Deltacoronaviruses* are reported to have avian infectious bronchitis coronavirus and porcine *Deltacoronavirus,* respectively. All these viruses are enveloped, large, and + sense RNA viruses [4].

Structural Biology of COVID-19 Proteins

SARS-CoV-2 (NC_045512.2) contains 11 genes containing 11 ORFs, including ORF1ab, ORF2, ORF3a, ORF4, ORF5 ORF6, ORF7a, ORF7b, ORF8, ORF9, and ORF10. The proteins of SARS-CoV-2 contain 02 large polyproteins, *e.g.,* ORF 1a and ORF1ab, which proteolytically slash to form 16 non-structural proteins. Besides these, ORF2, ORF4, ORF5, and ORF9 encode 4 proteins of the structural category of proteins of the SARS-CoV-2 (Table **1**) abbreviated S, E, M, and N proteins, respectively. Additionally, SARS-CoV-2 also possesses 06 proteins a category of "accessory" including ORF3a; ORF6; ORF7a; ORF7b; ORF8; and ORF10 [10] (Table **2**). These proteins are derived from certain genes and contain a specific number of amino acids, as shown in Table **1**.

Table 1. The genes expressed by SARS-CoV-2 with their encoded proteins.

S. No.	Gene	Gene ID	No. of Amino Acids	Protein	References
1.	ORF1ab	43,740,578	7,096	ORF1ab poly protein*	[3, 4]
1.	ORF1a	43,740,578	4,405	ORF1a poly protein*	[10]
2.	ORF2 (S)	43,740,568	1,273	Spike protein (S)	[11]
3.	ORF3a	43,740,569	275	ORF3a protein	[10, 12]
4.	ORF4 (E)	43,740,570	75	Envelope protein (E)	[7]
5.	ORF5 (M)	43,740,571	222	Membrane protein (M)	[5]
6.	ORF6	43,740,572	61	ORF6 protein	[13]
7.	ORF7a	43,740,573	121	ORF7a protein	[10, 14]
8.	ORF7b	43,740,574	43	ORF7b protein	[10, 14]
9.	ORF8	43,740,577	121	ORF8 protein	[10] [15]
10.	ORF9 (N)	43,740,575	419	Nucleocapsid protein (N)	[16, 17]
11.	ORF10	43,740,576	38	ORF10 protein	[10]

* polyproteins slash to form 16 non-structural proteins NSP1-16.

The Structural Proteins

This protein category comprises 4 candidates named S, E, M, and N proteins.

Spike Protein

S protein (surface glycoprotein) is a transmembrane protein having a molecular weight of about 150 kDa, containing 1273 amino acids. It is responsible for the adherence of the pathogen to the host cell. S protein makes large bulges from the virus surface out of all structural proteins to give the crown-shaped appearance to coronaviruses. Besides facilitating entry to the virus, the spike is a determining severe factor for the host range of virus and tissue tropism and chiefly responsible for activating host immune responses. Spike consists of 3 segments: a) large ectodomain, b) single-pass transmembrane anchor, and c) short intracellular tail. Former consists of S1 as receptor-binding subunit while S2 serves as membrane-fusion subunit. Spike has been found as a clove-shaped trimmer with 3 S1 heads while one trimeric S2 stalk as identified by electron microscopy [10]. S protein of SARS-CoV-2 owns two subunits S1 and S2. The former subunit is accountable for virus-host range and tropism; however, the latter subunit is helping the fusion of membranes of host and the viral permitting entrance of the genome to the host cells. These proteins identify the human ACE2 receptor to predilected cell surfaces of humans [18]. S protein-derived entry into cells is strongly prevented by SARS-CoV spike mouse polyclonal antibodies. Remarkably, the furin cleavage site presents the S protein of SARS-CoV-2 (Fig. **3**) which is not found in the S protein of pathogen SARS-CoV. This modification here can probably describe the variance in the pathogenicity of these two viruses [10]. While the TMPRSS2 gene (Transmembrane protease, serine 2), a protease is present on the host cell and helps binding S protein after priming with it. Both furin and TMPRSS2 are necessary for activation of SARS-CoV-2 pathogen in human airway cells on one end to serve as promising drug targets for the treatment of COVID-19 cases. Linkage of S protein with ACE2 is playing important concern because it is responsible for starting the infection development. Cryo-electron microscopy structure analysis has discovered that S protein of SARS-CoV-2 has almost 10−20 times greater binding ability for ACE2 compared to SARS-CoV [6]. Due to this reason, transmissibility and contagiousness of the SARS-CoV-2 are higher than SARS-CoV [19].

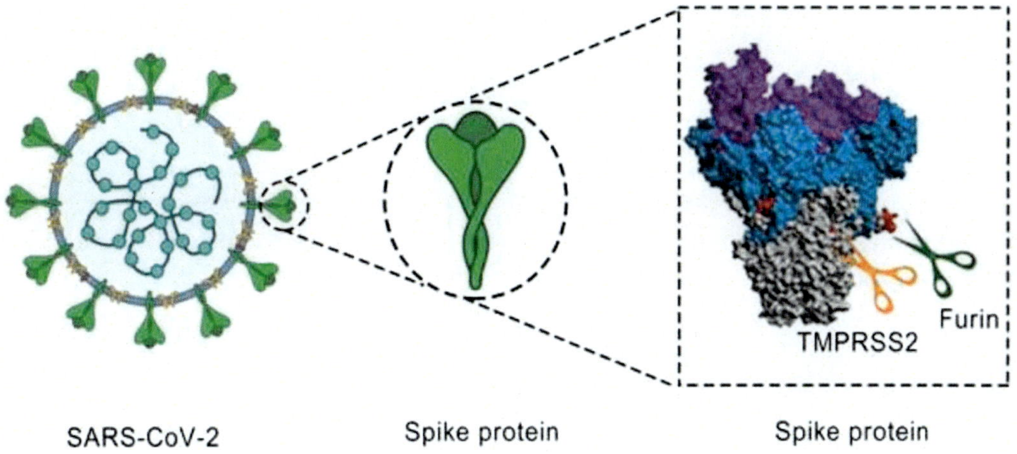

Fig. (3). Diagram of Spike (S) protein of SARS-CoV-2 showing trimeric segments.

Envelope Protein

This protein is a small central membrane protein in coronaviruses, containing 75 amino acids. It can oligomerize to develop an ion channel. The E protein of SARS-CoV-2 (Fig. **4**) is responsible for doing many functions in the viral replication cycle involving viral assembly, the release of the virion, and viral pathogenesis [7].

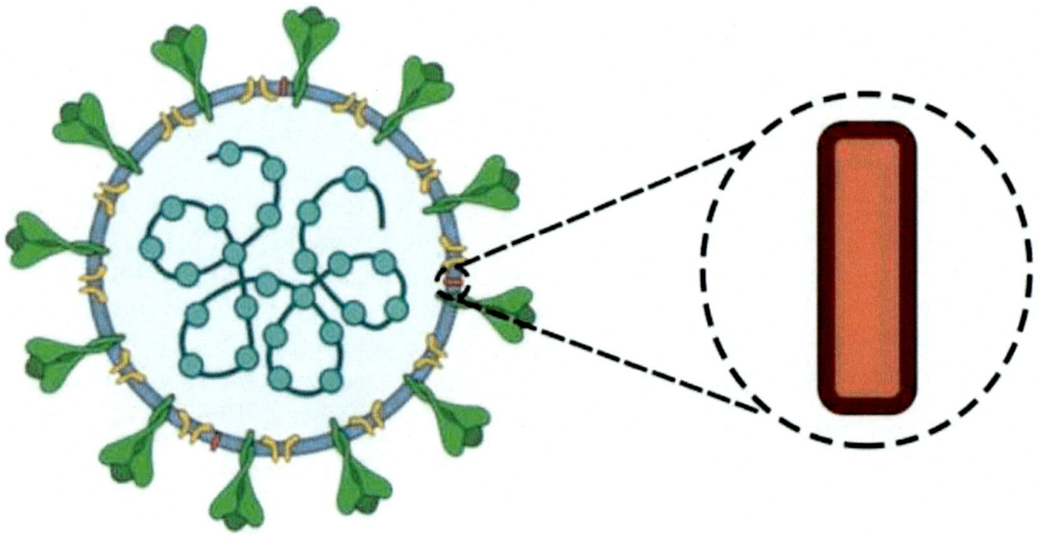

Fig. (4). Diagram of Envelope (E) protein of the SARS-CoV-2.

Interestingly, when sequence alignment of the E proteins from both types of SARS viruses was studied. It was observed that the SARS-CoV pathogen has a glutamate residue (E69) with a negative charge which resembles a positively charged arginine in SARS-CoV-2 (R69) [7].

Membrane Protein

The SARS coronavirus M protein is essential that plays a significant role in viral assembly. It contains 222 amino acids. M protein of SARS-CoV-2 is the most fundamental candidate of structured protein that presents a vital role in confirming the virus envelope (Fig. **5**). It extends the membrane bilayer three times leaving behind a short NH2-terminal domain external to the virus while keeping a lengthy COOH-terminus (cytoplasmic domain) inside it. This protein can bind to all other proteins of its category. N proteins stabilize by binding with M protein and promote the accomplishment of viral assembly by making the N protein-RNA complex inside the internal virion. Additionally, the SARS coronavirus M protein can also induce apoptosis. The M protein interrelates with the N protein to encapsulate the RNA genome [5].

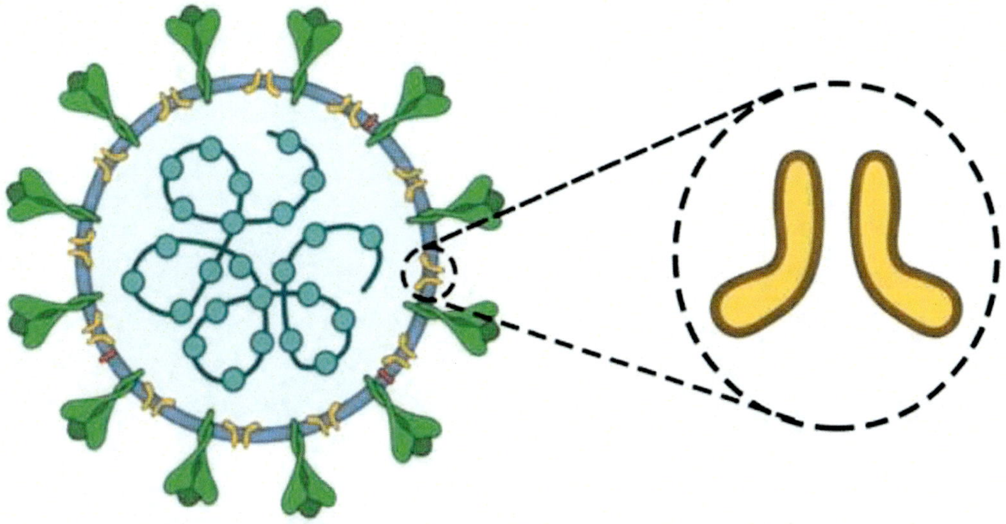

Fig. (5). Diagram of Membrane (M) protein of SARS-CoV-2.

Nucleocapsid Protein

N protein of coronaviruses comprised of 419 amino acids. The protein is an essential part of SARS-CoV-2 confining in the endoplasmic reticulum-Golgi region that is structurally adhered to the nucleic acid material of the virus. This protein adheres to RNA to perform functions relevant to the viral genome, viral replication cycle, and cellular reaction of host cells against infections inflicted by the virus [16]. N protein is also densely phosphorylated and predicted to result in structural changes increasing affinity for viral RNA [17]. It is very much immunogenic and expressed in large quantities during infection, binding directly to viral RNA and making it stable (Fig. **6**).

N protein enters the host cell with viral RNA to help the replication process, proceeded assembly, and release of virus particles. This protein contains 2 different RNA-binding domains (N-terminal domain NTD and C-terminal domain CTD) associated with an impoverished structure linkage region comprising a serine/arginine-rich domain [20]. The SARS-CoV N-NTD and the N-CTD can bind with the viral RNA genome because of positive amino acids [21]. It is expected to possess 2 well-folded domains in which both the terminals of N protein are fairly saturated in b-strands. However, CTD is comprised of some of the short helices [16].

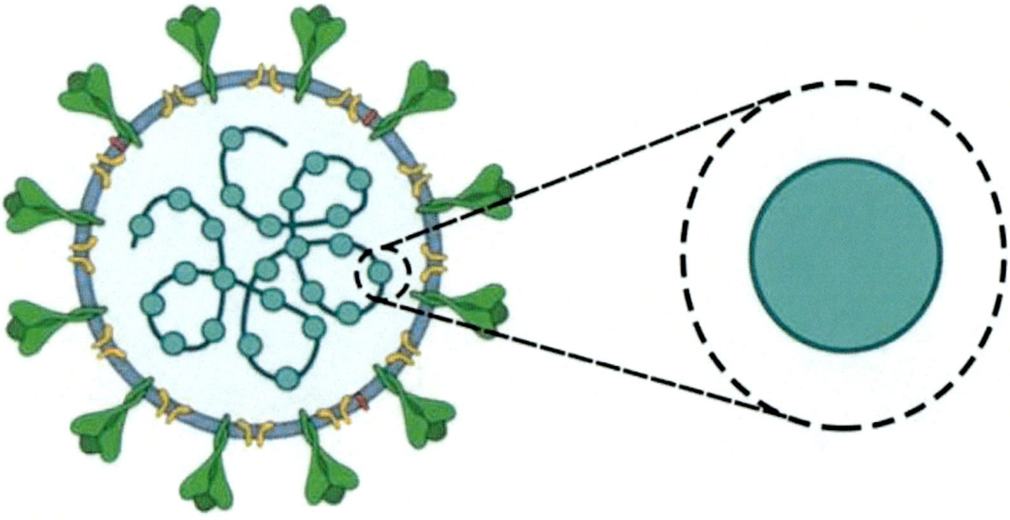

Fig. (6). Diagram of Nucleocapsid (N) protein bound to RNA of SARS-CoV-2.

Sequence analysis of N protein exhibited nearly 90% similarity with SARS-CoV because of most well-kept regions in two core domains and linker. Phylogenetic analysis of N proteins exhibited SARS-CoV-2 belonging to lineage B of *Betacoronavirus,* same as SARS-CoV and bat coronaviruses. Remarkably, the fusion of the SARS-CoV N protein is highly muddled. There are many disordered regions without bounding to nucleic acid in recombinant full-length N protein of the SARS-CoV-2 [22]. This particular disordered region can help the protein quickly bind to different allies and sustain an accurate structure of N protein [23]. Moreover, N protein has been found to provoke antiviral RNAi. In a new study, the N protein was found to prevent cyclin-CDK (cyclin-cyclin dependent kinase) complex that will ultimately cause hypophosphorylation of retinoblastoma protein resulting in inhibition of S phase (genome replication) development in the cell cycle.

Non-Structural Proteins (*NSPs*)

The ORF1ab of the COVID-19 virus expresses polyproteins which are made up of 16 NSPs. Their role in pathogenesis is being explained in the following subheadings.

NSP1 (Leader Protein)

NSP1 protein of SARS-CoV-2, also known as leader protein made up of 180 amino acids. This protein strongly inhibits host gene expression by binding to the 40S ribosome of the host cell to deactivate translation and stimulates selective degradation of host mRNA. In contrast, viral mRNA remains undamaged [24].

NSP2

NSP2 is the second protein of the polyprotein of SARS-CoV-2, containing 638 amino acids. This protein is well-maintained in SARS-CoV. It can bind to 02 host proteins named prohibitin 1 and prohibitin 2 (PHB1 and PHB2). Then it is responsible for cell cycle development, cell relocation, cellular differentiation, apoptosis, and mitochondrial biogenesis. In short, NSP2 acts to disturb the host cell environment [25].

NSP3 (Papain-like Protease)

NSP3 is the papain-like protease protein consisting of 1945 amino acids, the most significant encoded protein of SARS-CoV-2 having about 200 kDa. Due to its long sequence, it has numerous conserved domains, including ssRNA binding, ADP-ribosyl (ADPr) binding, G-quadruplex binding, ssRNA binding, protease (papain-like protease) and NSP4 binding, and transmembrane domain [25]. PL1 protease (papain-like protease 1) can cut the site between NSP2 and NSP3. Additionally, the PL1 domain can provoke the release of the first 03 non-structural proteins (NSP1, NSP2, and NSP3) from the N-terminal region of polyprotein1a and polyproteins 1ab of coronaviruses [26].

NSP4 (Contains Transmembrane Domain 2) and NSP5 (3C-like Proteinase)

NSP4 is made up of 500 amino acids and interrelates with NSP3. It probably has host proteins to reorganize the membrane in SARS-CoV-2, so it is necessary to replicate the virus [25]. NSP5 consists of 306 amino acids. It splits at 11 distinct sites to produce mature and intermediate non-structural proteins (NSPs) [25].

NSP6 (Putative Transmembrane Domain)

NSP6 contains 290 amino acids. NSP6 protein can produce autophagosomes from the endoplasmic reticulum to assist in the association of replicase proteins. Moreover, NSP6 restricts autophagosome/lysosome development, resulting in the inhibition of autophagosomes to distribute the viral constituents of disruption in lysosomes [10]. In the case of SARS-CoV, it has been reported to produce membrane vesicles [10].

NSP7, NSP8, and NSP9

NSP7 is made up of 83 amino acids. It forms a complex with NSP8 and NSP12 to produce the RNA polymerase activity of NSP8 [27]. NSP8 comprises 198 amino acids. It is a peptide cofactor that makes a heterodimer with NSP7. In addition to the NSP7-NSP8 heterodimer, an NSP8 monomer unit also make complexes with NSP12 to produce RNA polymerase complexes necessary for viral pathogenicity [27]. NSP9 contains 113 amino acids. It interrelates with the DEAD-box RNA helicase 5 (DDX5) cellular protein to make a complex essential for viral replication [13].

NSP10, NSP11, and NSP12 (RNA-dependent RNA polymerase)

NSP10 is made up of 139 amino acids. It interacts with NSP14 to enhance the activity of NSP14 as an S-adenosylmethionine (SAM)-dependent (guanine-N7) methyltransferase (N7-MTase) in SARS-CoV-2 and NSP16 (2′---methyltransferase) [3]. NSP11 contains 13 amino acids. The function of NSP11 is unclear until now. NSP12 makes replicas of viral RNA. It comprises 932 amino acids. NSP12 makes a complex with an NSP7-NSP8 heterodimer and shows reduced processing in RNA synthesis because NSP7 and NSP8 reduce the detachment rate of NSP12 from RNA [28].

NSP13 (Helicase)

NSP13 is made up of 601 amino acids that enhance the helicase enzyme activity of unwinding the RNA duplex in SARS-CoV-2. Furthermore, NSP13 of SARS-CoV-2 exhibits 5′-triphosphatase activity, which can introduce the 5′-terminal cap of the viral mRNA. This 5′-terminal cap is the site to recognize translation and necessary for splicing, nuclear export, translation, and help to stabilize mRNA [29].

NSP14 (3′ to 5′ Endonuclease, N7-Methyltransferase)

NSP14 is made up of 527 amino acids. NSP14 of coronaviruses can exhibit 3′-5′ exoribonuclease and N7-methyltransferase activity. The guanine-N--methyltransferase activity is part of introducing the 5′-cap of the SARS CoV-2, which defends mRNA degradation by using the host guanylyl transferase enzyme [30].

NSP15 (endoRNAse)

NSP15 (endoribonuclease), consisting of 346 amino acids, cuts RNA at uridylates at the 3′-position to form a 2′-3′ cyclic phosphodiester product in SARS CoV-2. This protein especially targets and damages the viral polyuridine structures to inhibit the immune sensing system of the host from identifying the virus. NSP15 uses manganese as a cofactor to stimulate endoribonuclease activity. It has been reported that NSP15 destroys viral dsRNA to avoid its recognition by the host [10].

NSP16 (2′-O-Ribose-Methyltransferase)

NSP16 contains 298 amino acids and forms a complex with NSP10 in SARS-CoV. There is 5′-cap in viral RNA, which defends it from mRNA degradation by 5′-exoribonucleases, stimulates mRNA translation, and inhibits the identification of viral RNA by the innate immune system [12].

Accessory Proteins

Apart from the above-mentioned proteins, there are 06 accessory proteins found in SARS-CoV-2, which are helpful to perform specific functions.

ORF3a Protein

The ORF3a protein in SARS-CoV-2 is an ion channel protein that causes activation of NLRP3 inflammasome (NOD, LRR- and pyrin domain-containing protein 3). It is made up of 1381 amino acids. ORF3a interrelates with TNF receptor associated-factor 3 (TRAF3), resulting in activation of apoptosis-associated speck-like protein (ASC) ubiquitination. It can finally cause activation of caspase 1 and IL-1β maturation [12].

ORF6 Protein

The ORF6 protein is an accessory protein having 61 amino acids and exhibits a significant role in the pathogenesis of SARS-CoV-2. ORF6 can interact with the NSP8 to stimulate the activity of RNA polymerase [13].

ORF7a and ORF7b Protein

ORF7a is an accessory type I transmembrane protein of SARS coronavirus comprising 122 amino acids [14]. The ORF7b accessory protein of SARS-CoV is present in the Golgi section, containing 41 amino acids [14].

ORF8 Protein

SARS-CoV-2 has a single ORF8 protein, while SARS-CoV has 2 ORF8 proteins: ORF8a and ORF8b. ORF8 protein contains 41 amino acids. In SARS-CoV, the ORF8b protein attaches to the associated domain of interferon regulatory factor 3 (IRF3) to deactivate interferon signaling [15].

ORF10 Protein

ORF10 protein is made up of 38 amino acids, and its function is unidentified. Remarkably, SARS-CoV contains an ORF9b protein (NP_828859.1) absent in SARS-CoV-2 [10].

Pathogenesis in Real-Time Replication of COVID-19

There are 26 proteins of different categories, *i.e.,* structural, non-structural, and accessory, with their specific role in pathogenesis (Table **2**). Pathogenesis has been detailed into various subsections with underlying mechanisms where these proteins play their role.

Table 2. Summary of key proteins of SARS-CoV-2 and their role in the pathogenesis of COVID-19.

S. No.	Protein	Full Name	Number of Amino Acids	Role in Pathogenesis	References
1.	S protein	Spike protein	1273	Binding of virus to host cell receptor ACE2	[10]
2.	E protein	Envelope protein	75	Virus assembly, release, and pathogenesis	[7]
3.	M protein	Membrane protein	222	Responsible for virus assembly	[5]
4.	N protein	Nucleocapsid protein	419	Binds directly to viral RNA and provide stability	[10, 16, 17]
5.	NSP1	Leader Protein	180	Responsible for inhibiting signaling of IFN and causes blockage of host innate immune response by promoting cellular deprivation and ultimately causes blockage of host RNA translation	[10, 24]
6.	NSP2	-	638	Binds to PHBs 1, 2	[25]
7.	NSP3	Papain like Protease	1945	Stimulating expression of cytokines and cause breakage of the viral polyprotein	[26]
8.	NSP4	Contains Transmembrane Domain 2	500	Membrane rearrangement	[10, 25]
9.	NSP5	3C-like proteinase	306	Cleaves at 11 sites of (3C-like proteinase) NSP polyprotein	[10, 25]

(Table 2) cont.....

S. No.	Protein	Full Name	Number of Amino Acids	Role in Pathogenesis	References
10.	NSP6	Putative Transmembrane Domain	290	Contributes to the formation of double-membrane vesicles by trans membrane scaffold protein and generate autophagosomes	[10]
11.	NSP7	-	83	Processivity lock RNA polymerase by making a hexadecameric complex with NSP8	[10, 27]
12.	NSP8	-	198	Processivity lock for RNA polymerase by making the complex of hexadecameric shape	[10, 27]
13.	NSP9	RNA binding protein phosphatase	113	Binds to helicase	[13]
14.	NSP10	-	139	Stimulation of ExoN and 2-O-MT activity	[3, 10].
15.	NSP11	-	13	Not identified yet	[10, 28]
16.	NSP12	RNA Dependent RNA Polymerase	932	Copies viral RNA (RNA polymerase) methylation (guanine)	[10, 28]
17.	NSP13	Helicase	601	Unwinds duplex RNA (Helicase)	[29]
18.	NSP14	3′ to 5′ Endonuclease, N7-Methyltransferase	527	Stimulation of activity of ExoN and 2-O-MT	[10, 30]
19.	NSP15	endoRNAse	346	Degrades RNA to (endoRNAse/endoribonuclease) evade host defense	[10]
20.	NSP16	2′-O-Ribose-Methyltransferase	298	Avoids MDA5 recognition and inhibits innate immunity regulation	[12].
21.	ORF3a	-	1381	Activates NLRP3	[10, 12]
22.	ORF6	-	61	Interacts with NSP8 to activate RNA polymerase	[13]
23.	ORF7a	Type I transmembrane protein	122	Inhibits transmembrane protein BST-2 glycosylation	[10, 14]
24.	ORF7b	-	41	Present in the Golgi compartment and combined with viral particles	[10, 14]
25.	ORF8	-	41	Helps in the deactivation of interferon signaling	[10] [15]
26.	ORF10	-	38	Unidentified	[10]

Receptor Recognition by Spike Protein

Coronaviruses exhibit a problematic configuration to identify receptors [31]. *Alphacoronavirus* HCoV-NL63 and SARS-CoV both identify Zn peptidase ACE2 [32]. All coronavirus receptors show specific physiological functions in addition to their role in viral attachment. There are 2 major regions in coronavirus a) S1 N-terminal domain (S1-NTD) and S1 C-terminal domain (S1-CTD). They act as the receptor-binding domain (RBD) by binding alone or in combination with host receptors. S1-NTDs bind sugar in all coronaviruses except MHV S1-NTD of *Betacoronavirus*, which identifies as a protein receptor CEACAM1. S1-CTDs can identify protein receptors ACE2, APN, and dipeptidyl peptidase 4 (DPP4) [33].

Mechanism of Membrane Fusion by Spike Protein

Spike protein is included in class I viral membrane fusion proteins. *In vitro* activators like trypsin cleavage and urea incubation cause pre-fusion SARS-CoV spike protein to change to the post-fusion status where S1 separates while S2 converts into dumbbell-shaped having a rod-like appearance in the middle but globular form at every end. These trimeric S2 molecules further combine on one side to give rise to rosettes form in the solution. Compared to influenza virus HA, the six-helix bundle made by coronavirus is remarkably long, which is an indicator for the profuse collection of energy that can be distributed during the structural change of S2, and it helps in the membrane fusion process. Generally, it is reported that coronavirus spikes fusion membranes like those of other class I membrane fusion proteins. It has exceptional features including their bigger size, double cleavage sites, internal fusion peptide, and long six-helix bundle [34].

Activators for Membrane Fusion by Spike Protein

Spike protein comprises 2 functional units viz. S1 and S2. S1 unit contains N-terminal and a C-terminal RBD that directly interact with the host cells [32]. S2, on the other hand, facilitates the virus fusion (by the formation of homo-trimers) to host cellular membranes. S2 sub-unit, containing fusion machinery, converts to a stabilized perfusion state aided by RBD from S1 subunits [10]. The cleavage of both subunits occurs, leading to permanent conformational transformations with the help of host proteases. It has been reported that apart from spike glycoproteins, the clathrin-dependent and clathrin-independent endocytic pathways mediate SARS-CoV entry to host cells [35]. These pathways are yet to be investigated to play a key role in SARS-CoV-2 pathogenesis. The spike glycoproteins present at the outer membranes of the virus bring conformational changes leading to successful internalization in host cells after attaching with ACE2 host receptors facilitated by TMPRSS2 (Fig. **7**). Following this discovery, it has been recently established that the utilization of serine protease inhibitors can block the function of ACE2 and TMPRSS2 [36]. Using S proteins for immunogenetics is based on the ability to initiate T cell-mediated immune protection [37]. Therefore, there is an urgency to optimize receptor targets for antiviral and anti-COVID 19 vaccine strategies for animal models before use in clinical settings.

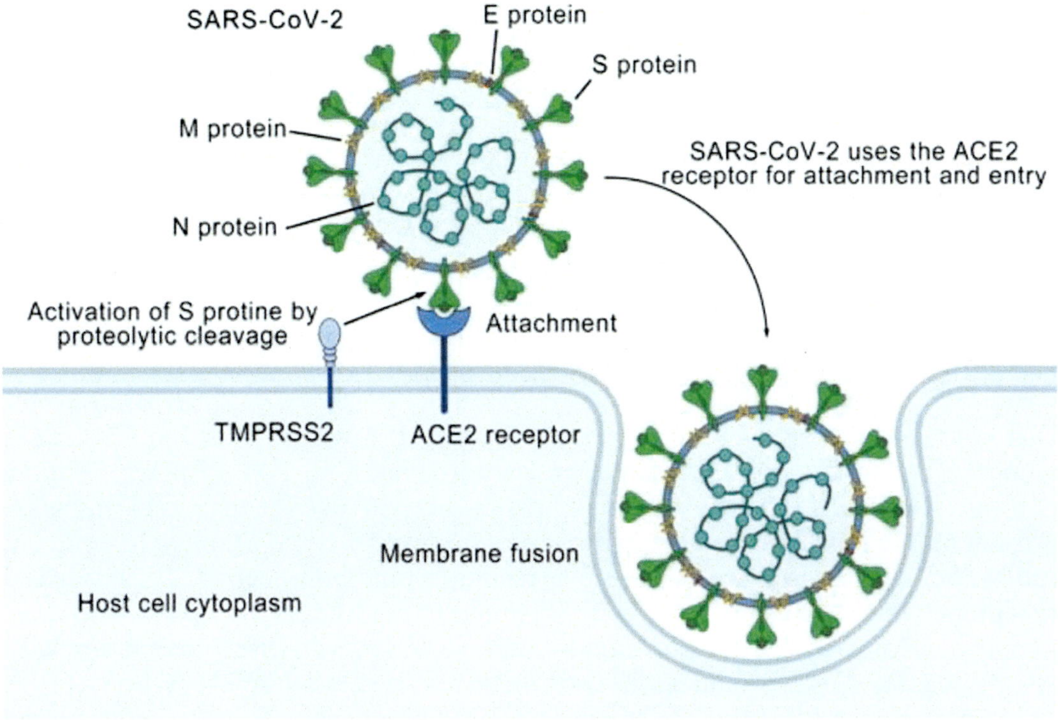

Fig. (7). Structural mechanism showing S protein attacks on the host cell and gets entry after activation and attachment. The virus is attaching it to the ACE2 receptor protein present on the superficial membrane of host cells. A protease, TMPRSS2, facilitates this attachment. The linkage of viral S protein with ACE2 on the host cell surface results in the entry of the virus into the host cell leading to the development of infection.

The gene enrichment analysis of ACE2 has revealed the mechanisms responsible for the successful viral attack and replication within host cells. It has been shown that alveolar type 2 (AT2) cells were highly expressed in COVID-19 patients, depicting the success of novel coronavirus in jeopardizing host cells for transmission and reproduction of virus [18]. The modeling of S proteins for risk factor analysis and target drug designing against SARS-CoV-2 has opened arenas for putative drug targets based on *in silico* analysis. The study reported that despite genetic diversity, the RBD domain of the S protein of COVID-19 supports strong electrostatic interactions with human ACE2. This finding highlighted the potential of SARS-CoV-2 to infect and transmit disease in humans [3].

Sufficiently low metastability of S2 sub-unit, supported by a low S1 affinity for target receptors, both depending on proteolytic ability, could halt the successful receptor binding and cell transfection. The vital role of S proteins in pathogenesis and infectivity within host cells has been sought for vaccine and treatment candidates against coronaviruses.

Evolution of Spike Proteins

S proteins are generally different from other coronaviruses generally, and Betacoronaviruses (including SARS-CoV) earns them a genetically distinguished nomenclature [38]. Residues from SARS-CoV-2 RBD, crucial for ACE2 binding, are highly conserved or share very similar properties as SARS-CoV. This homology highlights the convergent evolution between both SARS and SARS-CoV-2 coronaviruses [18]. The S protein mutations have been historically giving rise to mutant genetic variations. The typical examples of this phenomenon are feline infectious peritonitis virus (FIPV) serotype II and porcine epidemic diarrhea virus (PEDV). This recombination may not only alter the genetic makeover but modify the tropism for host species [39].

Different coronaviruses possess various binding sites within S1 subunits that are recognized for binding and host cell internalization. For instance, human coronavirus HKU1 and OC43 attach *via* S domain-A (S^A) to acetyl sialoside present on the host cell surface made of glycolipid and glycoproteins. In contrast, the MERS coronavirus utilizes the S^A domain to bind non-acetylated surfaces of receptors which probably promote S^B domain binding to receptors and host peptidase. However, SARS-CoV and SARS-r CoV undergo direct interaction with ACE2, mediated by S^B, to attack host cells. It is well noted that SARS-CoV-2 is as well adapted as SARS-CoV to selectively bind human ACE2 receptors for viral entry [10]. The S proteins of SARS-CoV-2 are trimers that are evolutionarily conserved and highly glycosylated in nature. Therefore, it is required to probe into the evolutionary patterns of S1 and S2 subunits of S proteins making binding to ACE2 receptors very distinct. This binding is highly significant as its detailed understanding could contribute to bringing forward some alterations in the 3D structure leading to attenuation of the virus particles.

Invasion and Replication of SARS-CoV-2

S protein belonging to coronavirus is an important contributing factor for invading viruses into host cells [40]. The SARS-CoV-2 may enter the host *via* the respiratory tract or mucosal surfaces such as the conjunctiva. SARS-CoV-2 binds to epithelial cells of the nasal cavity, whereas the upper respiratory tract is an efficient replication site of this novel coronavirus. SARS-CoV-2 causes a less abrupt onset of symptoms like other conventional human coronaviruses that are the extensive cause of common seasonal colds [2]. During the prodrome period, the infected patients produce a copious virus in the upper respiratory tract. SARS-CoV-2 can also replicate in the lower respiratory tract and causes radiological evidence of lower respiratory tract involvement in patients having no clinical pneumonia [41]. S protein attaches to cellular receptor ACE2 for SARS-CoV [42] and SARS-CoV-2 [43]. This is further evident by a fluorescent study that SARS-CoV-2 applies the ACE2 receptor the same way as the SARS-CoV [44]. Bronchoalveolar lavage fluid from a positive COVID-19 patient also confirmed the use of ACE2 as an entry receptor by SARS-CoV-2 [36]. ACE2 protein remarkably presents alveolar epithelial cells and gives rise to the regulation of transmission within humans and cross-species [43]. The S-glycoprotein on the SARS-CoV-2 surface attaches to the ACE2 cellular receptor of human cells and holds two subunits (S1 and S2). Subunit S1 is responsible for virus-host range and cellular tropism by RNA binding domain aiding the attachment, whereas S2 causes the virus-cell membrane fusion through heptad repeats 1 (HR1) and HR2, the tandem domains [3]. Lysine 31 residue present on the human ACE2 receptor identifies 394-glutamine residue located in the RBD region of the virus. Single N501T mutation in the virion S protein of SARS-CoV-2 may have shown a significant increase in binding affinity for ACE2. A study suggested that the binding efficiency of ACE2 and SARS-CoV-2 S protein is found 10-20 folds higher as compared with SARS-CoV. The attachment of SARS-CoV-2 into cells is being determined by fusions of membranes between virus and plasma [43]. A recent study on SARS-CoV-2 has reported that S protein priming is required to facilitate the process of entry, which is provided by the TMPRSS211 produced in the host cell (Fig. **7**) [43]. In addition to the mechanism of membrane fusion, entry of the virus is facilitated by clathrin-dependent endocytosis and independent endocytosis [45]. After membrane fusion, the virus eliminates the RNA genome into the cytoplasm as an ss+ RNA followed by the translation of two viral replicase polyproteins, pp-1a and pp-1ab, which encode the NSPs, finally giving rise to RTC (replication-transcription complex) in double-membrane vesicle [36]. Continuous replication of RTC gives rise to nests of sub-genomic RNAs that finally encode proteins from the structural category and those of the proteins' accessory category [43]. Additionally, the viral genome encodes some non-structural proteins, including RdRp, 3CLpro, and PLpro, which are slashed into effector proteins by using viral proteinases [46]. PLpro acts as a deubiquitinase that can cause immune suppression by deubiquitinating specific host cell proteins like interferon factor 3 (IF-3) and NF-κB [47]. 3CLpro causes proteolysis of viral polyprotein into functional units while RdRp makes a complete negative-stranded RNA template which can be used by RdRp to further produce RNA of viral genome. Newly developed envelope proteins are introduced into membrane of endoplasmic reticulum, and hence genomic RNA and nucleocapsid protein combine to form nucleocapsid that subsequently assemble into virions. The virus then grows in endoplasmic reticulum-Golgi intermediate compartment that finally releases from host cells *via* vesicles having enclosed with virus particles [43] as shown in Fig. (**8**).

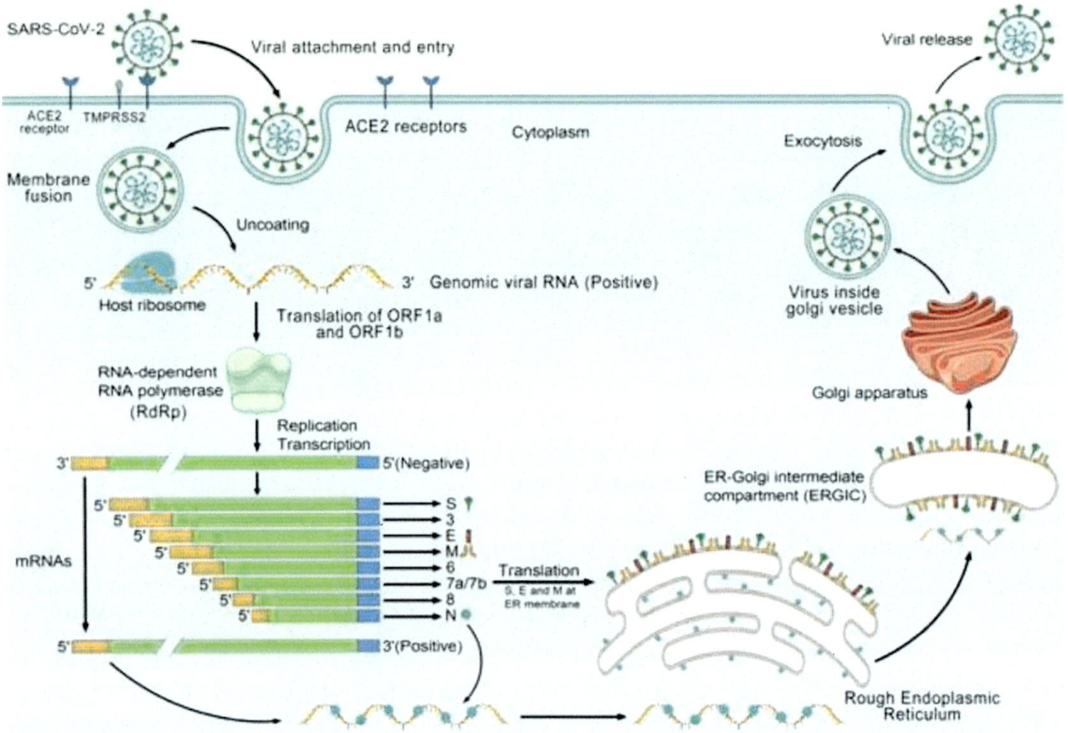

Fig. (8). The entire mechanism of action of proteins from attachment to viral release. Firstly, the S protein attaches to ACE2, followed by conformational alteration in S protein facilitating the union of viral envelop with cell membranes *via* the endosomal pathway. The virus eliminates RNA into the host cell to translate it into viral replicase polyproteins pp1a and pp1ab. These polyproteins are slashed by viral proteinase enzymes giving rise to small products. Polymerases also produce subgenomic mRNA sequences using intermittent transcription, translated into viral proteins of significant importance. Proteins further combine with the RNA genome to construct virions in the endoplasmic reticulum and Golgi bodies transported through vesicles. These vesicles finally attach to the host cell membrane to release the virus.

Antigen Appearance in COVID-19 Infection

Upon entering the virus into cells, the antigen-presenting cells (APC) take up the viral antigen necessary for the body's immunity against viruses. After this, peptides of antigenic nature are taken up by MHC or human leukocyte antigen and, after that, further reach virus-specific Tc lymphocytes [43].

Activation of Humoral and Cellular Immunity against Covid-19 Infection

The appearance of an antigen consequently activates all kinds of the body's immune responses with the help of virus-specific immune cells. Just like acute viral infections, antibodies including IgM and IgG produce against the SARS-CoV-2 virus. Shortly before the termination of the 12th week, SARS-specific IgM antibodies disappear, whereas IgG3 antibodies persist for a prolonged duration which is an indication of defensive character [48]. In contrast, S and N specific antibodies are considered SARS-related IgG antibodies [40]. Recent research has reported the reduced amount of cluster of differentiating immune cells (CD4+ and CD8+) T cells in the blood circulation of the patients. However, their amount are increased like human leukocyte antigen–DR isotype [3]. SARS-CoV patients exhibit a severe reduction of CD4+ and CD8+ T cells in acute kinds of disorders. Even in the absence of antigen, CD4+ and CD8+ memory T cells are observed for 4 years in some SARS recovered patients while playing viral share in the proliferation of T cell, delayed-type hypersensitivity response, and produce *interferon-gamma (*IFN-γ) [49].

Cytokine Storm in COVID-19

Acute respiratory distress syndrome (ARDS) is predicted to be the main reason for deaths in COVID-19 patients reported by Lancet [50]. ARDS is a general immunopathological event in SARS, COVID-19, and MERS infections [3]. The dominant mechanism for ARDS is cytokine storm which occurs due to excessive release of chemokine 2, (CCL2); chemokine 3, CCL3; chemokine 5, CCL5; chemokine 8, CXCL8; chemokine 9, CXCL9; chemokine 10, CXCL10), and the pro-inflammatory cytokines (IFNα; IFNγ; TGFβ; IL-1β; IL-6; IL-12; IL-18; IL-33;) by immune effector cells in SARS infections [51]. MERS-CoV infected patients also exhibit increased levels of some cytokines like IL-6, IFN-a, and chemokines CCL5, CXCL8, and CXCL-10 in serum similar to SARS-CoV infection [52]. However, SARS-CoV-2 infected patients with many T-lymphocytes, macrophages, and dendritic cells cause excessive release of pro-inflammatory cytokines, which can eventually lead to ARDS [53]. This cytokine storm can cause hyperactivation of the immune system in the body resulting in ARDS and failure of organs that finally result in the expiry of the COVID-19 of critical situations comparable to MERS and SARS infection [3].

Coronavirus Immune Evasion

The causative agents of SARS disease and MERS disease use various approaches to bypass immunity for better survival in host cells. Pathogen-associated molecular patterns are well-maintained microbial structures that pattern recognition receptors can identify. But, both pathogens, *i.e.,* SARS-CoV and

MERS-CoV, can stimulate the formation of double-membrane vesicles devoid of PRRs (pathogen recognition receptors), so they can multiply in these vesicles and avoid the host recognition of their ds RNA [54]. IFN-I (IFNα- and IFN-b) expresses a defensive response in the case of SARS-CoV and MERS-CoV infection [55]. Similarly, SARS-CoV-2 also uses passive and active mechanisms to avoid the IFN-1 response in which passive mechanisms involve forming double-membrane vesicles, as mentioned above. At the same time, active mechanism occurs due to the direct effect of proteins of the pathogen on transcription factors and intracellular signaling molecules that control the IFN cascade. Particularly the ORF6 proteins of SARS-CoV-2 play their role to prevent the effect of INF regulatory transcription [53].

Factors Affecting SARS-CoV-2 Pathogenesis

It is necessary to rule out the origin of pathogen and reservoir to develop preventive strategies to combat this disease. This formidable outbreak appeared in the Huanan Seafood Wholesale Market of Wuhan, Hubei, China. The market provided palm civets, bats, raccoon dogs, frogs, snakes, marmots, and other wild animals that are frequently sold [56]. Initially, it appeared as a perception that patients with COVID-19 may have visited the Huanan Seafood Market or may have eaten the infected birds or animals [57]. Primary studies also reported some COVID-19 positive environmental specimens in Wuhan, and the snake was considered a possible key reservoir, but some researchers disagreed. Afterward, the role of bats and some other wild animals, including pangolin, was speculated to support the rapid spillover events of COVID-19 [58]. Recent research expressed that the SARS-CoV-2 is related to subgroup *Betacoronavirus* having mostly identical genomic sequences to a SARS-like bat coronavirus (bat-CoV), indicating bat natural host of origin. Genomic analysis showed that the genome of SARS-CoV-2 shares nearly 96% identity to the bat-CoV RaTG13, while it is almost 80% identical to SARS-CoV [38]. These speculations were somehow supported by evidence of genetic homology in ACE2 receptor binding mechanisms. Also, the people that had traveled to or had any interaction with the workers/routine visitors of the market were reportedly contracting the disease. Still, later on, some people contracted the disease even without visiting the seafood market [59]. The exact origin, location, and potential natural reservoir of pathogen SARS-CoV-2 are still unclear, and they might come from some wild animal in the market. But it is thought that the virus has zoonotic nature, and bats may be suspected as key reservoirs because of the identical genome to the bat-CoV, and they might share the same ancestors [56]. It was previously presumed that COVID-19 might have transplacental or vertical transmission. This notion supported by various research cohorts-based results has been nullified [60]. Apart from these, some bad health habits, *i.e.,* tobacco smoking and alcohol consumption, may also be important risk factors. The disease has been confirmed in passive smokers; however, active smokers may be adversely affected, leading to inadequate immune response and viral containment. It could be concluded that smoking causes degeneration of protective cilia (alveolar injury) and suppresses the local immunity, eventually leading to more chances of viral internalization and subsequent disease [61].

Host Factors on the Genetic Basis

It was speculated that the COVID-19 infection severity and its outcomes in Asian, Caucasian, European populations might differ [56]. Similarly, it was presumed that there might be some difference in the susceptibility of males and females to contract coronavirus disease. Both notions have been supported and rejected by different research groups making these factors highly controversial [62]. Co-morbidity and immunosuppression in any individual can make the viral pathogenesis shorter and more severe [63]. The elderly or chronic disease (hepatitis, cancer, other renal or hepatic disorders) patients with low profile immune system functionality is also at higher risk of contracting the disease. This could be attributed to compromised immunity and weakened local responses to the virus [64]. Some preliminary examinations also suggested severe obesity and smoking as associated risk factors [65]. However, some researchers reported more risk in males than females in Italy, which may be due to a high incidence of smoking habits [9]. Studies found that SARS-CoV-2 infections lead to fatal pneumonia in old-aged patients, and bacterial infection may also cause secondary bacterial pneumonia [66].

Organ failure due to COVID-19 depends upon the percentage of expression of ACE2 receptors by different cells. These receptors make way for viruses to the organ. The proportion of ACE2 $<1\%$ is associated with a low risk of organ failure, while an increase in proportion is directly linked with a higher risk of getting the disease. Nasal and bronchi do not express ACE2; hence have low or no risk of getting organ failure. The highest proportion of ACE2 expression is noted in the ileum giving rise to nearly 30% of the expression of ACE2 receptors hence categorized as high-risk organ failure. The respiratory tract, urinary bladder, esophagus, kidney, and heart are categorized under high-risk organs because the expression of ACE2 appears to be 2%, 2.4%, $>1\%$, 4%, and 7.5%, respectively. Cardiac injury is the most important disease complication in the wake of COVID-19, where 13% of the increase in creatinine kinase [4]. Such patients are observed to have higher levels of mRNA and ACE2 expression that take the patient to organ failure. Kidney failure was found among 14.4% of COVID-19 patients presenting increased levels of serum creatine [61]. Hospital-based mortality becomes 16.1%, while patients showing higher baseline serum creatinine show double mortality than those who did not have a higher baseline creatinine issue. Effective cell adhering and uninterrupted virus entry, low chance of virus elimination, compromised T cell function, susceptibility against cytokine storms, and excessive inflammation are key steps of enhanced progression and pathogenesis of SARS-CoV-2. However, ACE2 expression decreases with insulin administration [67]. In contrast, ACE2 function is reduced by hypoglycemic candidates such as thiazolidinedione, glucagon-like peptide-1, ACE inhibitors, angiotensin receptor blockers, antihypertensive drugs, and statins up-regulated. Compared with the normal control group, the rodent diabetes model exhibited a strong expression of ACE2 in vital organs of the body in the study [68]. According to their Mendelian randomized study, the lungs of patients with diabetes mellitus (DM) determined in COVID-19 disease and characteristics showed increased expression of ACE2. It has also been found that protein concentrations of overexpressed protease enzymes (such as furin) are too high in diabetic patients, promoting the cleavage of spike proteins, hence permitting entry of the virus.

TMPRSS2 is a protease enzyme that is produced by the host and resultantly potentiates priming of S protein of SARS-CoV-2. This process facilitates binding with ACE2, and ultimately entry of virus in the tissue. Some TMPRSS2 inhibitors are approved for clinical application to block entry thus may be helpful in the treatment protocol. Camostat mesylate is a drug that inhibits the expression of this gene [36].

Viral Factors

SARS-CoV-2 is an air-borne virus capable of sustaining on inanimate objects for hours. The virus possesses great genetic diversity, having reported at least 7 distinct types to date. Important virulence factors like an invasion of immune checks from the host under double vesicle formation, inactivation of translational machinery by 8 different proteins of the virus, host cap machinery mimicry, blocking various STAT signaling pathways, and downregulation of gene expression for rendering antigen presentation unsuccessful. These pathways are mediated by both non-structural and structural proteins [69]. It is necessary to take care of and devise strategies for these targeted pathways of viral infection.

RNA-dependent RNA-polymerase (RdRp)

RdRp is responsible for the replication of the genome of COVID-19. Antiviral drugs like Ribavirin & Remdesivir are used for Ebola virus infection, Hepatitis C infection, and RSV infection with the hypothesis of the drug serving as nucleotides analog that restricts the process of replication by a virus that blocks nucleotide formation of SARS-CoV-2 virus. There are some reactions in terms of increased transaminases and renal injuries [5].

Papain-like Protease (PLpro)

These proteins result in the proteolysis of viral polyprotein into active viral protein. Lopinavir has been tried against HIV in combination with ritonavir that works to inhibit protease. Adverse reactions were nausea, vomiting, GIT disturbances, pancreatitis, and cardiac abnormalities [70].

Coronavirus Protease (3CLpro)

This protein causes proteolysis of polyprotein into an active protein. Lopinavir antiviral drugs previously have been used in combination with ritonavir to inhibit protease. Nausea, GIT issues, pancreatitis, vomiting, and cardiac abnormalities were limiting factors [70].

Spike Protein (S Protein)

These proteins help adhere the virus to the host receptor, which facilitates the entrance of the virus. Otherwise, ACE2 catalyzes angiotensin II to angiotensin1–7and angiotensin1–9, which serve as anti-inflammatory and antioxidants, to play a vital role in treating acute respiratory distress. Arbidol antiviral drug is supposed to prevent binding of S protein to the host cell, thus blocking the entry of bacteria into host tissues. The drug has been used against Influenza while elevated transaminase, allergic response, and GIT disorder are observable side effects [58].

Comparison of Different Coronaviruses

Novel virus belongs to the same *Betacoronavirus* that owns bat SARS-like coronaviruses, and MERS-CoV. However, SARS-CoV differs in some respects from other coronaviruses [23]. It causes milder infection and is transmitted much more in the community, whereas MERS-CoV and SARS-CoV spread is nosocomial [71].

Virology and Genome

Phylogenetic analysis reveals SARS-CoV-2 (belonging to Clad I and Clad IIa; bats are animal reservoirs; the intermediate host is unknown) to be more related to SARS-CoV (belonging to Clad I and Clad IIb; bats are animal reservoirs; the intermediate host is palm civets) and bat SARS-like coronavirus [69]. Phylogenetic association between pangolin CoVs and SARS-CoV-2, although they share a common animal origin. Phylogenetic studies are still scarce to correctly state pangolin as an intermediate host of SARS-COVs. There are amino acid differences between SARS-CoV and SARS-CoV-2, while their mode of binding to ACE2 nearly remains similar. The SARS-CoV-2 shares 96.2% similarity to the bat-CoV RaTG13. This similarity reaches 79.5% with SARS-CoV and 82% identical to MERS-CoV pathogen (belonging to Clad II; bats are animal reservoirs; intermediate host camels) in genomic sequence [60]. MERS virus shows up stable genome since the time of origin in 2012 while other viruses of this genus keep on evolving with new combinations.

S1/S2 of S protein has been proved to be a controlling loop to stabilize the virus when structural cleavage is intact, reaching the downstream S2′ site, which monitors exposure to peptide fusion and their functionality. SARS-CoV-2 S protein contains clear insertion in a genome that maps the S1/S2 priming loop, and this distinction is not found in any other coronaviruses in *Betacoronavirus* lineage B. This distinct insert in the genome of SARS-CoV-2 gives rise to potential changes in the virus every time. Moreover, SARS-CoV-2 S1/S2 site is considered an exposed flexible loop that makes an easily approachable site for protease cleavage, which presents a bigger share in the S protein function of the SARS-CoV-2 pathogen. The priming loop is predicted to alter the pathway of entry of the pathogen predominantly. There is no attribute found in any other virus belonging to *Betacoronavirus* lineage B. Cleavage of S protein by furin (Golgi-resident protein) while virus assembly and delivery to cell surfaces. Another source of change in structure is FCoV, a loop that is a proteolytically sensitive structural loop present in the hypervariable region of the spike. This makes the spike region a significant driver of virus evolution [16]. Cryo-electron microscopy found SARS-CoV receptor-binding motif (RBM) down confirmation to be packed closer to the NTD of the S protein. At the same time, that of SARS-CoV-2 RBD angled to the center of the trimmer in down conformation. While similar binding modes for both SARS-CoV and SARS-CoV-2 RBDs compensate for the difference of amino acids in the proteins of both CoVs [18].

The SARS-CoV-2 amino acid sequence of S protein resembles 76.47% of SARS-CoV, showing the same structural configuration and electrostatic properties in the interaction interface [3]. Substitution of only 380 amino acids between SARS-CoV and SARS-CoV-2, which are commonly found in genes of non-structural proteins, has been found by genomic comparison between SARS-CoV-2 and SARS. In contrast, 27 mutations have been found in S protein are liable for receptor adherence and entry into the host cell [43]. This might explain the low pathogenic nature of SARS-CoV-2 pathogen than SARS-CoV but needs more investigations [72]. SARS-CoV-2 has emerged as a human pathogen by a mutation in S protein at RBD, resulting in increased pathogenicity by increased affinity to the receptor and determining the tropism. Therefore, it is assumed that SARS-CoV-2 behaves similarly [73]. Genomic studies revealed that the same human cell receptor, ACE2, is being shared by SARS-CoV-2 and SARS-CoV to enter the cell. However, the primary receptor that MERS-CoV uses is DPP4 for cell entry. The ACE2 receptors are ectoenzymes that are found anchored to various tissues' cell membranes, especially in the lower respiratory tract, gastrointestinal tract, kidney, and heart [66]. SARS-CoV-2 holds 6 major amino acid changes in the RBD region of S glycoprotein at position 344, position 360, position 472, position 479, position 480, and position 487 compared to SARS-CoV where no substitution of amino acids was present in RBD that interacts directly with ACE2 human receptor [74].

Epidemiology

COVID-19 transmission among humans is the greatest challenge to control this disease. Studies have shown that asymptomatic carriers have a high virus load in the upper respiratory tract which participates in a high prevalence of COVID-19. The transmission of a virus is indicated by R0 (reproductive number), indicating the average no. of new infections produced by an infected person from a mass that has never seen the disease before. $R_0>1$ indicates that the infection is likely to enhance whereas, $R_0<1$ indicates that the outbreak will decline. The World Health Organization has estimated higher R_0 of SARS-CoV-2 (2-2.5) compared to MERS (<1) and SARS (1.7-1.9), suggesting the higher pandemic potential of novel infection [69]. Serial interval (time of onset of disease and time of onset of disease in secondary case) in SARS-CoV-2 is less than 4 days that suggest transmission of disease before the clinical case. Lower serial interval and higher reproductive number lead to a higher spread of COVID-19. Whereas the death rate of SARS-CoV-2 has been recorded to be 2.3%, SARS-CoV gives rise to 9.5%, while the MERS virus results in 34.4% deaths of patients as reported by the Chinese Centre for Disease Control and Prevention in China [65]. The binding attraction of the SARS-CoV-2 S-protein & ACE2 receptor is higher than the SARS disease virus (2003 strain). This might explain the rapid development and transmission among humans by the SARS-CoV-2 pathogen. It is also predicted that if one nucleotide mutation in RBD of SARS-CoV-2 happens, it would further enhance pathogenesis [73]. The *in vitro* inoculation of SARS-CoV-2 on the epithelial cell surface of human airways causes cessation of cilia movement and cytopathic effect [60]. In type I and type II pneumocytes as well as enterocytes, there is higher replication of SARS-CoV-2. In the lungs epithelium, downregulation of ACE2 receptors due to SARS-CoV results in the pathogenesis of lung injury and finally expresses as ARDS clinical presentation [66]. However, MERS-CoV recognizes DPP4 as a receptor [75].

Key Protein Differences in Clinical Findings

There are similarities in coronaviruses' clinical manifestation, which included fever, dyspnea, dry cough, and CT scans of different anomalies. Nevertheless, there exist some differences too. Earlier studies revealed increased serum pro-inflammatory cytokines; IP10, MCPI, IFNγ, IL1B, IL6, and IL12 in SARS-CoV patients leading to extensive lung damage *via* pulmonary inflammation [76]. The increased serum concentration of pro-inflammatory cytokines; TNFα, IFNγ, IL15, and IL17 are associated with MERS-CoV infection. In contrast, COVID-19 patients revealed a higher amount of IFNγ, MCP1, IL1B, and IP10 that might lead to activated T-helper-1 (Th1) cell responses. Patients admitted to ICU show higher TNFα, IP10, MCPI, GCSF, and MIP1A concentrations than those who do not need intensive care, which shows an association of cytokine storm with the lethality of disease [24]. Furthermore, in COVID-19 patients, initiation of increased Th2 cytokine (IL4 and IL10) secretion has been found that suppress inflammation different from SARS [76]. Increased incidence of liver injury in patients that are suffering from SARS and MERS has been reported. Whereas liver anomalies with mild to moderately increased transaminase, prolongation of prothrombin time, and hypoalbuminemia have also been noted in SARS-CoV-2 infection patients [77]. Other clinical findings include increase lactic dehydrogenase, creatine kinase, aminotransferase, C-reactive protein level, and WBCs count (mainly neutrophils), along with the decreased number of lymphocytes. However, RBCs and platelets were similar to that of SARS and MERS infections [78].

CONCLUSION

SARS-CoV-2 that resulted in the pandemic COVID-19, possesses 26 key proteins of three categories named structural proteins (4 members), non-structural proteins (16 members), and accessory category of proteins (6 members). The SARS-Co--2 and SARS-CoV share similar host ACE2 receptors, while MERS coronavirus uses DPP4 for cell entry. The genomic structural comparison shows the substitution of 380 amino acid mutations in SARS-CoV-2 compared to other SARS-like coronaviruses that play a key role in infectious ability and potential differentiation mechanisms of SARS-CoV-2 to cause formidable infection. Besides the role of these key proteins, some viral and host factors are also important for developing COVID-19 infection. These proteins and protein subunits necessarily are targeted to develop treatment or control measures against COVID-19.

CONSENT FOR PUBLICATION

Not Applicable.

CONFLICT OF INTEREST

The author confirms that this chapter contents have no conflict of interest.

ACKNOWLEDGEMENT

Declared none.

REFERENCES

[1] Udugama B, Kadhiresan P, Kozlowski HN, *et al.* Diagnosing COVID-19: The Disease and Tools for Detection. ACS Nano 2020; 14(4): 3822-35. [http://dx.doi.org/10.1021/acsnano.0c02624] [PMID: 32223179]

[2] Soufi GJ, Hekmatnia A, Nasrollahzadeh M, Shafiei N, Sajjadi M, Iravani P, *et al.* SARS-CoV-2 (COVID-19): New discoveries and current challenges. Applied Sciences (Switzerland) 2020; 10 [http://dx.doi.org/10.3390/app10103641]

[3] Xu Z, Shi L, Wang Y, *et al.* Pathological findings of COVID-19 associated with acute respiratory distress syndrome. Lancet Respir Med 2020; 8(4): 420-2. [http://dx.doi.org/10.1016/S2213-2600(20)30076-X] [PMID: 32085846]

[4] Zhou P, Yang XL, Wang XG, *et al.* A pneumonia outbreak associated with a new coronavirus of probable bat origin. Nature 2020; 579(7798): 270-3. [http://dx.doi.org/10.1038/s41586-020-2012-7] [PMID: 32015507]

[5] Chan JF-W, Yip CC-Y, To KK-W, Tang TH-C, Wong SC-Y, Leung K-H, *et al.* Improved molecular diagnosis of COVID-19 by the novel, highly sensitive and specific COVID-19-RdRp/Hel real-time reverse transcription-polymerase chain reaction assay validated <em>*in vitro* </em> and with clinical specimens. Journal of Clinical Microbiology 2020; JCM.00310-20. [http://dx.doi.org/10.1128/JCM.00310-20]

[6] Lu R, Zhao X, Li J, *et al.* Genomic characterisation and epidemiology of 2019 novel coronavirus: implications for virus origins and receptor binding. Lancet 2020; 395(10224): 565-74. [http://dx.doi.org/10.1016/S0140-6736(20)30251-8] [PMID: 32007145]

[7] Nieto-torres JL, Alcaraz A, Dediego ML, Verdia C. Since January 2020 Elsevier has created a COVID-19 resource centre with free information in English and Mandarin on the novel coronavirus COVID- 19 . The COVID-19 resource centre is hosted on Elsevier Connect , the company' s public news and information 2020.

[8] Mu J, Xu J, Zhang L, *et al.* SARS-CoV-2-encoded nucleocapsid protein acts as a viral suppressor of RNA interference in cells. Sci China Life Sci 2020; 63(9): 1413-6. [http://dx.doi.org/10.1007/s11427-020-1692-1] [PMID: 32291557]

[9] Wu D, Wu T, Liu Q, Yang Z. The SARS-CoV-2 outbreak: What we know. Int J Infect Dis 2020; 94: 44-8. [http://dx.doi.org/10.1016/j.ijid.2020.03.004] [PMID: 32171952]

[10] Yoshimoto FK. The proteins of severe acute respiratory syndrome coronavirus-2 (SARS CoV-2 or n-COV19), the cause of COVID-19. Protein J 2020; 39(3): 198-216. [http://dx.doi.org/10.1007/s10930-020-09901-4] [PMID: 32447571]

[11] Walls AC, Park YJ, Tortorici MA, Wall A, McGuire AT, Veesler D. Structure, function, and antigenicity of the SARS-CoV-2 spike glycoprotein. Cell 2020; 181(2): 281-292.e6. [http://dx.doi.org/10.1016/j.cell.2020.02.058] [PMID: 32155444]

[12] Decroly E, Debarnot C, Ferron F, *et al.* Crystal structure and functional analysis of the SARS-coronavirus RNA cap 2′-O-methyltransferase nsp10/nsp16 complex. PLoS Pathog 2011; 7(5): e1002059.

[http://dx.doi.org/10.1371/journal.ppat.1002059] [PMID: 21637813]

[13] Zhao S, Ge X, Wang X, Liu A, Guo X, Zhou L. Since January 2020 Elsevier has created a COVID-19 resource centre with free information in English and Mandarin on the novel coronavirus COVID- 19. The COVID-19 resource centre is hosted on Elsevier Connect, the company' s public news and information. 2020.

[14] Nelson CA, Pekosz A, Lee CA, Diamond MS, Fremont DH. Structure and intracellular targeting of the SARS-coronavirus Orf7a accessory protein. Structure 2005; 13(1): 75-85. [http://dx.doi.org/10.1016/j.str.2004.10.010] [PMID: 15642263]

[15] Le TM, Wong HH, Tay FPL, *et al.* Expression, post-translational modification and biochemical characterization of proteins encoded by subgenomic mRNA8 of the severe acute respiratory syndrome coronavirus. FEBS J 2007; 274(16): 4211-22. [http://dx.doi.org/10.1111/j.1742-4658.2007.05947.x] [PMID: 17645546]

[16] Tai W, He L, Zhang X, *et al.* Characterization of the receptor-binding domain (RBD) of 2019 novel coronavirus: implication for development of RBD protein as a viral attachment inhibitor and vaccine. Cell Mol Immunol 2020; 17(6): 613-20. [http://dx.doi.org/10.1038/s41423-020-0400-4] [PMID: 32203189]

[17] Maier HJ, Bickerton E, Britton P. Coronaviruses: Methods and protocols. Coronaviruses: Methods and Protocols 2015; 1282: 1-282. [http://dx.doi.org/10.1007/978-1-4939-2438-7] [PMID: 25870870]

[18] Lan J, Ge J, Yu J, *et al.* Structure of the SARS-CoV-2 spike receptor-binding domain bound to the ACE2 receptor. Nature 2020; 581(7807): 215-20. [http://dx.doi.org/10.1038/s41586-020-2180-5] [PMID: 32225176]

[19] Tang YW, Schmitz JE, Persing DH, Stratton CW. Laboratory Diagnosis of COVID-19: Current Issues and Challenges. J Clin Microbiol 2020; 58(6): 1-22. [http://dx.doi.org/10.1128/JCM.00512-20] [PMID: 32245835]

[20] Hurst KR, Koetzner CA, Masters PS. Identification of *in vivo*-interacting domains of the murine coronavirus nucleocapsid protein. J Virol 2009; 83(14): 7221-34. [http://dx.doi.org/10.1128/JVI.00440-09] [PMID: 19420077]

[21] Chen CY, Chang CK, Chang YW, *et al.* Structure of the SARS coronavirus nucleocapsid protein RNA-binding dimerization domain suggests a mechanism for helical packaging of viral RNA. J Mol Biol 2007; 368(4): 1075-86. [http://dx.doi.org/10.1016/j.jmb.2007.02.069] [PMID: 17379242]

[22] Zeng W, Liu G, Ma H, Zhao D, Yang Y, Liu M. Since January 2020 Elsevier has created a COVID-19 resource centre with free information in English and Mandarin on the novel coronavirus COVID- 19. The COVID-19 resource centre is hosted on Elsevier Connect, the company's public news and information. 2020.

[23] Chang CK, Sue SC, Yu TH, *et al.* Modular organization of SARS coronavirus nucleocapsid protein. J Biomed Sci 2006; 13(1): 59-72. [http://dx.doi.org/10.1007/s11373-005-9035-9] [PMID: 16228284]

[24] Huang C, Wang Y, Li X, *et al.* Articles Clinical features of patients infected with 2019 novel coronavirus in Wuhan China 2020; 6736: 1-10. [http://dx.doi.org/10.1016/S0140-6736(20)30183-5]

[25] Sakai Y, Kawachi K, Terada Y, Omori H, Matsuura Y. Since January 2020 Elsevier has created a COVID-19 resource centre with free information in English and Mandarin on the novel coronavirus COVID-19. The COVID-19 resource centre is hosted on Elsevier Connect, the company's public news and information 2020.

[26] Lei J, Kusov Y, Hilgenfeld R. Since January 2020 Elsevier has created a COVID-19 resource centre with free information in English and Mandarin on the novel coronavirus COVID- 19 . The COVID-19

resource centre is hosted on Elsevier Connect , the company' s public news and information 2020.

[27] te Velthuis AJW, van den Worm SHE, Snijder EJ. The SARS-coronavirus nsp7+nsp8 complex is a unique multimeric RNA polymerase capable of both *de novo* initiation and primer extension. Nucleic Acids Res 2012; 40(4): 1737-47.
[http://dx.doi.org/10.1093/nar/gkr893] [PMID: 22039154]

[28] Subissi L, Posthuma CC, Collet A, *et al.* One severe acute respiratory syndrome coronavirus protein complex integrates processive RNA polymerase and exonuclease activities. Proc Natl Acad Sci USA 2014; 111(37): E3900-9.
[http://dx.doi.org/10.1073/pnas.1323705111] [PMID: 25197083]

[29] Jang KJ, Jeong S, Kang DY, Sp N, Yang YM, Kim DE. A high ATP concentration enhances the cooperative translocation of the SARS coronavirus helicase nsP13 in the unwinding of duplex RNA. Sci Rep 2020; 10(1): 4481.
[http://dx.doi.org/10.1038/s41598-020-61432-1] [PMID: 32161317]

[30] Nakagawa K, Lokugamage KG, Makino S. Viral and Cellular mRNA Translation in Coronavirus-Infected Cells. Adv Virus Res 2016; 96: 165-92.
[http://dx.doi.org/10.1016/bs.aivir.2016.08.001] [PMID: 27712623]

[31] Li F. Receptor recognition mechanisms of coronaviruses: a decade of structural studies. J Virol 2015; 89(4): 1954-64.
[http://dx.doi.org/10.1128/JVI.02615-14] [PMID: 25428871]

[32] Li F. Since January 2020 Elsevier has created a COVID-19 resource centre with free information in English and Mandarin on the novel coronavirus COVID- 19. The COVID-19 resource centre is hosted on Elsevier Connect , the company' s public news and information 2020.

[33] Su S, Wong G, Shi W, *et al.* Epidemiology, genetic recombination, and pathogenesis of coronaviruses. Trends Microbiol 2016; 24(6): 490-502.
[http://dx.doi.org/10.1016/j.tim.2016.03.003] [PMID: 27012512]

[34] Li F, Berardi M, Li W, Farzan M, Dormitzer PR, Harrison SC. Conformational states of the severe acute respiratory syndrome coronavirus spike protein ectodomain. J Virol 2006; 80(14): 6794-800.
[http://dx.doi.org/10.1128/JVI.02744-05] [PMID: 16809285]

[35] Kuba K, Imai Y, Ohto-Nakanishi T, Penninger JM. Trilogy of ACE2: a peptidase in the renin-angiotensin system, a SARS receptor, and a partner for amino acid transporters. Pharmacol Ther 2010; 128(1): 119-28.
[http://dx.doi.org/10.1016/j.pharmthera.2010.06.003] [PMID: 20599443]

[36] Hoffmann M, Kleine-Weber H, Schroeder S, *et al.* SARS-CoV-2 cell entry depends on ACE2 and TMPRSS2 and is blocked by a clinically proven protease inhibitor. Cell 2020; 181(2): 271-280.e8.
[http://dx.doi.org/10.1016/j.cell.2020.02.052] [PMID: 32142651]

[37] Astuti I. Since January 2020 Elsevier has created a COVID-19 resource centre with free information in English and Mandarin on the novel coronavirus COVID- 19 . The COVID-19 resource centre is hosted on Elsevier Connect , the company' s public news and information 2020.

[38] Lu R, Zhao X, Li J, *et al.* Genomic characterisation and epidemiology of 2019 novel coronavirus: implications for virus origins and receptor binding. Lancet 2020; 395(10224): 565-74.
[http://dx.doi.org/10.1016/S0140-6736(20)30251-8] [PMID: 32007145]

[39] Pérard-viret J, Quteishat L, Alsalim R. Free information in English and Mandarin on the novel coronavirus COVID- 2020.

[40] de Wit E, van Doremalen N, Falzarano D, Munster VJ. SARS and MERS: recent insights into emerging coronaviruses. Nat Rev Microbiol 2016; 14(8): 523-34.
[http://dx.doi.org/10.1038/nrmicro.2016.81] [PMID: 27344959]

[41] Chan JF, Yuan S, Kok K, To KK, Chu H, Yang J, *et al.* Since January 2020 Elsevier has created a COVID-19 resource centre with free information in English and Mandarin on the novel coronavirus

COVID- research that is available on the COVID-19 resource centre - including this for unrestricted research re-use a 2020.

[42] Li W, Moore MJ, Vasilieva N, Sui J. Angiotensin-converting enzyme 2 is a functional receptor for the SARS coronavirus. Nature 2003; 2003: 426.

[43] Wu F, Zhao S, Yu B, Chen YM, Wang W, Song ZG, *et al.* Author Correction: A new coronavirus associated with human respiratory disease in China (Nature, (2020), 579, 7798, (265-269), 10.1038/s41586-020-2008-3). Nature 2020;580:E7. [http://dx.doi.org/10.1038/s41586-020-2008-3]

[44] Guo YR, Cao QD, Hong ZS, *et al.* The origin, transmission and clinical therapies on coronavirus disease 2019 (COVID-19) outbreak - an update on the status. Mil Med Res 2020; 7(1): 11. [http://dx.doi.org/10.1186/s40779-020-00240-0] [PMID: 32169119]

[45] Wang H, Yang P, Liu K, *et al.* SARS coronavirus entry into host cells through a novel clathrin- and caveolae-independent endocytic pathway. Cell Res 2008; 18(2): 290-301. [http://dx.doi.org/10.1038/cr.2008.15] [PMID: 18227861]

[46] Báez-santos YM, John SES, Mesecar AD. The SARS-coronavirus papain-like protease: Structure, functionand inhibition by designed antiviral compounds COVID-19 resource centre is hosted on Elsevier Connect, the company's public news and information website. Elsevier hereby grants permission t. Antiviral Res 2015; 115: 21-38. [http://dx.doi.org/10.1016/j.antiviral.2014.12.015] [PMID: 25554382]

[47] Lee TW, Cherney MM, Huitema C, *et al.* Crystal structures of the main peptidase from the SARS coronavirus inhibited by a substrate-like aza-peptide epoxide. J Mol Biol 2005; 353(5): 1137-51. [http://dx.doi.org/10.1016/j.jmb.2005.09.004] [PMID: 16219322]

[48] Li G, Chen X, Xu A. Profile of specific antibodies to the SARS-associated coronavirus. N Engl J Med 2003; 349(5): 508-9. [http://dx.doi.org/10.1056/NEJM200307313490520] [PMID: 12890855]

[49] Fan YY, Huang ZT, Li L, *et al.* Characterization of SARS-CoV-specific memory T cells from recovered individuals 4 years after infection. Arch Virol 2009; 154(7): 1093-9. [http://dx.doi.org/10.1007/s00705-009-0409-6] [PMID: 19526193]

[50] Huang C, Wang Y, Li X, *et al.* Clinical features of patients infected with 2019 novel coronavirus in Wuhan, China. Lancet 2020; 395(10223): 497-506. [http://dx.doi.org/10.1016/S0140-6736(20)30183-5] [PMID: 31986264]

[51] Channappanavar R, Perlman S. Pathogenic human coronavirus infections: causes and consequences of cytokine storm and immunopathology. Semin Immunopathol 2017; 39(5): 529-39. [http://dx.doi.org/10.1007/s00281-017-0629-x] [PMID: 28466096]

[52] Min CK, Cheon S, Ha NY, *et al.* Comparative and kinetic analysis of viral shedding and immunological responses in MERS patients representing a broad spectrum of disease severity. Sci Rep 2016; 6: 25359. [http://dx.doi.org/10.1038/srep25359] [PMID: 27146253]

[53] Coperchini F, Chiovato L, Croce L, Magri F, Rotondi M. The cytokine storm in COVID-19: An overview of the involvement of the chemokine/chemokine-receptor system. Cytokine Growth Factor Rev 2020; 53: 25-32. [http://dx.doi.org/10.1016/j.cytogfr.2020.05.003] [PMID: 32446778]

[54] Snijder EJ, van der Meer Y, Zevenhoven-Dobbe J, *et al.* Ultrastructure and origin of membrane vesicles associated with the severe acute respiratory syndrome coronavirus replication complex. J Virol 2006; 80(12): 5927-40. [http://dx.doi.org/10.1128/JVI.02501-05] [PMID: 16731931]

[55] Channappanavar R, Fehr AR, Zheng J, *et al.* IFN-I response timing relative to virus replication determines MERS coronavirus infection outcomes. J Clin Invest 2019; 129(9): 3625-39.

[http://dx.doi.org/10.1172/JCI126363] [PMID: 31355779]

[56] Wang Y, Wang Y, Chen Y, Qin Q. Unique epidemiological and clinical features of the emerging 2019 novel coronavirus pneumonia (COVID-19) implicate special control measures. J Med Virol 2020; 92(6): 568-76.
[http://dx.doi.org/10.1002/jmv.25748] [PMID: 32134116]

[57] Bassetti M, Vena A, Giacobbe DR. The novel Chinese coronavirus (2019-nCoV) infections: Challenges for fighting the storm. Eur J Clin Invest 2020; 50(3): e13209.
[http://dx.doi.org/10.1111/eci.13209] [PMID: 32003000]

[58] Jin YH, Cai L, Cheng ZS, *et al.* A rapid advice guideline for the diagnosis and treatment of 2019 novel coronavirus (2019-nCoV) infected pneumonia (standard version). Mil Med Res 2020; 7(1): 4.
[http://dx.doi.org/10.1186/s40779-020-0233-6] [PMID: 32029004]

[59] Phelan AL, Katz R, Gostin LO. The novel coronavirus originating in Wwuhan, China: challenges for global health governance. JAMA 2020; 323(8): 709-10.
[http://dx.doi.org/10.1001/jama.2020.1097] [PMID: 31999307]

[60] Zhu N, Zhang D, Wang W, *et al.* A novel coronavirus from patients with pneumonia in China, 2019. N Engl J Med 2020; 382(8): 727-33.
[http://dx.doi.org/10.1056/NEJMoa2001017] [PMID: 31978945]

[61] Chen Y, Liu Q, Guo D. Emerging coronaviruses: Genome structure, replication, and pathogenesis. J Med Virol 2020; 92(4): 418-23.
[http://dx.doi.org/10.1002/jmv.25681] [PMID: 31967327]

[62] Dai WC, Zhang HW, Yu J, *et al.* CT imaging and differential diagnosis of COVID-19. Can Assoc Radiol J 2020; 71(2): 195-200.
[http://dx.doi.org/10.1177/0846537120913033] [PMID: 32129670]

[63] Cai G. Bulk and single-cell transcriptomics identify tobacco-use disparity in lung gene expression of ACE2, the receptor of 2019-nCov MedRxiv 2020.
[http://dx.doi.org/10.20944/preprints202002.0051.v1]

[64] Ferrari R, Pasquale G, Di , Rapezzi C. Since January 2020 Elsevier has created a COVID-19 resource centre with free information in English and Mandarin on the novel coronavirus COVID- 19. The COVID-19 resource centre is hosted on Elsevier Connect , the company' s public news and information 2020.

[65] Wang C, Horby PW, Hayden FG, Gao GF. A novel coronavirus outbreak of global health concern. Lancet 2020; 395(10223): 470-3.
[http://dx.doi.org/10.1016/S0140-6736(20)30185-9] [PMID: 31986257]

[66] Petrosillo N, Viceconte G, Ergonul O, Ippolito G, Petersen E. COVID-19, SARS and MERS: are they closely related? Clin Microbiol Infect 2020; 26(6): 729-34.
[http://dx.doi.org/10.1016/j.cmi.2020.03.026] [PMID: 32234451]

[67] Roca-Ho H, Riera M, Palau V, Pascual J, Soler MJ. Characterization of ACE and ACE2 expression within different organs of the NOD mouse. Int J Mol Sci 2017; 18(3): E563.
[http://dx.doi.org/10.3390/ijms18030563] [PMID: 28273875]

[68] Rao S, Lau A, So H-C. Exploring Diseases/Traits and Blood Proteins Causally Related to Expression of ACE2, the Putative Receptor of SARS-CoV-2: A Mendelian Randomization Analysis Highlights Tentative Relevance of Diabetes-Related Traits. Diabetes Care 2020; 43(7): 1416-26.
[http://dx.doi.org/10.2337/dc20-0643] [PMID: 32430459]

[69] Li Z, Yi Y, Luo X, *et al.* Development and clinical application of a rapid IgM-IgG combined antibody test for SARS-CoV-2 infection diagnosis. J Med Virol 2020; 92(9): 1518-24.
[http://dx.doi.org/10.1002/jmv.25727] [PMID: 32104917]

[70] Malik YS, Sircar S, Bhat S, *et al.* Emerging novel coronavirus (2019-nCoV)-current scenario, evolutionary perspective based on genome analysis and recent developments. Vet Q 2020; 40(1): 68-

76.
[http://dx.doi.org/10.1080/01652176.2020.1727993] [PMID: 32036774]

[71] Munster VJ, Koopmans M, van Doremalen N, van Riel D, de Wit E. A novel coronavirus emerging in China - Key questions for impact assessment. N Engl J Med 2020; 382(8): 692-4.
[http://dx.doi.org/10.1056/NEJMp2000929] [PMID: 31978293]

[72] Benvenuto D, Giovanetti M, Ciccozzi A, Spoto S, Angeletti S, Ciccozzi M. The 2019-new coronavirus epidemic: Evidence for virus evolution. J Med Virol 2020; 92(4): 455-9.
[http://dx.doi.org/10.1002/jmv.25688] [PMID: 31994738]

[73] Chu DKW, Pan Y, Cheng SMS, *et al.* Molecular Diagnosis of a Novel Coronavirus (2019-nCoV) Causing an Outbreak of Pneumonia. Clin Chem 2020; 66(4): 549-55.
[http://dx.doi.org/10.1093/clinchem/hvaa029] [PMID: 32031583]

[74] Wu A, Peng Y, Huang B, *et al.* Commentary Genome Composition and Divergence of the Novel Coronavirus (2019-nCoV). Originating in China 2020.

[75] Al Johani S, Hajeer AH. MERS-CoV diagnosis: An update. J Infect Public Health 2016; 9(3): 216-9.
[http://dx.doi.org/10.1016/j.jiph.2016.04.005] [PMID: 27106390]

[76] Wong CK, Lam CWK, Wu AKL, *et al.* Plasma inflammatory cytokines and chemokines in severe acute respiratory syndrome. Clin Exp Immunol 2004; 136(1): 95-103.
[http://dx.doi.org/10.1111/j.1365-2249.2004.02415.x] [PMID: 15030519]

[77] Kukla M, Skonieczna-Żydecka K, Kotfis K, *et al.* COVID-19, MERS and SARS with Concomitant Liver Injury-Systematic Review of the Existing Literature. J Clin Med 2020; 9(5): 1420.
[http://dx.doi.org/10.3390/jcm9051420] [PMID: 32403255]

[78] Meo SA, Alhowikan AM, Al-Khlaiwi T, *et al.* Novel coronavirus 2019-nCoV: prevalence, biological and clinical characteristics comparison with SARS-CoV and MERS-CoV. Eur Rev Med Pharmacol Sci 2020; 24(4): 2012-9.
[http://dx.doi.org/10.26355/eurrev_202002_20379] [PMID: 32141570]

CHAPTER 5

Differential Diagnosis of COVID-19

Amjad Islam Aqib[1,*], Iqra Muzammil[2], Qaisar Tanveer[3], Sana Muzammal[4], Amna Ahmad[5], Firasat Hussain[6] and **Kashif Rahim[6]**

[1] Department of Medicine, Faculty of Veterinary Science, Cholistan University of Veterinary and Animal Sciences, Bahawalpur-63100, Pakistan

[2] Department of Clinical Medicine and Surgery, University of Agriculture, Faisalabad-38000, Pakistan

[3] Institute of Pharmacy, Physiology and Pharmacology, University of Agriculture, Faisalabad-38000, Pakistan

[4] Department of Mathematics, National College of Business Administration and Economics, Sub-Campus Bahawalpur, Pakistan

[5] Faculty of Veterinary Science, University of Agriculture, Faisalabad-38000, Pakistan

[6] Department of Microbiology, Faculty of Veterinary Science, Cholistan University of Veterinary and Animal Sciences, Bahawalpur-63100, Pakistan

Abstract: Differential diagnosis is a key step to treat and prevent any disease at current. Differential identification becomes more inevitable in diseases that become pandemic while their signs and symptoms overlap with many diseases. Coronavirus disease-19 shows resemblance in its pneumonic presentation with related coronaviruses (SARS virus, and MERS virus), adenovirus, influenza virus, human Metapneumovirus, parainfluenza, Respiratory Syncytial Virus, rhinovirus, bacterial pneumonia (*Streptococcus pneumonia, Haemophilus influenza pneumonia*, *Moraxella catarrhalis* pneumonia, and *Chlamydia pneumonia*), and *Mycoplasma pneumonia.* Contrary to the discussion of only diagnostic findings, a comprehensive approach of differences in aetiologies, transmission/epidemiology, pathogeneses, clinical signs, and response therapy is necessary to resolve pandemic corona infection. Additionally, mathematical predictive models calculate the reproductive number (R_0) to show the epidemic nature of the disease in comparison to other conditions, thus aids therapeutic and prevention measures. The current chapter differentiates minor and major differences of COVID-19 compared to viral and bacterial diseases that show similar signs and symptoms.

Keywords: Aetiologies, Clinical signs, Coronavirus disease-19, Diagnosis, Differential, Pathogenesis, Response therapy, Transmission/epidemiology.

* **Corresponding author Dr. Amjad Islam Aqib:** Department of Medicine, Faculty of Veterinary Science, Cholistan University of Veterinary and Animal Sciences, Bahawalpur-63100, Pakistan. Tel.: +92 343 7474 583; E-mail: amjadwaseer@cuvas.edu.pk

Kamal Niaz & Muhammad Farrukh Nisar (Eds.)

INTRODUCTION

Common human coronaviruses are *Alphacoronaviruses* (HCoV-229E, and HCoV-NL63) and *Betacoronaviruses* (HCoV-OC43, and HCoV-HKU1). They are a source of the Common cold and some upper respiratory tract infections in humans. Severe acute respiratory syndrome-coronavirus disease (SARS-CoV), Middle East respiratory syndrome-coronavirus disease (MERS-CoV), and coronavirus disease-19 (COVID-19) belong to the genus *Betacoronavirus*. They are a source of major epidemics and cause severe respiratory and other systemic infections [1]. Differential diagnosis must include the probability of various widespread respiratory diseases. Patients remain asymptomatic while the symptomatic may be categorized as mild, moderate, and severe, seasonal flu symptoms. Few people show more severe symptoms of pneumonia and sometimes acute respiratory distress syndrome (ARDS) and septic shock to be hospitalized immediately [2]. Detection of COVID-19 at the earliest is a necessary step to treat patients on accurate guidelines. For suspected cases, rapid antigen detection and other examinations should be done to evaluate common respiratory pathogens and non-infectious disorders. A COVID-19 diagnostic testing kit has been developed and is available in clinical testing labs.

Reverse Transcription-Polymerase Chain Reaction (RT-PCR) is used as a gold standard for testing COVID-19 [3]. A computed tomography (CT) scan has a greater value in initial detection and differential diagnosis of COVID-19 [1]. There are various imaging expressions in COVID-19 at distinct stages primarily associated with pathogenesis. At the initial stages of COVID-19, inflammation of lungs penetrated to the subpleural areas of one or both lungs showing irregular or segmented pure ground-glass opacities (GGOs) along with dilation of vessels. A short number of cases are also noticed with negative CT findings at the initial stages. But in the advanced stage, CT shows chiefly an enhanced amount of pure ground-glass opacities in lungs, consolidations of particular lesions, and GGOs surrounding consolidated lesions, which are the prominent characters of advanced stage COVID-19 infection [4]. Imaging diagnosis for COVID-19 is considered difficult to differentiate for viral pneumonia, including influenza viruses, adenovirus, Respiratory Syncytial Virus, SARS-CoV, MERS-CoV, and bacterial pneumonia [5]. Viral pneumonia, except COVID-19, is chiefly associated with interstitial inflammation of peribronchial and perivascular regions, spreading toward the inner part of the pulmonary interstitium. Their CT expressions are manifold interweaved due to infiltration of the interlobular septa [6].

COVID 2019 must also be differentiated from bacterial pneumonia and *Mycoplasma pneumonia (M. pneumonia)* (separated from bacterial pneumonia) is the smallest and atypical bacteria that causes mild respiratory symptoms) [7].

Bacterial pneumonia occurs in the lung parenchyma, and there is bronchial or lobar pneumonia and numerous inflammatory secretions. Its CT expressions exhibit widespread irregular consolidations of the lung parenchyma, while GGOs are rare [8]. *M. pneumonia* usually occurs in children and young people but seldom occurs in adults. The chest CT manifestations of *M. pneumonia* in adults are commonly bronchial wall thickening, an indicator of lobar pneumonia, and centrilobular nodules, which are small airway lesions. In contrast, the CT scan of COVID-19 shows mostly pure GGOs at the initial stage and observable consolidations in the center of the lesions at the advanced stage [9]. The current chapter will describe in detail about pathogenicity, clinical signs, diagnostic procedures, and treatment of COVID-19 as differential indications keeping relevant viral and bacterial diseases of the respiratory system in an intact discussion (Fig. **1**).

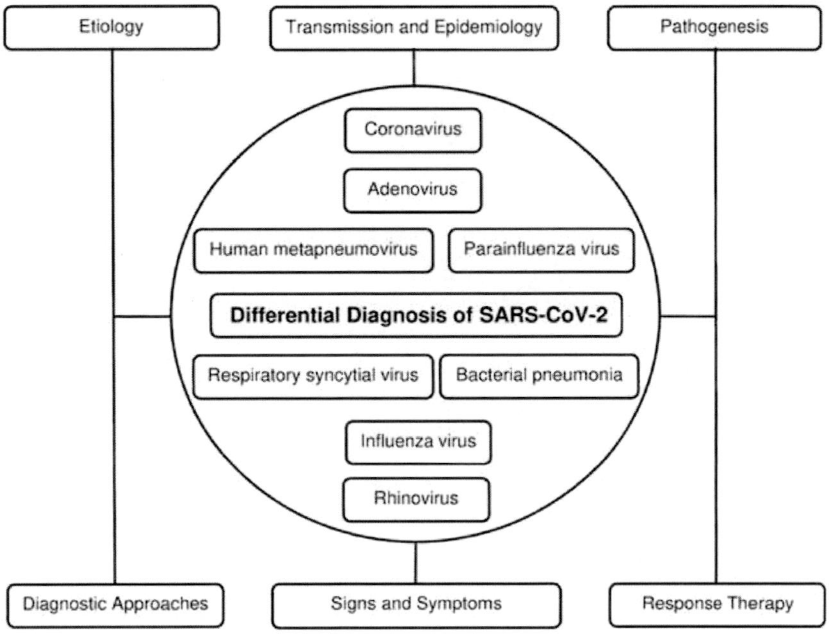

Fig. (1). Differential diagnosis of SARS-CoV-2 with different diseases based on different factors/characteristics.

Differential Diagnosis of COVID-19

Differential diagnosis involves confirmation of a disease condition whose signs and symptoms somehow show similarities with other diseases or disease conditions. To treat or prevent any disease at current and to avoid another illness with similar signs and symptoms, it is imperative to have sound knowledge of the differential diagnosis. Complete knowledge of differences in etiology, transmission/epidemiology, pathogenesis, clinical findings, diagnostic tests, and treatment protocols should be considered to achieve this. The differential diagnosis in this chapter covers differences concerning etiology, epidemiology & transmission, pathogenesis, clinical signs & symptoms, diagnostic outcomes, and response therapies.

COVID-19 will be differentiated with the following diseases in this book chapter:

- Other Coronaviruses (SARS, MERS)
- Adenovirus
- Influenza Virus
- Human Metapneumovirus (HMPV)
- Parainfluenza Virus
- Respiratory Syncytial Virus (RSV)
- Rhinovirus (Common cold)
- Bacterial pneumonia (*Streptococcus pneumonia, Haemophilus influenza pneumonia, Moraxella catarrhalis* pneumonia, and *Chlamydia pneumonia)* and
- *M. pneumonia*

Differential Etiology

COVID-19 and other Coronaviruses

Coronavirus belongs to genus *Betacoronavirus*, subfamily *Orthocoronaviridae*, family *Coronaviridae* and order Nidovirales. Phylogenetic analysis reveals SARS-CoV-2 belonging to Clad I and Clad IIa. The reservoir host of these viruses are bats, while the intermediate host is yet not known. Some studies suspect pangolin as an intermediate host while authenticity is yet questionable [10]. The virus is 50–200 nanometres in diameter, having positive-sense single-stranded RNA (+ssRNA) with a single linear RNA segment that accounts for approximately a genome size of 29,903 bases (2.9kb) and 11 open reading frames (ORFs). SARS-CoV (belonging to Clad I and Clad IIb; bats are animal reservoirs; the intermediate host is palm civets) is single-stranded positive-sense viral RNA having 13–15 ORFs while consists of a total of nearly 3kb (30,000 nucleotides) [11]. Both SARS-CoV and SARS-CoV-2 bind to ACE 2 of the host to get into the human body. Genomic comparison between SARS-CoV and SARS-CoV-2 presents a difference of only 380 amino acid substitutions, which are concentrated mainly in the non-structural protein genes. Viral spike protein, S protein, responsible for binding to the ACE receptor, shows 27 mutations in genes that encode it.

On the other hand, MERS-CoV belongs to Clad II; bats are animal reservoirs; camels are intermediate hosts. The virus binds to the host cellular receptor dipeptidyl peptidase 4 (DPP4) to enter the host cells. The virus is also a positive-sense single-stranded consisting of 301-31kb genome with the versatility of adopting a new environment and transmission across species.

Adenovirus

Adenoviruses result in upper and lower respiratory tract infections, keratoconjunctivitis, pharyngitis, pneumonia, and many other infections in humans. Adenoviruses are named so because they were isolated from human adenoids. They belong to the family *Adenoviridae* and genus *Mastadenovirus*. They are non-enveloped, having non-segmented double-stranded DNA. They have icosahedral nucleocapsid, formed by 252 capsomeres: 240 haxons form the face, and 12 forms the vertices. A fiber protrudes from each vertex of the capsid, and it is the organ of attachment and hemagglutinin. More than 100 different serotypes of adenoviruses have been identified. Of which about half infects the human host. Human adenoviruses serotypes are classified into seven sub-genera or species [12]. A: 12, 18, and 31, B: B_1 (3, 7, 16, 21, and 51); B_2 (11, 14, 34, and 35); C: 1, 2, 5, and 6; D: 8, 9, 10, 13, 15, 17, 19, 20, 22-30, 32, 33, 36-39, 42-49, and 50; E: 4; F: 40, 41; G: 52.

Influenza Virus

Influenza viruses are considered significant due to several epidemics and pandemics. They belong to the family *Orthomyxoviridae.* They have enveloped RNA viruses with segmented genomes, helical nucleocapsid, and lipoprotein envelopes and are small (about 110nm in diameter). Hemagglutinin and neuraminidase protein spikes are present on their surface.

Human Metapneumovirus (HMPV)

Human Metapneumovirus (HMPV), a ubiquitous infection present in all age groups, has similarities to avian metapneumovirus. HMPV is a negative-strand RNA virus known to cause lower respiratory tract infection [13]. It belongs to the family *Paramyxoviridae* sub-family *Pneumovirinae* and genus *Metapneumovirus*. The virus was first isolated from children in 2001 in Netherland, showing symptoms identical to human Respiratory Syncytial Virus (hRSV) infections. The mechanism of the virus recognizing host cell and target receptor is not widely known. However, an experiment showed that the cell lines that cannot synthesize glycosaminoglycans (GAGs), especially heparan sulfate proteoglycans (HSPGs), were resistant to binding and infection HMPV.

Parainfluenza Virus

Parainfluenza virus causes laryngitis, bronchiolitis, laryngotracheobronchitis (croup), and pneumonia in children and adults. The virus belongs to the *Paramyxoviridae* family and has a negative sense of single-stranded enveloped RNA. Hemagglutinin (H), neuraminidase (N), and fusion (F) protein are present as spikes on the surface of the virus. Parainfluenza viruses also infect animals, but strains that cause diseases cannot infect humans [14].

Respiratory Syncytial Virus (RSV)

Respiratory Syncytial Virus (RSV) belongs to the *Paramyxoviridae* family and is known to cause pneumonia, otitis media, and bronchiolitis in infants and old people [15]. Its nucleocapsid is helical, and the outer envelope consists of lipoprotein molecules covered with spikes of the fusion protein. Fusion proteins present on the surface fuse to form multinucleated giant cells (syncytia), so the virus is named a syncytial virus. The virus has two serotypes named A and B.

Rhinovirus (Common Cold)

Rhinovirus is an important cause of the Common cold, a recurrent but otherwise comparatively insignificant and self-limited disease. It can cause infection of the lower respiratory tract and activate asthma exacerbations in both adults and children. The virus belongs to the family *Picornaviridae* and genus *Enterovirus* while appears to be positive-sense, single-stranded-RNA (ssRNA) of about 7,200 bp. The single gene-based whole viral genome is cleaved to translate and produce 11 proteins [16]. These viruses gain entry into the host cell by three major types of cellular membrane glycoproteins, including low-density lipoprotein receptor (LDLR) family members (12 RV-A types), intercellular adhesion molecule-1 (ICAM-1), and cadherin-related family member 3 (CDHR3).

Bacterial Pneumonia

Streptococcus Pneumoniae

Streptococcus pneumoniae (S. pneumoniae), also termed *pneumococcus*, is a Gram-positive and catalase-negative organism resulting in pneumococcal infections. This bacterium is a leading candidate for community-acquired pneumonia, bacterial meningitis, otitis media, septic arthritis, sinusitis, endocarditis, osteomyelitis, and peritonitis [17].

Haemophilus Influenza

This is a gram-negative coccobacillus facultative anaerobe bacterium. This bacterium inhabits the respiratory tract leads to infection of various body systems for producing bacteremia, meningitis, epiglottitis, endocarditis, septic arthritis, or cellulitis [18].

Moraxella Catarrhalis Pneumonia

Moraxella catarrhalis is responsible for causing chronic bronchitis leading to pneumonia. *Moraxella* organisms are small, Gram-negative diplococci or bacilli. It is the most significant pathogen of the *Moraxella* genus [19].

Chlamydial Pneumonia

The causative pathogen is *Chlamydial pneumonia*, a Gram-negative, small, and obligate intracellular bacterium that leads to community-acquired pneumonia or lung infections [20].

M. Pneumonia

M. pneumonia is a microscopic pathogen that belongs to the class Mollicutes. It damages the lining of the respiratory system (throat, lungs, and windpipe), and sometimes it is referred to as "walking pneumonia" because it causes milder pneumonia than other bacterial pneumonia. It was first isolated in cattle species with pleuropneumonia in 1898 [21].

The differential etiology of COVID-19 with other bacterial and viral respiratory diseases is summarized in Table **1**.

Table 1. Differential aetiologies of COVID-19 with viral and bacterial diseases.

Virus/bacteria	Disease Name	Order, Family, Genus	Size and Nature of Nucleic Acid	Animal Reservoir	Intermediate Host	Host Receptor
SARS-CoV2	COVID-19	Order: Nidovirales Clad I and Clad IIa Genus: *Betacoronavirus* Subfamily: *Orthocoronaviridae* Family: *Coronaviridae*	Positive-sense single-stranded RNA (+ssRNA) 29,903 bases (2.9kb)	Bats	Not known yet	ACE-2
SARS-CoV	SARS (Severe acute respiratory syndrome)	Clad I and Clad IIb	Single-stranded positive-sense viral RNA 30,000 nucleotides (3kb)	Bats	Palm civets	ACE-2

(Table 1) cont.....

Virus/bacteria	Disease Name	Order, Family, Genus	Size and Nature of Nucleic Acid	Animal Reservoir	Intermediate Host	Host Receptor
MERS	Middle East respiratory syndrome	Clad II	Positive-sense single-stranded RNA 301-31kb	Bats	Camel	Cellular receptor dipeptidyl peptidase 4 (DPP4
Adenovirus	Pharyngitis, pneumonia	Genus: *Mastadenovirus* Family: *Adenoviridae*	Non-enveloped non-segmented double-stranded DNA 34-36kb	-	-	Coxsackie virus and adenovirus receptor (CAR)
Influenza virus	Influenza	Family *Orthomyxoviridae*	Negative-sense single-stranded enveloped RNA 13kb	-	-	Neuraminic acid. sialic acid
human Metapneumovirus (HMPV)	HMPV infection	Genus: *Metapneumovirus* Family: *Paramyxoviridae* Sub-family: *Pneumovirinae*	Negative-sense single-strand RNA 13.3kb	-	-	Heparan sulfate
Parainfluenza virus	Croup	Family: *Paramyxoviridae*	Negative-sense single-stranded enveloped RNA 15kb	-	-	Sialyl (2-3) GAL receptor
Respiratory Syncytial Virus (RSV)	Bronchiolitis	Genus: *Pneumovirus* Family: *Paramyxoviridae*	Negative-sense single-stranded RNA 15kb	-	-	CX3CR1
Rhinovirus (Common cold)	Common cold	Family *Picornavirida* and genus *Enterovirus*	Positive-sense, single-stranded RNA (ssRNA) 7.2 kb	-	-	LDLR, ICAM-1, CDHR3

(Table 1) cont.....

Virus/bacteria	Disease Name	Order, Family, Genus	Size and Nature of Nucleic Acid	Animal Reservoir	Intermediate Host	Host Receptor
Bacterial Pneumonia	Bacterial pneumonia	1- Genus: *Streptococcus* Family: *Streptococcaceae.* 2- Genus: *Haemophilus* Family: *Pasteurellaceae* 3- Genus: *Moraxella* Family: *Moraxellaceae* 4- Order: *Chlamydiae* Family: *Chlamydiaceae* Genus: *Chlamydia*	1- Gram-positive bacterium 2.1 Mb 2- Gram-negative, facultative anaerobe 1.8 Mb 3- Gram-negative commensal 1.89 Mb 4- Gram-negative DNA 1234 kb	-	-	-
M. pneumonia	Atypical pneumonia	Class: *Mollicutes* Order: *Mycoplasma tales*	816kb	-	-	-

COMPARATIVE MODES OF TRANSMISSION AND EPIDEMIOLOGY

COVID-19 and other Coronaviruses (SARS, MERS)

SARS-CoV-2 is contagious and spread by aerosol droplets from infected people and fomites. Human-to-human transmission causes its pandemic. Incubation ranges from 2-14 days. Basic case reproduction rate (BCR)–the number of people infected from a single patient- in the case of COVID-19 is 2-6.47 [22]. It was 2 and 1.3 in the case of SARS and influenza H_1N_1 respectively. Coronavirus infections are limited to cells of mucosa in the respiratory tract. Sometimes, in about 50% of cases, the infection can be asymptomatic yet spread the virus. Reinfection can occur after recovery due to low-cut immunity. SARS disease is spread by the SARS-CoV virus, which is transmitted by respiratory aerosol droplets. Human to human transmission is the major source of disease spread and outbreak. The incubation period for SARS is 2-10 days, in which 5 days are considered to be the average. The death rate is 3-4% and primarily due to respiratory failure. MERS-CoV's transmission of MERS caused by MERS-CoV, also named human coronavirus-EMC (HCoV-EMC), occurs through camel-to-human as the virus is shed in body fluids, mainly respiratory and rectal discharge; and human-to-human [2]. The mortality rate of SARS, MERS, and COVID-19 is 11%, 34%, and 2-3% respectively.

Adenovirus

Adenovirus may have direct transmission from person to person or indirect transmission from the environment. Transmission of adenovirus occurs by aerosol droplet, feco-oral route, and direct inoculation by fingers or contact with fomites [23]. The incubation period is 5-7 days, with fever starts from 2-3 days. The virus continues to excrete for several months from an initial infection. That's why the feco-oral route is thought to be a major route of viral transmission. Feco-oral route of transmission is common among young children and their families. Usually, adenovirus infections are endemic, but outbreaks occur in the military probably because of close living conditions. Adenovirus infections are ubiquitous and generally common in children and cause 2-5% of total respiratory tract infections to occur in them. Severe complications seldom occur. More specifically, Ad3 and Ad7 from species B, Ad1, Ad2, and Ad5 from species C are common agents associated with respiratory tract infections that may persist in children without causing symptoms for years. Ad8, Ad19, and Ad37 from species D cause conjunctivitis. Ad4 from species E causes both respiratory and ocular infections. Ad40 and Ad41 from species F and Ad52 from species G cause severe gastroenteritis [12].

Influenza Virus

Influenza virus is contagious, and transmission occurs through airborne respiratory droplets. The morbidity rate of influenza is very high, especially in children and elders. Outbreaks occur every year, especially in winters. The incubation period is usually 24-48 hours. Immunocompromised patients, pregnant women, children >2 years of age, and elders are more prone to infection. **Influenza A virus** is the most virulent human pathogen can cause severe disease and the source of most pandemics. They are capable of infecting both humans and animals. These viruses are categorized into different serotypes keeping in view response to the antibody against the virus. They have 16 antigenically distinct types of hemagglutinin and 9 antigenically distinct types of neuraminidase. Changes in antigenicity occur due to hemagglutinin and neuraminidase proteins. Also, the non-existence of pre-existing antibodies in humans against them causes pandemics of Influenza type A. **Influenza B virus** is present only in humans. It mutates less than influenza type A virus and causes several outbreaks but not pandemic. **Influenza C virus** can infect humans, dogs, and pigs. It is a less common type of Influenza virus and causes mild respiratory tract infections.

Human Metapneumovirus (HMPV)

HMPV cases have been reported worldwide. It is prevalent in the winter season and followed by the Respiratory Syncytial Virus (RSV). They show two genotypes named A and B as defined by genomic sequence and phylogenetic analysis [24]. Infection with HMPV is common in childhood. It can cause severe lower respiratory infections such as pneumonitis and bronchospasm in very young children, premature born, people with underlying heart and lung disease, immune-compromised patients, and elders [13].

Parainfluenza Virus

The virus was first isolated in 1955 from children having croup. The disease is present worldwide and mostly occurs during the winter months. Transmission occurs through respiratory droplets [25].

Respiratory Syncytial Virus (RSV)

Transmission of RSV occurs through respiratory droplets and direct contact of contaminated hands with the face. Transmission of the disease is worldwide, and everyone is thought to be infected by 3 years. Children, hospitalized infants, the elderly, and patients with chronic cardiopulmonary diseases are at greater risk. The disease is more prevalent during winters [15].

Rhinovirus (Common cold)

Rhinovirus is responsible for 1/3 to 1/2 of cases in adults per annum. More than 100 serotypes have been recognized. Normally two to three colds per year occur in adults and 8 to 12 colds per year in children because they serve as a chief reservoir for rhinovirus [26]. Aerosols, fomites, and direct contact with infected nasal secretions are common sources of spread. However, the main route has not been identified yet. However, this virus can persist in the environment >8 hours and infect people's hands and consequently transfer to their eyes or nose to develop infection [27].

Bacterial Pneumonia

Streptococcus pneumonia: *S. pneumoniae* is the source of a wider range of clinical symptoms. It causes disease in surrounding anatomic structures by extending from either direct extension from the nasopharynx and vascular invasion *via* hematogenous spread. Children with age <5 years and adults aged>55-65 years are considered high-risk patients. Comorbidities like HIV infection, diabetes, and malignancy normally impair the immune system hence infection caused by *S. pneumonia* is aggravated. Similarly, the synergistic effect of the appearance of clinical symptoms lies with asthma, chronic bronchitis, or chronic obstructive pulmonary disease [17].

Haemophilus influenzae pneumonia: Accurate prevalence and incidence are yet not known. This bacterium can live in the nasopharynx of both children and adults. Almost 3 to 5% of newborns have *Haemophilus influenze (H. influenzae)* type b in their nasopharynx before vaccination. Children who have been vaccinated against *H. influenzae* type b have fewer chances to get infected with this organism. But the risk for getting an infection is almost 600 times higher in non-vaccinated persons than the risk in the age-adjusted general population. Transmission is executed due to direct contact with nasopharyngeal respiratory droplets excreted by the carrier or patient. Aspiration of amniotic fluid or contact with contaminated genital tract secretions causes infection in newborns. The disease maximally spread due to lack of vaccination in children <5 years of age and adults with >65. Household contacts, day-care fellows having influenza b infection are salient risk factors. Comorbidities like sickle cell disease, immunoglobulin & complement component deficiencies, HIV, and malignant cancers are situations that are synergistic to strengthen clinical signs [28].

Moraxella catarrhalis pneumonia: *M. catarrhalis* is a commensal organism generally that transmits from person to person, mostly in hospitals. This infection is more prevalently reported in individuals with respiratory complications like COPD or infants having underdeveloped immune systems [29].

Chlamydial pneumonia: This infection follows the same transmission routes as other respiratory infections, like as it spreads through sneezing or coughing and by touching the surfaces having droplets containing the bacteria [30].

Mycoplasma pneumonia

This type of bacteria spreads through coughing or sneezing from person to person, which produces small respiratory droplets in the air containing bacteria. People surrounding infected people breathe in the bacteria. Asymptomatic individuals may carry bacteria in their nose or throat at one time or another. Most people who spend a very short time with *C. pneumoniae* infected individuals do not get the disease. The incubation period of *C. pneumoniae* infection is very long, varying from 1 to 4 weeks [31].

The summary of comparative modes of transmission and epidemiology of COVID-19 to other bacterial and viral respiratory diseases is discussed in Table **2**.

Table 2. Characteristic features of viral and bacterial diseases.

Disease	Transmission	Incubation Period	Risk Factors
COVID-19	Aerosol droplets and fomites	2-14 days	Comorbidities like the cardiac and respiratory problems, Immune compromised patients at higher risk
SARS	Aerosol droplets	2-10 days	
MERS	Aerosol droplets	2-14 days	
Adenovirus	Aerosol droplets, feco-oral and direct inoculation	5-7 days	
Influenza virus	Aerosol droplets	24-48 hour	
human Metapneumovirus (HMPV)	Aerosol droplets	5-21 days	Young children, premature born, people with underlying heart and lung disease, elders, and immunocompromised patients
Parainfluenza virus	Respiratory droplets	2-6 days	Immunocompromised patients, people after hematopoietic stem cell transplantation (HCT) are at high risk
Respiratory Syncytial Virus (RSV)	Respiratory droplets and direct contact of contaminated hands with face	4-6 days	Children, hospitalized infants, the elderly, and patients with chronic cardiopulmonary diseases are at higher risk
Rhinovirus (Common cold)	Aerosols, fomites, and direct contact with infected nasal secretions	12-72 hr	Chronic medical condition, cancer, smoking
Bacterial Pneumonia	Direct extension from the nasopharynx, coughing, sneezing, or touching the surfaces infected with bacteria while vascular invasion *via* blood spread	*Streptococcus pneumonia:* 1-3 days *Haemophilus influenzae pneumonia:* 7 days *Moraxella catarrhalis* pneumonia: Unknown *Chlamydial pneumonia:* 3-4 weeks	Age <5 years and adults of age >55-65 years, presence of other diseases like asthma, chronic bronchitis, diabetes, and malignancy, non-vaccinated people are at higher risk, nosocomial infection
M. pneumonia	Spread through coughing or sneezing droplets in the air containing bacteria	Very long, varying from 1 to 4 weeks	People working at crowded places are at higher risk

COMPARATIVE PATHOGENESIS

COVID-19 and Other Coronaviruses (SARS, MERS)

Coronaviruses enter the host by inhaling the infected person's aerosol droplets and then get attached to their specific receptors. These viruses release their RNA after binding to its receptor and initiate infection development [32]. SARS-CoV-2 may enter the host through the respiratory tract or mucosal surfaces such as the conjunctiva. The inhaled SARS-CoV-2 virus binds to nasal cavity epithelial cells, while the upper respiratory tract is found to be an efficient replication site for this novel coronavirus. This can also replicate in the lower respiratory tract and causes radiological evidence of lower respiratory tract involvement in patients with no clinical pneumonia [33]. In a fluorescent trial, the evidence indicates that the SARS-CoV-2 uses angiotensin-converting enzyme 2, the same entrance receptor as SARS-CoV [2]. Bronchoalveolar lavage fluid from a positive COVID-19 patient reported SARS-CoV-2 use of ACE2 as an entrance receptor [34]. Angiotensin-converting enzyme protein is notable on alveolar epithelial cells and causes regulation and transmission of both human-to-human and cross-species [35].

The S-glycoprotein present on the surface of SARS-CoV-2 that has S1 and S2 subunits binds to ACE2. S1 is responsible for RNA binding domain (RBD), supporting the attachment for both virus-host and cell tropism, while S2 causes the fusion of virus-cell membrane [36]. The critical residue of lysine 31 present on the human receptor ACE2 recognizes the 394-glutamine residue located in the SARS-CoV-2's RBD region. The viral RNA is released into the host's cell cytoplasm after membrane fusion, followed by the translation of two viral replicase polyproteins, pp-1a and pp-1ab, which encode the NSPs, ultimately forming a double-membrane vesicle that is replication-transcription complex (RTC). RTC continuously replicates and synthesizes nests of sub-genomic RNAs, which finally encodes structural proteins and accessory relevant proteins. Subsequently, genomic RNA, glycoproteins envelope, and nucleocapsid proteins assemble into the endoplasmic reticulum's virion, followed by Golgi. Finally, the newly formed vesicles that contain virion are fused with the plasma membrane of the host to release new viruses [37]. SARS's pathogenesis is highly complex, with several factors leading to severe lung injury and the virus transmitted to several other organs [38]. Like SARS-CoV-2, the proteins and RNA of the specific virus are synthesized after binding with ACE2 receptor and fusion of plasma membrane, probably entirely within the cytoplasm. The expression of the virus begins with the translation of polyproteins including ppla and pplb, which undergo proteolytic co-translational manufacturing of proteins. Newly synthesized virions are accumulated into the intracellular membranes by budding and released through vesicles by cell secretory mechanisms [39]. While in comparison to SARS-CoV-2 and SARS-CoV, MERS-CoV interacts with cellular receptor DPP4 (dipeptidyl peptidase 4) to enter permissive host cells [40]. After entry, MERS-CoV follows the same steps as other CoVs.

Adenovirus

Adenoviruses infect the epithelial layer of different organs particularly the respiratory tract, conjunctiva, and gastrointestinal tract. Type-specific and life-long immunity is based on neutralizing antibodies being produced. Destruction of bronchial epithelium and bronchial glands is observed in severe cases. Tissues involved show cellular infiltrates. Tissue necrosis, cellular infiltrates, and basophilic inclusions are observed in the liver affected by adenovirus. The persistence of the antigen-antibody complex present in the body instigates an inflammatory response that causes damage to the cornea. Adenoviruses cause acute infection and latent infection. In the case of latent infection, their predilection sites are adenoid and tonsillar tissues in the throat. The adenoviruses become less infective when exposed to 56°C or above for 10 minutes. They are insensitive to lipid solvents and stable when exposed to mild acids [41].

Influenza Virus

After the inhalation of the virus, neuraminidase present on its surface degrades the protective mucus layer and helps the virus penetrate the virus to upper and lower respiratory tract cells. The influenza virus is limited to the respiratory tract due to the presence of proteases that cleave hemagglutinin. A virus causes inflammation of the respiratory tract (nose, pharynx, larynx, trachea, bronchi). Necrosis of superficial respiratory tract epithelium can occur. Pneumonia may also be occurred due to circulating cytokines and myalgia. Influenza rarely leads to viremia. Immunity depends on IgA and cytotoxic T-cells' presence.

Human Metapneumovirus (HMPV)

An experimental study was performed on BALB/c mice and cotton rats to understand the pathogenesis of HMPV. After the intranasal administration of virus culture, its replication occurs in the lungs leading to lung inflammation, weight loss, and respiratory distress. Virus titer was recorded at peak at day 5 post-infection, and on day 21 no viruses were recovered. Peak pulmonary inflammation was observed on day 5 and then started to decline and was not observed on day 21. Inflammatory changes include interstitial inflammation, alveolitis, and peri bronchiolitis. Inflammatory cells (neutrophils and macrophages) increased from day 1 post-infection and then gradually slow down. Cytokines level, *e.g.*, interferon-gamma (IFN-γ), macrophage inflammatory protein-1 alpha (MIP-1α), and interleukin-4 (IL-4) increased immediately post-infection at day 1 [42].

Parainfluenza Virus

Based on pathogenicity, parainfluenza viruses are divided into 4 types. Most of the infections are subclinical. However, the clinical disease involves upper and lowers respiratory disease depending on the type of virus that causes it. Type 1 and 2 causes laryngotracheobronchitis or croup. Type 3 virus causes lower respiratory tract infection and is more prevalent in infants. Type 4 causes a Common cold [43].

Respiratory Syncytial Virus (RSV)

RSV does not cause viremia and is localized in the respiratory tract. The disease is more adverse in babies than in elders and older children and involves the lower respiratory tract. Immunity in the recovered patients is incomplete, and infection can be recurring. An IgA antibody lowers the frequency of infection as a personage.

Rhinovirus (Common Cold)

Rhinovirus (RV) infection uses nasal epithelium as a primary site. About 90% of well-known RV stereotypes, HRV-A, and HRV-B families use ICAM-1 as the receptor for cell entry. In contrast, the other 10 serotypes use small group receptors, which is low-density lipoprotein [44]. ICAM-1 uses as a binding site for HRV. After binding, the virus loses its capsid of protein. Virus uptake occurs through micropinocytosis, independent endocytosis, and clathrin-dependent [45]. The virions consequently go through some structural alterations for producing hydrophobic subviral particles. In endosomes, this process is started *via* ICAM-1 and/or the low-pH environment. Negative strand RNA is replicated and undergoes translation to form structural and non-structural proteins. The virion is accumulated before cellular export and packed *via* cell lysis [16]. The cold symptoms begin one day after entry of the virus and highest on the third or fourth day. It is unknown whether rhinitis is caused by the direct cytocidal effect of virus replication or mediator release. Symptoms of RV infection are generally confined to the upper respiratory tract in non-asthmatic individuals. The most prominent rhinorrhoea and nasal obstruction symptoms are linked with an inflammatory neutrophilic response associated with enlarged permeability of vessels and activation of increased secretion of mucous [46].

Bacterial Pneumonia

***Streptococcus pneumoniae*:** The *pneumococcus* is the traditional extracellular bacterial, Gram-positive pathogen. A wide range of *pneumococcal* virulence factors tailored effectively to specific host niches. The nasopharynx is the ecological niche that *pneumococcus* employs. When bacteria enter the lower respiratory tract, the mucous defense must be escaped, and bacteria must reach the alveoli [47]. Bacteria strongly attaches to the alveolar epithelium, followed by replication and beginning of host damage leading to classic lobar pneumonia. This process is driven by the collaboration of secretions and attached bacterial constituents of the cell surface with the alveolar epithelium and innate immune defenses. The pore-forming toxin pneumolysin and hydrogen peroxide produced by the bacteria in large amounts interferes with the alveolar epithelium and accumulates edema fluid in the alveolar space [48]. This infection can become severe due to other invasive diseases like pneumonia, meningitis, and septicemia [49].

Haemophilus influenzae pneumonia: The bacterium *H. influenzae* lives in the human nasopharynx and conjunctiva may spread to cause pneumonia, otitis media, or meningitis. The *H. Influenzae* is classified into encapsulated and non-encapsulated strains. Infections caused by encapsulated strains invade the bloodstream to cause hematogenic spread. A capsular polysaccharide is a crucial factor that facilitates invasion by virulence [18]. The initial stage in the pathogenesis of non-typeable *H. Influenzae* is an invasion of the upper respiratory tract. Multiple virulence factors mediate colonization and infection, including adhesives, nutrient absorption systems, host-resistant molecules, and others [18].

Moraxella catarrhalis pneumonia: *M. catarrhalis* is found mainly in the respiratory tract of humans. This organism sticks to mucosal cells with the help of pili. It spreads from colonization to the infection site due to more infectious strains to which the host does not possess immunity. *M. catarrhalis* can occur in respiratory secretions along with *H. influenza* because the outer membrane vesicles of *M. catarrhalis* deactivate complement to increase the latter's existence. *M. catarrhalis* is linked to various infections, including upper and lower respiratory tract infections, bacteraemia, septic complications, endocarditis, meningitis, and brain abscess in addition to wound infections [50].

***Chlamydia pneumoniae*:** *C. pneumoniae* has been shown to replicate and thrive within the vascular walls (macrophages, smooth muscle cells, endothelial cells, and epithelial cells) and the airway of most cell types. These types of cells can lead to both acute infection and chronic respiratory disease progression. The pathogenesis of *C. pneumoniae* is a complicated process that relies on the population of an invaded cell, initiation of a genetic state of replicative and non-replicative pathogens, and the effector molecules of host cells [51]. In adolescents and young adults, *C. pneumoniae* causes sinusitis, pharyngitis, bronchitis, and pneumonia. Older adults can experience more severe illnesses and recurrent infections. An increased risk of vascular lesions, asthma, and COPD was associated with frequent or recurrent infections [52].

Mycoplasma pneumonia

M. pneumonia attachment to the respiratory epithelium (Cytadherence) is a precondition for subsequent changes resulting in the development of diseases. The P1 adhesin is a concentrated 170-kDa protein at the tip of the attachment responsible for attachment of *M. pneumonia* with host cells [53]. Extrapulmonary complications that involve the systems of all the major organs may happen in association with *M. pneumoniae* infection by an autoimmune response or direct invasion. Sometimes the extra-pulmonary occurrences are more lethal and clinically important than the primary infection of the respiratory system [54]. In association with *M. pneumoniae* infection, pro-inflammatory cytokines release has been involved as a possible mechanism for underlying chronic pulmonary diseases such as asthma. Evidence of the contributory role of mechanism in the chronic condition of lungs such as asthma is gradually building [53]. The differential pathogenesis of COVID-19 with viral and bacterial respiratory diseases is summarized in Table **3**.

Table 3. Differential pathogenesis of COVID-19 with viral and bacterial diseases.

Disease	Pathogenesis
COVID-19	Virus attachment and entry → Binding to ACE 2 receptors for COVID-19 and SARS and DPP4 for MERS → Replication of virus → Translatiom → Assembly and budding → Exocytosis → Virus release and infect alveolar II cells and lungs
SARS	
MERS	
Adenovirus	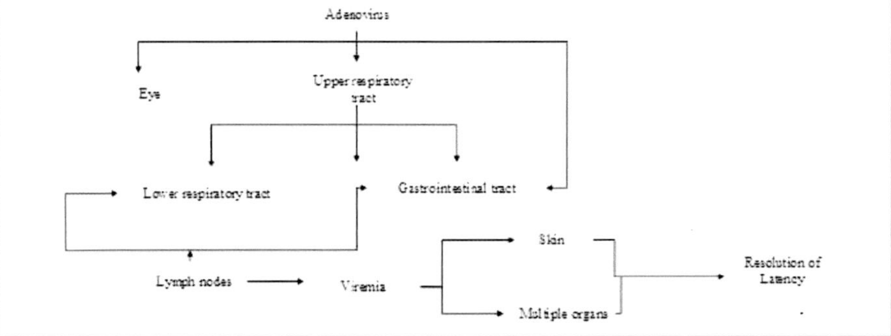

(Table 3) cont.....

Disease	Pathogenesis
Influenza virus	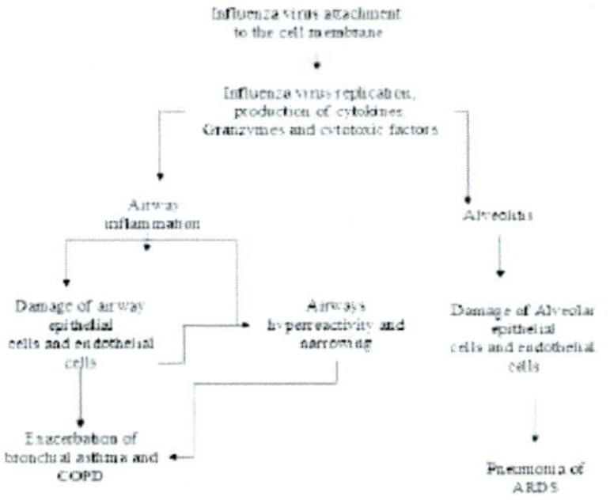
Human Metapneumovirus (HMPV)	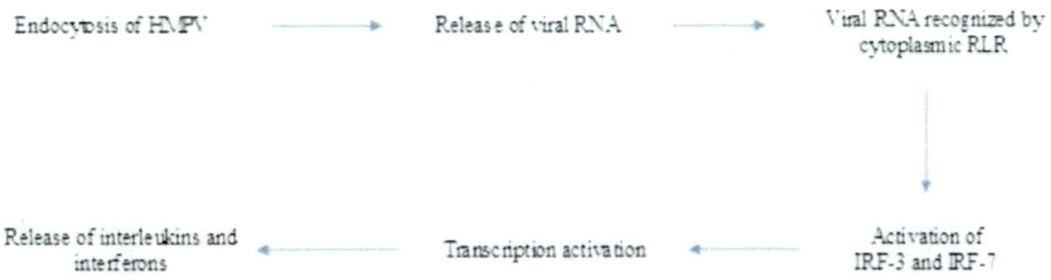
Parainfluenza	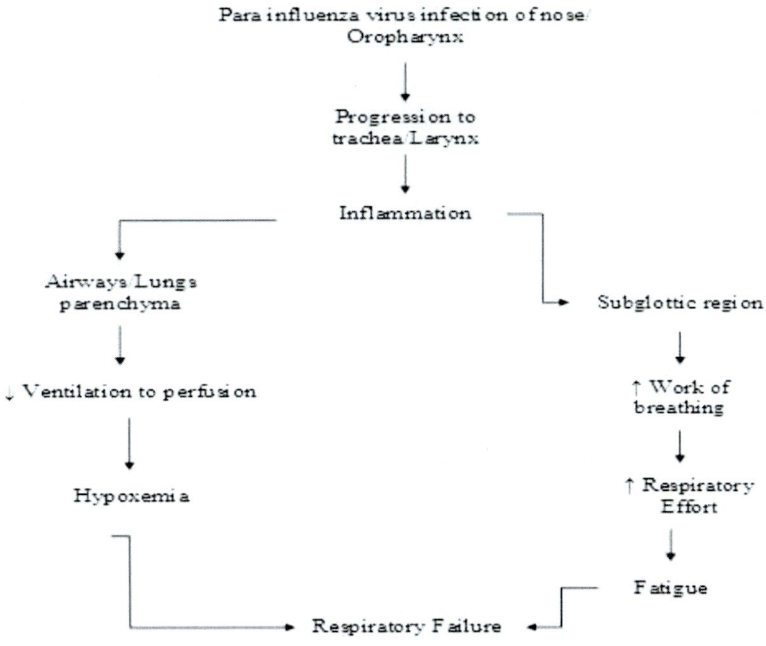

(Table 3) cont.....

Disease	Pathogenesis
Respiratory Syncytial Virus (RSV)	RSV attaches via F and G protein → RSV penetration in cell membrane for injecting RNA → Replication of viral RNA → Release of newly synthesized virus particles → Sloughing of cells and reduced ciliary action → Cell infiltration mucus production leading to bronchiolitis
Bacterial Pneumonia	Infection of lungs by bacteria → Initiation of inflammatory response → Alveolar edema and exudate formation → Filling of alveoli and respiratory bronchioles serous exudate, blood cell, fibrin and bacteria → Consolidation of lung tissues
M. pneumonia	Mycoplasma Pneumonia infection → NLRP3 + Inflammasome → Activation of NLRP3 inflammasome complex → Procaspase-1 → Caspase-1 → Pro-IL-Iβ → Active-IL-Iβ → Airway Inflammation

Differential Signs and Symptoms

COVID-19 and other Coronaviruses (SARS, MERS)

COVID-19 may involve multiple body systems such as respiratory, gastrointestinal, musculoskeletal, and nervous systems. High-grade fever, shortness of breath, cough, body aches, fatigue, headache, the new loss of taste or smell, sore throat, congestion, vomiting, and diarrhea are salient symptoms of COVID-19. They progressively lead to acute respiratory distress syndrome (ARDS) and multiple organ failure. The disease is also remaining asymptomatic in most patients. The common cold caused by coronavirus is identified as coryza (rhinorrhoea, and runny nose), sore throat, bronchitis, and low-grade fever. The illness continues for several days. Clinical finding for SARS and MERS is similar. They cause severe but atypical pneumonia characterized by fever (38°C), dyspnoea, non-productive cough, and hypoxia. Chills, rigors, malaise, and headaches are commonly seen. Sore throat and rhinorrhoea are generally not observed.

Adenovirus

About half of the adenovirus infections are asymptomatic. And from the remaining symptomatic infections, most of them settle spontaneously. Severe infections occur only in children or immunocompromised patients such as AIDS, organ, or stem cell transplant in which patients already intake immune-suppressing drugs. Adenoviruses in the upper respiratory tract cause pharyngitis and pharyngoconjunctival fever (PCF), an acute respiratory disease characterized by fever, nonproductive cough, headache, and sore throat, coryza, and conjunctivitis. In the lower respiratory tract, they cause bronchitis and atypical pneumonia with dyspnoea, ulceration, and scarring of bronchial epithelium, and destruction of bronchial glands. Post-infection bronchiectasis is also observed in patients, especially children recovering from pneumonia [55].

Influenza Virus

Influenza is characterized by severe myalgia with respiratory signs (sore throat, cough), fever, and headache. Vomiting and diarrhea are uncommon. If no secondary bacterial infection is involved, symptoms usually limit to 4-7 days. The involvement of bacterial infection (generally *Staphylococcus aureus* or *Streptococcus pneumoniae*) can worsen the condition by developing pneumonia. Reye's syndrome is a life-threatening condition, categorized by encephalopathy and liver degeneration, usually occurring in children as sequelae of some viral infections.

Human Metapneumovirus (HMPV)

Cough and wheezing, dyspnoea, sputum production, bronchitis, and pneumonia are also present. Fever is uncommon: a differential feature from influenza infection. Unlike human Respiratory Syncytial Virus (hRSV), young adults generally have asymptomatic infection [15]. HMPV is more likely to cause bronchiolitis and less likely to cause pneumonia than influenza and RSV. Mostly lower respiratory tract infection, but upper respiratory tract infection can also be present uncommonly. Patients with HMPV upper respiratory infection show otitis media (OM) because inflammatory response against virus causes blockage of the

Eustachian tube, bacteria get entry and cause osteomyelitis. Disease by HMPV is not severe unless it coincides with other infections [42].

Parainfluenza Virus

Parainfluenza virus infection is characterized as croup in children <5 years of age. Croup is indicated by hoarseness and harsh cough. Other clinical findings include respiratory conditions such as Common cold, pharyngitis, laryngitis, bronchitis, pneumonia, and osteomyelitis [14].

Respiratory Syncytial Virus (RSV)

The severity of the infection varies depending on the age group. RSV is one of the major causes of pneumonia and bronchiolitis in infants. Young children develop otitis media due to RSV, while older children, young and healthy adults develop respiratory tract infections like Common cold and bronchitis. In old age and patients with cardiopulmonary diseases, RSV can cause severe diseases such as severe lower respiratory tract infections and pneumonia [56].

Rhinovirus (Common cold)

Characteristic signs of cold are cough, runny nose, sneezing, nasal congestion, sore throat, muscle ache, fatigue, headache, and loss of appetite. There are 40% of cases suffering from sore throat while 50% are presented with cough. Fever usually does not occur in adults but common in newborns and young children. In the case of rhinovirus, mild cough is present as compared to influenza. Mostly Common cold viruses exhibit asymptomatic infections [57].

Bacterial Pneumonia

***Streptococcus pneumonia*:** Conjunctivitis, otitis media, sinusitis, acute exacerbations of chronic bronchitis, pneumonia, meningitis, bacteremia, osteomyelitis, septic arthritis, myositis, periorbital cellulitis, abscess, peritonitis, and endocarditis [17].

Haemophilus influenzae pneumonia: Clinical signs of *H. influenzae* include fever, cough, and lobar consolidation in the radiographic examination. Sometimes parapneumonic effusions or empyema may also occur [18].

Moraxella catarrhalis pneumonia: *M. catarrhalis* causes chronic bronchitis, pneumonia, chronic obstructive pulmonary disease, and comorbidities like diabetes mellitus. Additionally, *M. catarrhalis* can cause nosocomial pneumonia due to the person-to-person spread of the organism [58].

Chlamydial pneumonia: General signs are runny nose, tiredness, low-grade fever, harshness or loss of voice, sore throat, slowly increasing cough, and headache. Lower respiratory tract infections include bronchitis and pneumonia, which can take 3 to 4 weeks for symptoms to appear after the invasion of bacteria [59].

Mycoplasma pneumonia

Signs of *M. pneumoniae* infections are very similar to cold pneumonia in children. Generally, *M. pneumoniae* causes mild disease symptoms that appear and worsen within 1 to 4 weeks. This bacterium can cause tracheobronchitis (chest cold) in children, including sore throat symptoms, fatigue, fever, slowly worsening cough that can last for weeks or months, and headache. It is estimated that 1/10 people develop pneumonia due to an *M. pneumoniae* infection. General symptoms of pneumonia include productive cough, fever and chills, shortness of breath, chest pain, and fatigue [21]. Table **4** summarizes the differential clinical signs of COVID-19 with other viral and bacterial respiratory diseases.

Table 4. Differential clinical signs of COVID-19 with other viral and bacterial diseases.

Symptoms	COVID-19	SARS	MERS	Adenovirus	Influenza Virus	human Metapneumovirus (HMPV)	Para Influenza Virus	Respiratory Syncytial Virus (RSV)	Rhinovirus (Common cold)	Bacterial Pneumonia	*M. pneumonia*
Cough	Present	Present	Present	Present	Present	Present	Absent	Present	Present	Absent	Present
Fever	Present	Present	Present	Present	Present	Occasional	Absent	Occasional	Absent	Occasional	Present
Dsypnoea	Present	Present	Present	Present	Present	Present	Absent	Absent	Absent	Absent	Absent
Flu	Absent	Present	Present	Present	Present	Present	Present	Absent	Present	Present	Occasional
Pneumonia	Present	Present	Present	Present	Present	Present	Present	Present	Absent	Present	Present
Headache	Present	Present	Present	Present	Present	Occasional	Absent	Absent	Absent	Absent	Present
Sore throat	Present	Present	Present	Present	Present	Absent	Present	Absent	Absent	Present	Present
Others	Loss of taste or smell, nasal congestion, vomiting, diarrhea	Not specific	Chills, rigors, malaise	coryza and conjunctivitis	Severe myalgia	Sputum production, bronchitis	Croup, pharyngitis, laryngitis, bronchitis	Otitis media, bronchitis	Mostly asymptomatic infections occur	Conjunctivitis, otitis media, sinusitis, meningitis, bacteremia	Fatigue

Differential Diagnostic Approaches

COVID-19 and other Coronaviruses (SARS, MERS)

Chest radiograph shows multifocal alveolar opacities leading to complete pleural opacity in severe cases. At the initial stages of infection, no significant alveolar changes can be depicted in a chest radiograph. It is not a sensitive means in disease diagnosis, although it can help in the diagnostic process or follow-up events of disease [60]. Chest computed tomography scan (CT-scan) is abnormal even in asymptomatic patients and shows infiltrates, sub-segmental consolidation, and ground-glass opacities. Diagnosis with CT-scan can be made even in the patients with the negative molecular tests. In reported cases, abnormal CT-scan with negative molecular test showed positive molecular test on repeat testing [61]. Cavitations, calcifications, pleural effusion, and lymphadenopathies are also found during the chest CT-scan. None of them has specifically been associated with the novel coronavirus disease. These findings are equally present in other respiratory tract infections that cause pneumonia-like SARS, MERS, influenza, CMV, and bacterial infections *Mycoplasma, Chlamydia*, and *Streptococcus* [62]. **Lung ultrasonography** shows a focal interstitial pattern ("White lung") with subpleural consolidations or nodules [63]. **Laboratory findings:** Leucopenia, lymphopenia, high neutrophil-to-lymphocyte, and platelet to lymphocyte count ratio. Raised levels of liver enzymes like lactate dehydrogenase (LDH), muscle enzymes, and C-reactive protein. Elevated D-dimer, particularly in severe cases [64]. A **serological assay,** commonly called an antibody test is conducted to detect the presence or absence of the level of antibodies present in an individual against a specific disease. Each antibody present in a testing individual is against a specific disease. The presence of antibodies does not always indicate the ongoing infection as it is also used to detect the previous infection and immunity against that infection. Serological testing can be used to detect the previous or ongoing infection and the level of antibodies detected depends upon the timing of the infection started and test performed. However, it is not specific or sensitive to diagnose COVID-19. The **molecular assay** is the recommended test by WHO for the diagnosis of COVID-19. It is also named a viral test or test for current infection by CDC. A cotton swab collects the sample for the test from an oropharyngeal or nasopharyngeal site. Other samples such as bronchoalveolar lavage (BAL), expectorated sputum, or endotracheal aspirates can also be used for patients on ventilators. The sample is then processed for the presence or absence of a viral pathogen by RT-PCR. The mechanism of the molecular assay is the first conversion of single-stranded viral RNA into double-stranded DNA by reverse transcriptase enzyme. It amplifies the genomic material up to the extent that it's sufficient to detect the specific genetic code of the virus that is already conserved by gene sequencing of the specific virus. Typical commercially available primers are used for this purpose. It is the only confirmatory test available and should be repeated to check the viral clearance in the recovered patients [3]. Other coronaviruses are primarily diagnosed on a clinical basis. If suspected, SARS and MERS can be confirmed by RT-PCR and antibody-based tests [11]. Seroconversion of SARS-CoV was observed when grown on Vero cells for virus isolation. Viral RNA was also detected in plasma during the acute phase of infection and feces during the late convalescent phase. Still, concentration was low, and high concentration was seen in sputum.

Adenovirus

Clinical diagnosis can be made on characteristic clinical signs: ARD and conjunctivitis. Throat, nasal, anal, or conjunctival scraping samples are used for isolation of virus on cell culture, and detection of the antibody titer (4-fold or greater rise) is the frequently used method of diagnosis. ELISA is an improved and quicker technique to detect antibodies. However, some serologic tests can be used as confirmatory tests, such as fluorescence microscopy, complement fixation test (CFT), and hemagglutination-inhibition (HI). Electron microscopic image shows a procrystalline array of adenovirus particles [65].

Influenza Virus

Generally, diagnosis is made on clinical findings. However, some tests can be used for this purpose, like ELISA for detecting viral antigen using nasal or throat swab/washing or sputum sample. Some rapid clinic tests involved FLU OIA and QuickVue Influenza Test to detect viral antigen by monoclonal antibodies, ZSTATFLU for detection of viral neuraminidase by using the color-changing substrate. Diagnosis can be made by evaluating the increase in antibody titer up to fourfold early in the illness and 10 days after. For this purpose, HI or CFT can be used. Other tests used are fluorescent antibody and polymerase chain reaction (PCR).

Human Metapneumovirus (HMPV)

Chest radiograph shows patchy densities in the lower lobes due to infiltration, peribronchial cuffing, and hyperinflation [24]. This virus grows poorly on cell culture as it requires trypsin for its propagation. Immunofluorescence is a quick method to detect respiratory virus antibodies but not as sensitive as RT-PCR. RT-PCR can detect viruses from subgroups of both genotypes of HMPV using different primers [42].

Parainfluenza Virus

Most infections are diagnosed based on clinical signs. Other diagnostic tools like virus isolation and detection of increased antibody titer can also be used. PCR is available for confirmatory diagnosis [14].

Respiratory Syncytial Virus (RSV)

Antigen detection by isolation in cell culture, Rapid antigen test, or immunofluorescence can be performed to diagnose the disease. A four-fold or more significant rise in antibody titer can also be used as a diagnostic tool. However, RT-PCR is also available [56].

Rhinovirus (Common cold)

The difference between viral upper respiratory tract infections is made based on visible signs like rhinitis, pharyngitis, and bronchitis. Sometimes an infection may occur in more than one area. The Common cold is generally well-defined as nasal inflammation along with throat inflammation. Self-diagnosis is common. Mostly virus isolation is not done, and sometimes it is not possible to recognize the virus type through symptoms [66].

Bacterial Pneumonia

***Streptococcus pneumonia*:** Potential specimens may be taken from blood, cerebrospinal fluid, sputum, pleural, Joint fluid, bone, and other abscess or tissue specimens to perform PCR. Imaging studies include chest radiography, ultrasonography, and CT-scans of the chest, sinuses, face, bones or joints, and magnetic resonance imaging (MRI) of the brain, bones, and joints [67].

Haemophilus influenzae pneumonia: The most common testing method uses blood or spinal fluid sample to diagnose *H. influenzae* infection. Gram-negative, small, *pleomorphic coccobacilli* with polymorphonuclear cells are the strongest indication of infection that is usually obtained by the test results on the body fluids from different sites of infection. Detection of organisms in blood culture or any other body fluid is the most valid diagnostic method [18].

Moraxella catarrhalis pneumoniae: *M. catarrhalis* may be differentiated from other bacteria by reducing nitrates, loss of colony pigmentation, and production of deoxyribonuclease [50]. Hydrolysis of DNA (detected using DNAse test agar with methyl green) and tributyrin are valuable differentiating tests for *M. catarrhalis*. Valuable methods like polymerase chain reaction are under the development phase to identify *M. catarrhalis* and other bacterial pathogens of respiratory secretions [19].

Chlamydial pneumoniae: Diagnosis of *Chlamydia pneumoniae* infection can be done using culture, serology, or molecular methods by taking a sample of sputum (phlegm) or a swab from the nose or throat or blood test. Culture is particular, but it is technically expensive, requires more time and transport. Direct fluorescent antibody assay and immunoassay enzymes are the detection tests that may provide a quick diagnosis without the need for rigid transport conditions. RT-PCR is the desired method for diagnosing acute testing of *C. Pneumoniae* infection, assuming an appropriate type of specimen is available [51]. For recurrent and acute diagnosis of *C. Pneumoniae* infection, the kinetics of antibody expression must consider. After 2-3 weeks of infection in a patient, and remain detectable and elevated for up to 2 to 6 months [52]. So far, there has been no proper reference test to validate persistent and chronic infection *via* serological testing. Persistent elevation of IgA and IgG antibodies has been used as a serological indicator. Numerous studies have recommended that IgA titers can be a good indicator of chronic infection than IgG [51].

Mycoplasma Pneumonia

Diagnosis of *M. pneumonia* is difficult due to its fastidious nature and the possibility of transitory asymptomatic carriage [68]. Diagnosis is made clinically; PCR of the nasopharyngeal swab, aspirate or sputum, or cultures can confirm the diagnosis. A serological method like CFT is most used. PCR is now used as a method of choice to detect pathogens directly, which provides greater sensitivity than ELISA [69]. The entire summary of differential diagnostic approaches of COVID-19 with other viral and bacterial respiratory diseases is discussed in Table **5**.

Table 5. Differential diagnostic approaches of COVID-19 with other viral and bacterial diseases.

Diagnostic Technique	COVID-19	SARS	MERS	Adenovirus	Influenza Virus	Human Metapneumovirus (HMPV)	Parainfluenza Virus	Respiratory Syncytial Virus (RSV)	Rhinovirus (Common cold)	Bacterial Pneumonia	*M. pneumonia*
Chest Radiograph	Bilateral peripheral consolidation	Focal opacity	Lung consolidation	Multifocal or diffuse opacity	Basal and axial alveolar consolidation	Parahilar opacities	Bilateral perihilar peribronchial thickening and interstitial infiltrates	Central pneumonia or peribronchitis	Bilateral perihilar peribronchial thickening	Focal segmental or lobar opacities in lungs	Bilateral lesions, pleural effusion, and hilar lymphadenopathy
Chest CT scan	Sub pleural, posterior consolidations, bilateral ground-glass opacities	Multifocal opacity, ground-glass opacities	Ground glass opacity, fibrosis of lungs	Bilateral GGO and consolidation with or without pleural effusion	Unilateral or bilateral multifocal ground-glass opacities	Hyperinflation, atelectasis, and consolidation of lungs	Multiple small peribronchial nodules, ground-glass opacities, and airspace consolidation	Multiple small peribronchial nodules and ground-glass opacities	Interlobular septal thickening, nodules, and consolidation of lungs	Abscesses or pleural effusions and enlarged lymph nodes	Combination of bronchial wall thickening and centrilobular nodules
ELISA	COVID-19 Nucleocapsid (NP) IgG/IgM anibodies	rN-type IgM and IgG antibodies	IgG antibodies detection	IgM antibody detection	Anti-*Influenza virus* A IgG antibodies	detection of hMPV antigens	IgG antibodies detection	IgG antibodies detection	Specific antibody IgA detection in serum and nasal secretion	C-polysaccharide (PnC) antigen detection	IgM antibodies detection
PCR	Qualitative detection of nucleic acid from SARS-CoV-2	Identification of SARS CoV genome	Target MERS- CoV nucleocapsid (N) gene	Detect DNA of adenovirus	Detect RNA from respiratory samples	89.6% sensitivity	Viral genome detection	Detect RNA of RSV	Detect HRV RNA from respiratory samples	Detect bacterial genome	A highly sensitive method for detection of mycoplasma

Differential Response Therapy

COVID-19 and other Coronaviruses (SARS, MERS)

There is currently no recommended drug by the U.S. Food and Drug Administration (FDA) against COVID-19.

Antiviral drugs: Chloroquine/hydroxychloroquine acts as an immunomodulant by lowering the viral load. They show a synergistic effect when used with macrolides

(Azithromycin) with anti-inflammatory and immunomodulatory effects [2]. It should be used in low doses as higher doses cause toxicity and QT-prolongation, and cardiac arrhythmia. Remdesivir- a potent RNA polymerase inhibitor that obstructs viral RNA multiplication [70]. Unselective antibiotic intake should not be practiced. ***Immunotherapy:*** Anti-Interleukin 6 (Tocilizumab) is a monoclonal antibody directed against interleukin-6 receptors, reduces mortality in COVID-19 patients by improving respiratory function and reducing inflammatory storm-pathogenic T-cells and inflammatory monocytes with an increased level of interleukin-6 due to host immune response [2]. ***Antithrombotic therapy:*** Patients infected with COVID-19 show an increase in fibrin, fibrin degradation products, fibrinogen, and D-dimers that results in increased chances of thromboembolic diseases (like venous thromboembolism VTE). Antithrombotic agents (*e.g.*, Enoxaparin) are directed to reduce the chances [71]. ***Systemic corticosteroids*** (*e.g.*, methylprednisolone) should not be used except in critically ventilated patients. ***Oxygen therapy:*** Oxygen fast challenge, non-invasive ventilation, intubation, and protective mechanical ventilation, extracorporeal membrane oxygenation (ECMO) should be used in patients with multiple organ dysfunctions (MOD) to support organ function with respiratory support. There is no specific antiviral therapy and vaccine available. However, combined therapy of antiviral drugs (ribavirin) and glucocorticosteroids is helpful, but their efficacy is uncertain [64].

Adenovirus

Epidemic keratoconjunctivitis (EKC) is an iatrogenic disease and can be prevented by strict asepsis [12]. There is not any specific antiviral therapy for it. The treatment used is symptomatic and supportive. Infection can be prevented by using vaccines. Live non-attenuated, monovalent vaccines against AdV4, 7, and 21 are available in the form of enteric-coated capsules. But these vaccines are used only by the military.

Influenza Virus

Commonly used drugs for the treatment of Influenza are Oseltamivir (Tamiflu) taken orally and zanamivir (Relenza) inhaled into the nose. Treatment is effective when taken within 48 hours from the onset of symptoms and helps to reduce the duration of symptoms by 1 to 2 days.

Human Metapneumovirus (HMPV)

Peramivir (Rapivab) is administered intravenously and became available in 2015. They are neuraminidase inhibitors that inhibit the release of the virus from infected cells and limit the infection by reducing the spread of the virus. They are effective against both influenza A and B viruses. Rimantadine (Flumadine), a derivative of amantadine, is used instead of amantadine to treat and prevent influenza A because of its higher efficacy and lower side effects than amantadine. The best way to control the influenza infection is by preventing it from using vaccines. About every year, influenza vaccines are formulated using new prevalent strains to get better immunity. Killed (flu shot), live attenuated vaccine (nasal spray), and recombinant vaccines are available having hemagglutinin as a major antigen. Vaccination is not always effective due to a wide variety of antigens.

Parainfluenza Virus

No specific treatment and vaccine are available for treatment and as a prophylaxis measure [14].

Respiratory Syncytial Virus (RSV)

The use of aerosolized ribavirin is recommended in critically ill infants. However, it is more useful due to its uncertain effectiveness, a combination of hyperimmune antibodies and ribavirin. There is no vaccine available to prevent the disease. However, passive immunization with monoclonal antibodies and hyperimmune globulins is available for prophylaxis in premature or immunocompromised infants and chronic pulmonary disease children. Hand wash and gloves should be used to prevent nosocomial transmission [72].

Rhinovirus (Common cold)

Till now, no effective antiviral drugs for the Common cold, even though some initial research has shown benefits [65].

Bacterial pneumonia

Streptococcus pneumonia: Empirical antibiotics including β-lactams, Macrolides, and Fluoroquinolones are used, but bacteria develop resistance against these agents, specifically multidrug resistance, which causes treatment failure [73]. However, penicillin and β-lactam compounds can be selected to treat invasive pneumococcal diseases [74].

Haemophilus influenzae pneumonia: Third-generation cephalosporins are used to treat *H. influenzae* infections like meningitis or epiglottitis. Treatment with ceftriaxone or cefotaxime should be given to patients with confirmed or suspected *H. influenzae* infection. It must be continued till complete susceptibility data are available [28].

Moraxella catarrhalis **pneumonia:** Oral antibiotics like β-lactamase stable antibiotics such as amoxicillin-clavulanate are used to treat *M. catarrhalis* infections because of the presence of induced β-lactamases in many isolates. Besides, cephalosporin (cefaclor), or a non–β-lactam antibiotic such as trimethoprim-sulfamethoxazole should be introduced awaiting susceptibility test results [19].

Chlamydial pneumonia: Most clinicians prescribe macrolides (azithromycin) as first-line therapy, tetracyclines (tetracycline and doxycycline), and fluoroquinolones [59]. Tetracyclines and erythromycin show good activity *in vitro* and have been the most frequently used drugs in treating *C. pneumonia* infection. The most active macrolide is clarithromycin. The fluoroquinolones demonstrate good activity. Levofloxacin is much more active than ofloxacin and ciprofloxacin [75].

Mycoplasma pneumonia

M. pneumoniae infections are mostly mild, and they do not require any medicine, but some patients may need to become hospitalized if they develop pneumonia due to *M. pneumoniae*. In the case of hospitalization, azithromycin is commonly recommended [76]. Table **6** summarizes the differential response therapy of COVID-19 with other viral and bacterial respiratory diseases.

Table 6. Differential response therapy of COVID-19 with other viral and bacterial diseases.

Disease	Antiviral	Antibacterial	Steroids	NSAIDS	Others
COVID-19 **SARS** **MERS**	Chloroquine/ hydroxychloroquine	Macrolides (Azithromycin)	Methylprednisolone	Ibuprofen, Aspirin	Anti-Interleukin 6 (Tocilizumab)
Adenovirus	Cidofovir	-	-	Paracetamol, Ibuprofen	-
Influenza virus	Oseltamivir (Tamiflu), zanamivir (Relenza)	-	Dexamethasone	Naproxen	-
Human Metapneumovirus (HMPV)	Peramivir (Rapivab)	-	Prednisone	Ibuprofen, Naproxen	-
Parainfluenza	Ribavirin (Virazole)	-	Dexamethasone, Prednisone	Paracetamol, Ibuprofen	Adrenalin
Respiratory Syncytial Virus (RSV)	Ribavirin	-	Glucocorticoids	Acetaminophen	-

(Table 6) cont.....

Disease	Antiviral	Antibacterial	Steroids	NSAIDS	Others
Rhinovirus (Common cold)	-	-	-	Paracetamol, Ibuprofen	Pseudoephedrine
Bacterial Pneumonia	-	β-lactams, Macrolides, and Fluoroquinolones	Corticosteroids	-	-
M. pneumonia	-	Azithromycin, Tetracycline	Prednisolone	Ibuprofen, Naproxen	-

Mathematical Modelling in the Prediction of COVID-19

Simulations and modeling are proven predictive diagnostic tools that are helpful to control the human and animal diseases. Each disease exhibits typical biological properties; hence models are adapted accordingly to tackle the malaise in actual situations [77]. An accurate model for COVID-19 demands its ability of estimation, consideration of varying scenarios, many positive cases, death tolls & hospitalized patients, and COVID-19 territories in health-compromising areas. Several other models may be developed to help the control of the disease. Such models give rise to a product number of diseases which indicates the trend of the disease. A comparison of reproductive number R_0 of SARS-CoV-2 (2-2.5) compared to MERS (<1) and SARS (1.7-1.9) suggesting the higher pandemic potential of novel infection.

Salient and Latest Models Applied

Some short forecast phenomenological models that are real-time forecast models have already been used in various outbreaks of infectious diseases, *e.g.*, SARS, Ebola, dengue, and pandemic influenza in the past. These three phenomenological models include the generalized logistic growth model, Richard model, and sub-epidemic wave model [78]. Generalized logistic growth models accommodate sub-exponential growth dynamics using p-value, but the process extends a simple logistic growth model. Richard model uses *scaling* model to permit deviation from asymmetric logistic curve. The latter model helps in complex epidemics having multiple peaks, *e.g.*, SARS cases in Singapore. The resultant curve of this model is assumed as an aggregation of multiple primary sub-epidemics.

Mathematical equations can describe details about the spread rate of COVID-19 in a time-dependent analytical function with units of days [79]. For a country or region having population , it claimed that the time rate of change (spread rate) of H (Number of individuals contracting the disease) is proportional to the multiplication of no. of people who are infected with the disease and those did not infect. It is stated that "the time-dependent change (Spreading) rate of the H; the number of individuals who have caught a contagious disease is proportional to the multiplication of the numbers of those who have caught the disease and those who have not" [80]. Here only one equation is given while there are a series of equations that are kept on the resolution to reach the final equation., Further reading and explanation may be obtained from Cakir and Savas [79], keeping in view the domain of the book chapter.

$dH / dt = \mu H(P\text{-}H)$

$H(0) = H_0$

$H(t_1) = t_1$

where

t denotes unit days as an independent time variable

(t) represent dependent variable showing no. of the patient at "t" time

dH / dt represents derivatives corresponding to "t" dependent variation rat of disease

μ is a parameter covering the sum of factors that affect the spreading rate. Supposition to these equations include initially $t = 0$, no. of the patient (0) = $H0$, no. of patients at time $t = \boldsymbol{t1}$ provided as additional information ($t1$) = $\boldsymbol{H1}$, and no. of people open at risk to the diseases be P .

The currently applicable model for SARS-CoV2 is the θ-SEIHRD model, a novel model that has passed previous experiments over the Ebola virus outbreak from 2014-2016 and 2018-2020 in Congo with successful forecasts. This model is now applied in an adapted form on COVID-19, and an example was taken from China where corona outbreak occurr. It relates disease fatality percentage and percentage detected over real infected to find out the importance of outcome on the impact of the disease. The model utilizes assumptions inclusive of which are a) Susceptible (S) which are not infected by pathogen; b) Exposed (E) which are going through incubation period with no clinical signs but have ability to infect other with low probability however they may shift to next infectious category once show signs; c) Infectious (I) which are now showing clinical signs that in turn may be hospitalized or may keep spreading if SOPs are not adopted; d) Infectious but undetected (I u) are the group of people with clinical signs which are not severe enough to be considered for hospitalization or authorities may have overlooked, and are source of spread of pathogen in the absence of SOPs; e) Hospitalized or in quarantine at home (denoted by H_R) are group of people who are identified by authorities, shifted to hospital or quarantine at home, but may spread disease in the absence of observation of SOPs, f) Hospitalized that will die (H_D) are the group of people who are hospitalized in life threatening condition, and are still able to infect people, g) Dead by COVID-19 (D) are the group of people who did not survive, f) Recovered (R_d) are the group of people who recovered after being hospitalized, and have developed immunity but are not source of spread of infection to others, NB: days a person spend in hospital for convalescent period are "C" days, g) Recovered from infectious but stayed undetected (R_u) is the group of people who got infected previously but stayed undetected and have recovered with no threat to spread disease to others. Explanation of further variables and details to use this model can be studied from Ivorra et al. [77].

CONCLUSION

COVID-19, pandemic disease, differentially attaches to ACE-2 with substitution of 380 amino acids in non-structural kinds of proteins while 27 mutations in spike protein compared to that of SARS disease virus. High fever, shortness of breathing, dry cough, body aches are typical differential signs of this disease. CT-scan shows infiltrate sub-segmental consolidation and ground-glass opacities even in patients with false-negative molecular tests. RT-PCR is a gold standard test to quarantine/admission the patient to the hospital, while the coupling of this molecular test with other diagnostic approaches paves the road to treat the malaise. Azithromycin and chloroquine as immunomodulant and plasma therapy are used as response treatment and symptomatic treatment of the patient. The mathematical predictive model identifies 2-2.5 as the reproductive number (R_0) of this disease as differentially higher than related coronaviruses. The chapter thus acknowledges all aspects of disease before reaching confirmatory diagnosis to help effective treatment, control, and prevent pandemic coronavirus infection.

CONSENT FOR PUBLICATION

Not Applicable.

CONFLICT OF INTEREST

The author confirms that this chapter contents have no conflict of interest.

ACKNOWLEDGEMENT

Declared none.

REFERENCES

[1] Chung M, Zeng X, Jacobi A. CT Imaging Features of 2019 Novel Coronavirus 2020.

[2] Guo YR, Cao QD, Hong ZS, *et al.* The origin, transmission and clinical therapies on coronavirus disease 2019 (COVID-19) outbreak - an update on the status. Mil Med Res 2020; 7(1): 11. [http://dx.doi.org/10.1186/s40779-020-00240-0] [PMID: 32169119]

[3] Corman VM, Landt O, Kaiser M, *et al.* Detection of 2019 novel coronavirus (2019-nCoV) by real-time RT-PCR. Euro Surveill 2020; 25(3): 1-8. [http://dx.doi.org/10.2807/1560-7917.ES.2020.25.3.2000045] [PMID: 31992387]

[4] Bassetti M, Vena A, Giacobbe DR. The novel Chinese coronavirus (2019-nCoV) infections: Challenges for fighting the storm. Eur J Clin Invest 2020; 50(3): e13209. [http://dx.doi.org/10.1111/eci.13209] [PMID: 32003000]

[5] Corman VM, Landt O, Kaiser M, *et al.* Detection of 2019 novel coronavirus (2019-nCoV) by real-time RT-PCR. Euro Surveill 2020; 25(3). [http://dx.doi.org/10.2807/1560-7917.ES.2020.25.3.2000045] [PMID: 31992387]

[6] Kishaba T. Community-acquired pneumonia caused by *Mycoplasma pneumoniae*: How physical and radiological examination contribute to successful diagnosis. Front Med (Lausanne) 2016; 3: 28. [http://dx.doi.org/10.3389/fmed.2016.00028] [PMID: 27379238]

[7] Ishiguro T, Kobayashi Y, Uozumi R, *et al.* Viral pneumonia requiring differentiation from acute and progressive diffuse interstitial lung diseases. Intern Med 2019; 58(24): 3509-19. [http://dx.doi.org/10.2169/internalmedicine.2696-19] [PMID: 31839671]

[8] Dai H, Zhang X, Xia J, Zhang T, Shang Y, Huang R, *et al.* High-resolution chest CT features and clinical characteristics of patients infected with COVID-19 in Jiangsu, China. International Journal of Infectious Diseases 2020; 95: 106-2. [http://dx.doi.org/10.1016/j.ijid.2020.04.003]

[9] Dai WC, Zhang HW, Yu J, *et al.* CT imaging and differential diagnosis of COVID-19. Can Assoc Radiol J 2020; 71(2): 195-200. [http://dx.doi.org/10.1177/0846537120913033] [PMID: 32129670]

[10] Ji W, Wang W, Zhao X, Zai J, Li X. Cross-species transmission of the newly identified coronavirus 2019-nCoV. J Med Virol 2020; 92(4): 433-40. [http://dx.doi.org/10.1002/jmv.25682] [PMID: 31967321]

[11] Ksiazek TG, Erdman D, Goldsmith CS, *et al.* SARS Working Group. A novel coronavirus associated with severe acute respiratory syndrome. N Engl J Med 2003; 348(20): 1953-66. [http://dx.doi.org/10.1056/NEJMoa030781] [PMID: 12690092]

[12] Ebner K, Suda M, Watzinger F, Lion T. Molecular detection and quantitative analysis of the entire spectrum of human adenoviruses by a two-reaction real-time PCR assay. J Clin Microbiol 2005; 43(7): 3049-53. [http://dx.doi.org/10.1128/JCM.43.7.3049-3053.2005] [PMID: 16000414]

[13] Stockton J, Stephenson I, Fleming D, Zambon M. human metapneumovirus as a cause of community-acquired respiratory illness. Emerg Infect Dis 2002; 8(9): 897-901. [http://dx.doi.org/10.3201/eid0809.020084] [PMID: 12194763]

[14] Karron RA, Collins PL. Parainfluenza viruses. In Fields Virology: Sixth Edition. Wolters Kluwer Health Adis (ESP) 2013; 1. [http://dx.doi.org/10.1159/000393651]

[15] Hall CB. Respiratory Syncitial Virus and Parainflueza Virus1. Hall CB. Respiratory Syncitial Virus and Parainflueza Virus. English J. 2011;344(25):1917-1928. N Engl J Med 2001; 344: 1917-28. [http://dx.doi.org/10.1056/NEJM200106213442507] [PMID: 11419430]

[16] Palmenberg AC, Rathe JA, Liggett SB. Analysis of the complete genome sequences of human rhinovirus. J Allergy Clin Immunol 2010; 125(6): 1190-9. [http://dx.doi.org/10.1016/j.jaci.2010.04.010] [PMID: 20471068]

[17] Østergaard C, Konradsen HB, Samuelsson S. Clinical presentation and prognostic factors of *Streptococcus pneumoniae* meningitis according to the focus of infection. BMC Infect Dis 2005; 5: 93. [http://dx.doi.org/10.1186/1471-2334-5-93] [PMID: 16253143]

[18] Agrawal A, Murphy TF. Haemophilus influenzae infections in the H. influenzae type b conjugate vaccine era. J Clin Microbiol 2011; 49(11): 3728-32.
[http://dx.doi.org/10.1128/JCM.05476-11] [PMID: 21900515]

[19] Murphy TF, Parameswaran GI. *Moraxella catarrhalis*, a human respiratory tract pathogen. Clin Infect Dis 2009; 49(1): 124-31.
[http://dx.doi.org/10.1086/599375] [PMID: 19480579]

[20] Megran David, Peeling Rosanna W, Marrie Thomas J. Chlamydia Pneumoniae Pneumonia: An Evolving Clinical Spectrum. Canadian J Infectious Diseases 1995; 6: 191-5.

[21] Kashyap S, Sarkar M. Mycoplasma pneumonia: Clinical features and management. Lung India 2010; 27(2): 75-85.
[http://dx.doi.org/10.4103/0970-2113.63611] [PMID: 20616940]

[22] Wang C, Horby PW, Hayden FG, Gao GF. A novel coronavirus outbreak of global health concern. Lancet 2020; 395(10223): 470-3.
[http://dx.doi.org/10.1016/S0140-6736(20)30185-9] [PMID: 31986257]

[23] Ramanathan K, Antognini D, Combes A, Paden M, Zakhary B, Ogino M, *et al.* Since January 2020 Elsevier has created a COVID-19 resource centre with free information in English and Mandarin on the novel coronavirus COVID research that is available on the COVID-19 resource centre - including this for unrestricted research re-use 2020; 19-21.

[24] Biacchesi S, Skiadopoulos MH, Boivin G, *et al.* Genetic diversity between human Metapneumovirus subgroups. Virology 2003; 315(1): 1-9.
[http://dx.doi.org/10.1016/S0042-6822(03)00528-2] [PMID: 14592754]

[25] Ansari SA, Springthorpe VS, Sattar SA, Rivard S, Rahman M. Potential role of hands in the spread of respiratory viral infections: studies with human parainfluenza virus 3 and rhinovirus 14. J Clin Microbiol 1991; 29(10): 2115-9.
[http://dx.doi.org/10.1128/jcm.29.10.2115-2119.1991] [PMID: 1658033]

[26] Peltola V, Waris M, Österback R, Susi P, Ruuskanen O, Hyypiä T. Rhinovirus transmission within families with children: incidence of symptomatic and asymptomatic infections. J Infect Dis 2008; 197(3): 382-9.
[http://dx.doi.org/10.1086/525542] [PMID: 18248302]

[27] Saraya T, Kurai D, Ishii H, *et al.* Epidemiology of virus-induced asthma exacerbations: with special reference to the role of human rhinovirus. Front Microbiol 2014; 5: 226.
[http://dx.doi.org/10.3389/fmicb.2014.00226] [PMID: 24904541]

[28] MacNeil JR, Cohn AC, Farley M, *et al.* Current epidemiology and trends in invasive Haemophilus influenzae disease--United States, 1989-2008. Clin Infect Dis 2011; 53(12): 1230-6.
[http://dx.doi.org/10.1093/cid/cir735] [PMID: 22080119]

[29] Richards SJ, Greening AP, Enright MC, Morgan MG, McKenzie H. Outbreak of *Moraxella catarrhalis* in a respiratory unit. Thorax 1993; 48(1): 91-2.
[http://dx.doi.org/10.1136/thx.48.1.91] [PMID: 8434362]

[30] Porritt RA, Crother TR. *Chlamydia pneumoniae* infection and inflammatory diseases. For Immunopathol Dis Therap 2016; 7(3-4): 237-54.
[http://dx.doi.org/10.1615/ForumImmunDisTher.2017020161] [PMID: 30687565]

[31] Dawood FS, Ambrose JF, Russell BP, *et al.* Outbreak of pneumonia in the setting of fatal pneumococcal meningitis among US Army trainees: potential role of *Chlamydia pneumoniae* infection. BMC Infect Dis 2011; 11: 157.
[http://dx.doi.org/10.1186/1471-2334-11-157] [PMID: 21635754]

[32] Perlman S, Netland J. Coronaviruses post-SARS: update on replication and pathogenesis. Nat Rev Microbiol 2009; 7(6): 439-50.
[http://dx.doi.org/10.1038/nrmicro2147] [PMID: 19430490]

[33] Chan JF-W, Yip CC-Y, To KK-W, Tang TH-C, Wong SC-Y, Leung K-H, *et al.* Improved molecular diagnosis of COVID-19 by the novel, highly sensitive and specific COVID-19-RdRp/Hel real-time reverse transcription-PCR assay validated *in vitro* and with clinical specimen. J Clin Microbiol 2020; 23;58(5): e00310-20.
[http://dx.doi.org/10.1128/JCM.00310-20]

[34] Hoffmann M, Kleine-Weber H, Schroeder S, *et al.* SARS-CoV-2 cell entry depends on ace2 and tmprss2 and is blocked by a clinically proven protease inhibitor. Cell 2020; 181(2): 271-280.e8.
[http://dx.doi.org/10.1016/j.cell.2020.02.052] [PMID: 32142651]

[35] Chu DKW, Pan Y, Cheng SMS, *et al.* Molecular diagnosis of a novel coronavirus (2019-nCoV) causing an outbreak of pneumonia. Clin Chem 2020; 66(4): 549-55.
[http://dx.doi.org/10.1093/clinchem/hvaa029] [PMID: 32031583]

[36] Wu F, Zhao S, Yu B, Chen YM, Wang W, Song ZG, *et al.* Author correction: A new coronavirus associated with human respiratory disease in China. Nature 2020; 580(7803): E7.
[http://dx.doi.org/10.1038/s41586-020-2008-3]

[37] Zhao S, Ge X, Wang X, Liu A, Guo X, Zhou L. Since January 2020 Elsevier has created a COVID-19 resource centre with free information in English and Mandarin on the novel coronavirus COVID-19.The COVID-19 resource centre is hosted on Elsevier Connect , the company ' s public news and information 2020.

[38] Lam CWK, Chan MHM, Wong CK. Severe acute respiratory syndrome: clinical and laboratory manifestations. Clin Biochem Rev 2004; 25(2): 121-32.
[PMID: 18458712]

[39] Lan J, Ge J, Yu J, *et al.* Structure of the SARS-CoV-2 spike receptor-binding domain bound to the ACE2 receptor. Nature 2020; 581(7807): 215-20.
[http://dx.doi.org/10.1038/s41586-020-2180-5] [PMID: 32225176]

[40] Kukla M, Skonieczna-Żydecka K, Kotfis K, *et al.* COVID-19, MERS and SARS with Concomitant Liver Injury-Systematic Review of the Existing Literature. J Clin Med 2020; 9(5): 1420.
[http://dx.doi.org/10.3390/jcm9051420] [PMID: 32403255]

[41] Lefkowitz EJ, Dempsey DM, Hendrickson RC, Orton RJ, Siddell SG, Smith DB. Virus taxonomy: the database of the International Committee on Taxonomy of Viruses (ICTV). Nucleic Acids Res 2018; 46(D1): D708-17.
[http://dx.doi.org/10.1093/nar/gkx932] [PMID: 29040670]

[42] Hamelin M-È, Yim K, Kuhn KH, *et al.* Pathogenesis of human Metapneumovirus lung infection in BALB/c mice and cotton rats. J Virol 2005; 79(14): 8894-903.
[http://dx.doi.org/10.1128/JVI.79.14.8894-8903.2005] [PMID: 15994783]

[43] Schomacker H, Schaap-Nutt A, Collins PL, Schmidt AC. Pathogenesis of acute respiratory illness caused by human parainfluenza viruses. Curr Opin Virol 2012; 2(3): 294-9.
[http://dx.doi.org/10.1016/j.coviro.2012.02.001] [PMID: 22709516]

[44] Sonja A. Rasmussen, MD, MS JCS. Since January 2020 Elsevier has created a COVID-19 resource centre with free information in English and Mandarin on the novel coronavirus COVID-. Ann Oncol 2020; 19–21
[http://dx.doi.org/10.1007/s00134-020-05991-x.Bizzarro]

[45] Vlasak M, Roivainen M, Reithmayer M, *et al.* The minor receptor group of human rhinovirus (HRV) includes HRV23 and HRV25, but the presence of a lysine in the VP1 HI loop is not sufficient for receptor binding. J Virol 2005; 79(12): 7389-95.
[http://dx.doi.org/10.1128/JVI.79.12.7389-7395.2005] [PMID: 15919894]

[46] Kennedy JL, Turner RB, Braciale T, Heymann PW, Borish L. Pathogenesis of rhinovirus infection. Curr Opin Virol 2012; 2(3): 287-93.
[http://dx.doi.org/10.1016/j.coviro.2012.03.008] [PMID: 22542099]

[47] Henriques-Normark B, Tuomanen EI. The pneumococcus: epidemiology, microbiology, and pathogenesis. Cold Spring Harb Perspect Med 2013; 3(7): 1-16. [http://dx.doi.org/10.1101/cshperspect.a010215] [PMID: 23818515]

[48] Subramanian K, Henriques-Normark B, Normark S. Emerging concepts in the pathogenesis of the *Streptococcus pneumoniae*: From nasopharyngeal colonizer to intracellular pathogen. Cell Microbiol 2019; 21(11): e13077. [http://dx.doi.org/10.1111/cmi.13077] [PMID: 31251447]

[49] Hammerschmidt S, Bergmann S, Paterson GK, Mitchell TJ. Pathogenesis of Streptococcus pneumoniae infections:adaptive immunity, innate immunity, cell biology, virulence factors. Community-Acquired Pneumonia 2007; pp. 139-81. [http://dx.doi.org/10.1007/978-3-7643-7563-8_8]

[50] Al-Anazi K, Al-Fraih F, Chaudhri N, Al-Mohareb F. Pneumonia caused by *Moraxella catarrhalis* in haematopoietic stem cell transplant patients. Report of two cases and review of the literature. Libyan J Med 2007; 2(3): 144-7. [http://dx.doi.org/10.3402/ljm.v2i3.4716] [PMID: 21503215]

[51] Krüll M, Suttorp N. Pathogenesis of Chlamydophila pneumoniae infections — epidemiology, immunity, cell biology, virulence factors. Community-Acquired Pneumonia 2007; pp. 83-110. [http://dx.doi.org/10.1007/978-3-7643-7563-8_6]

[52] Kern JM, Maass V, Maass M. Molecular pathogenesis of chronic *Chlamydia pneumoniae* infection: a brief overview. Clin Microbiol Infect 2009; 15(1): 36-41. [http://dx.doi.org/10.1111/j.1469-0691.2008.02631.x] [PMID: 19220338]

[53] Waites KB, Talkington DF. *Mycoplasma pneumoniae* and its role as a human pathogen. Clin Microbiol Rev 2004; 17(4): 697-728. [http://dx.doi.org/10.1128/CMR.17.4.697-728.2004] [PMID: 15489344]

[54] Atkinson TP, Balish MF, Waites KB. Epidemiology, clinical manifestations, pathogenesis and laboratory detection of *Mycoplasma pneumoniae* infections. FEMS Microbiol Rev 2008; 32(6): 956-73. [http://dx.doi.org/10.1111/j.1574-6976.2008.00129.x] [PMID: 18754792]

[55] Ellis1 BRADTB. The enigma of yellow fever in East Africa. Rev Med Virol 2009; 19: 57-64. [http://dx.doi.org/10.1002/rmv]

[56] Falsey AR, McElhaney JE, Beran J, *et al.* Respiratory Syncytial Virus and other respiratory viral infections in older adults with moderate to severe influenza-like illness. J Infect Dis 2014; 209(12): 1873-81. [http://dx.doi.org/10.1093/infdis/jit839] [PMID: 24482398]

[57] Heymann PW, Platts-Mills TAE, Johnston SL. Discussion. Pediatr Infect Dis J 2005; 24: 217-22. [http://dx.doi.org/10.1097/01.inf.0000188164.33856.f9] [PMID: 16378049]

[58] Pappas DE, Hendley JO, Hayden FG, Winther B. Symptom profile of Common colds in school-aged children. Pediatr Infect Dis J 2008; 27(1): 8-11. [http://dx.doi.org/10.1097/INF.0b013e31814847d9] [PMID: 18162930]

[59] Fajardo KA, Zorich SC, Voss JD, Thervil JW. Pneumonia outbreak caused by chlamydophila pneumoniae among US air force academy cadets, Colorado, USA. Emerg Infect Dis 2015; 21(6): 1049-51. [http://dx.doi.org/10.3201/eid2106.141394] [PMID: 25988545]

[60] Ai T, Yang Z, Hou H, *et al.* Correlation of Chest CT and RT-PCR Testing for Coronavirus Disease 2019 (COVID-19) in China: A Report of 1014 Cases. Radiology 2020; 296(2): E32-40. [http://dx.doi.org/10.1148/radiol.2020200642] [PMID: 32101510]

[61] Bernheim A, Mei X, Huang M, *et al.* Chest CT Findings in Coronavirus Disease-19 (COVID-19): Relationship to Duration of Infection. Radiology 2020; 295(3): 200463.

[http://dx.doi.org/10.1148/radiol.2020200463] [PMID: 32077789]

[62] Yang Y, Yang M, Shen C, Wang F, Yuan J, Li J, *et al.* Evaluating the accuracy of different respiratory specimens in the laboratory diagnosis and monitoring the viral shedding of 2019-nCoV infections. MedRxiv 2020.
[http://dx.doi.org/10.1101/2020.02.11.20021493]

[63] Wen Z, Chi Y, Zhang L, *et al.* Coronavirus disease 2019: initial detection on chest ct in a retrospective multicenter study of 103 chinese patients. Radiol Cardiothorac Imaging 2020; 2(2): e200092.
[http://dx.doi.org/10.1148/ryct.2020200092] [PMID: 33778564]

[64] Petrosillo N, Viceconte G, Ergonul O, Ippolito G, Petersen E. COVID-19, SARS and MERS: are they closely related? Clin Microbiol Infect 2020; 26(6): 729-34.
[http://dx.doi.org/10.1016/j.cmi.2020.03.026] [PMID: 32234451]

[65] Moore HC, Jacoby P, Taylor A, *et al.* Kalgoorlie Otitis Media Research Project Team. The interaction between respiratory viruses and pathogenic bacteria in the upper respiratory tract of asymptomatic Aboriginal and non-Aboriginal children. Pediatr Infect Dis J 2010; 29(6): 540-5.
[http://dx.doi.org/10.1097/INF.0b013e3181d067cb] [PMID: 20134359]

[66] Royston L, Tapparel C. Rhinoviruses and respiratory enteroviruses: Not as simple as ABC. Viruses 2016; 8(1): E16.
[http://dx.doi.org/10.3390/v8010016] [PMID: 26761027]

[67] Khan SS, Smith MS, Reda D, Suffredini AF, McCoy JP Jr. Multiplex bead array assays for detection of soluble cytokines: comparisons of sensitivity and quantitative values among kits from multiple manufacturers. Cytometry B Clin Cytom 2004; 61(1): 35-9.
[http://dx.doi.org/10.1002/cyto.b.20021] [PMID: 15351980]

[68] Daxboeck F, Krause R, Wenisch C. Laboratory diagnosis of *Mycoplasma pneumoniae* infection. Clin Microbiol Infect 2003; 9(4): 263-73.
[http://dx.doi.org/10.1046/j.1469-0691.2003.00590.x] [PMID: 12667235]

[69] Montagnani F, Rossetti B, Vannoni A, Cusi MG, De Luca A. Laboratory diagnosis of *Mycoplasma pneumoniae* infections: data analysis from clinical practice. New Microbiol 2018; 41(3): 203-7.
[PMID: 29874388]

[70] Lee N-Y, Li C-W, Tsai H-P, Chen P-L, Syue L-S, Li M-C, *et al.* A case of COVID-19 and pneumonia returning from Macau in Taiwan: Clinical course and anti-SARS-CoV-2 IgG dynamic. J Microbiol Immunol Infect 2020; 53(3): 485-7.
[http://dx.doi.org/10.1016/j.jmii.2020.03.003]

[71] Woelfel R, Corman VM, Guggemos W, Seilmaier M, Zange S, Mueller MA, *et al.* Clinical presentation and virological assessment of hospitalized cases of coronavirus disease 2019 in a travel-associated transmission cluster. MedRxiv 2020.
[http://dx.doi.org/10.1101/2020.03.05.20030502]

[72] Hall CB. Respiratory Syncytial Virus. 6th ed. Principles and Practice of Clinical Virology 2009; pp. 441-61.
[http://dx.doi.org/10.1002/9780470741405.ch18]

[73] Ramirez JA, Anzueto AR. Changing needs of community-acquired pneumonia. J Antimicrob Chemother 2011; 66 (Suppl. 3): iii3-9.
[http://dx.doi.org/10.1093/jac/dkr094] [PMID: 21482567]

[74] Wang CY, Chen YH, Fang C, *et al.* Antibiotic resistance profiles and multidrug resistance patterns of *Streptococcus pneumoniae* in pediatrics: A multicenter retrospective study in mainland China. Medicine (Baltimore) 2019; 98(24): e15942.
[http://dx.doi.org/10.1097/MD.0000000000015942] [PMID: 31192930]

[75] Apan TZ, Alpay D, Alpay Y. The possible association of *Chlamydia pneumoniae* infection with nasal polyps. Eur Arch Otorhinolaryngol 2007; 264(1): 27-31.

[http://dx.doi.org/10.1007/s00405-006-0140-9] [PMID: 16902779]

[76] Zhang W, Zhang S, Wang Q, Li Y, Jing H, Hu G, *et al.* Outbreak of macrolide-resistant mycoplasma pneumoniae in a primary school in Beijing China 2018; 4-10.

[77] Ivorra B, Ferrández MR, Vela-pérez M, Ramos AM. Since January 2020 Elsevier has created a COVID-19 resource centre with free information in English and Mandarin on the novel coronavirus COVID- 19 . The COVID-19 resource centre is hosted on Elsevier Connect , the company ' s public news and information 2020.

[78] Roosa K, Lee Y, Luo R, *et al.* Real-time forecasts of the COVID-19 epidemic in China from February 5th to February 24th, 2020. Infect Dis Model 2020; 5: 256-63.
[http://dx.doi.org/10.1016/j.idm.2020.02.002] [PMID: 32110742]

[79] Cakir Z, Savas HB. A mathematical modelling approach in the spread of the novel 2019 coronavirus SARS-COV-2 (COVID-19) pandemic. Electron J Gen Med 2020; 17: 1-3.
[http://dx.doi.org/10.29333/ejgm/7861]

[80] Edwards CH, Penney DE. Differential equations : computing and modeling 1996; 1(various pagings)

Part II: Treatment Strategies for COVID-19

CHAPTER 6

Different Antiviral Drugs against COVID-19 and Future Perspective

Iyad Ibrahim Shaqura[1,2], Ahmed Abdelmajed Alkhodary[2,3], Abdullah[4], Muhammad Ibrar[5] and **Fazlullah Khan[6,*]**

[1] *Department of Health Management and Economics, School of Public Health, Tehran University of Medical Sciences, Tehran, Iran*

[2] *Ministry of Health, Gaza Governorates, Palestine*

[3] *International Centre for Casemix and Clinical Coding, Faculty of Medicine, National University of Malaysia, Kuala Lumpur, Malaysia*

[4] *Department of Pharmacy, University of Malakand, Chakdara Dir Lower, KPK, Pakistan*

[5] *Department of Allied Health Sciences, Iqra University Peshawar, Swat Campus, KPK, Pakistan*

[6] *Department of Allied Health Sciences, Bashir Institute of Health Sciences, Bharakahu, Islamabad, Pakistan*

Abstract: The outbreak of coronavirus disease-19 (COVID-19) across the world has caused serious health issues in terms of physical and psychological damage to human health. The spread of this virus was rapid and shortly spread to almost every country in the world. Due to the high infection rate and occurrence of complications in the infected individuals, the research and development of anti- COVID-19 drugs became the utmost necessity of time as no specific drug is available to relieve the clinical symptoms of COVID-19. We reviewed reliable information on targeted severe acute respiratory syndrome-coronavirus-2 (SARS-CoV-2) candidate drugs in the present chapter. Also, we summarized novel insight into the future development of safe, effective, and less-toxic antiviral drugs available and employed for the management of COVID-19. Similarly, we focused on antiviral medications under investigation for this purpose; several medications with different mechanisms of action were noticed for the treatment of COVID-19.

Keywords: COVID-19, Drug repurposing, Hydroxychloroquine, Remdesivir, Umifenovir.

[*] **Corresponding author Fazlullah Khan:** Department of Allied Health Sciences, Bashir Institute of Health Sciences, Bharakahu, Islamabad, Pakistan; Tel: +92-3469433155; E-mail: fazlullahdr@gmail.com

Kamal Niaz & Muhammad Farrukh Nisar (Eds.)

INTRODUCTION

According to the International Committee on Taxonomy of Viruses, severe acute respiratory syndrome coronavirus-2 (SARS-CoV-2) is the virus causing COVID-19 disease. This virus is belonging to the Coronaviridae family of viruses [1]. Acute respiratory distress syndrome is considered the most widespread critical feature of this disease. It is well known that this category among viruses is responsible for severe acute respiratory syndrome with up to 10% mortality rate [2]. In focus, COVID-19 disease is significantly linked with notifiable morbidity and mortality [3]. As a severe and infectious respiratory disease, several suggested clinical guidelines are currently available for treating COVID-19 [4 - 6]. Within these treatment guides, various types of medications are indicated as a part of the treatment strategy. Among the literature, the most commonly investigated treatment choices for COVID-19 disease were antiviral agents, immunomodulatory agents, antibiotics, analgesics, antipyretics, herbal medications, and some other supportive medications [7–9]. Currently, over 38 medications are under investigation for being considered as a treatment for COVID-19 disease [7 - 8].

Several medications with different mechanisms of action were noticed for the treatment of COVID-19 disease. These mechanisms encompass acting as protease inhibitors; RNA polymerase inhibitors, cell membrane fusion inhibitors, ACE2 receptor connection inhibitors, serine protease receptor inhibitors for the TMPRSS2, host cell immunostimulatory agents against virus invasion, mesenchymal stromal cells therapies, monoclonal antibodies, and passive immunization plasma [7 - 10]. One of the most pivotal antiviral medication groups includes protease inhibitors, which affect the 3-chymotrypsin like proteinase and Papain-like protease enzymes that act directly on the processing of the viral polyprotein. The second group of antivirals encompasses RNA polymerase inhibitors which inhibit the viral genome replication through competing natural nucleosides of the virus RNA-dependent RNA polymerase active site and then block the virus RNA synthesis process. A third group works mainly on the inhibition of intracellular viral replication through alkalization of the intracellular medium to inhibit the uncoating process of the virus envelope. Fourthly, the group of medications acting particularly on the avoidance of virus entry and membrane fusion into host cells by several mechanisms, most explicitly, preventing the binding of virus spike protein to host cell wall receptors such as ACE2 and TMPRSS2 receptors. The fifth group including those medications which work mostly extracellularly exerts its effect through binding to interleukin-6 receptor and inhibition of cytokine release to protect from amplified immune response [10].

Many clinical experiments are under investigation to reveal the safety and efficacy of these medications in use for treating COVID-19 infection [7, 11 - 13]. The perspective beyond these trials focuses mainly on repurposing those approved medications that are already existing and utilized for other indications before COVD-19. It is noteworthy that any of the investigated medications have been approved for such indication so far [8, 12, 13]. In this chapter, our main focus will be on the antiviral drugs under study for COVID-19 treatment.

Mechanisms of Different Antivirals Actions in COVID-19 Treatments

Nonstructural proteins (NSPs) are conserved proteins that function in gene expression during virus replication. It is thought that NSPs are fundamentally associated with the replication and function of coronavirus. Structural and accessory proteins are the other two types that are less conserved than the NSPs and only embraced in the virion synthesis. Hence, the antivirals might be pivotal in controlling the proteins during viral transcription and replication as well, then they could be a likely choice to recuperate the emanating COVID-19 infections and clinical consequences [14, 15]. This information sounds crucial especially when talking about the mechanisms of antiviral agents' actions. A brief about these mechanisms of antiviral agents is illustrated in Fig. (**1**).

G-441524 is the active metabolite of remdesivir that veils viral RNA polymerase and shirks proofreading by viral exonuclease, lowering the production of viral RNA. Remdesivir works by slowing up chain discontinuation of nascent viral RNA and positively affects SARS-CoV, MERS-CoV, and bat-CoV strains [16]. Drawing on the repurposing concept, Umifenovir is one of the portentous antiviral drugs with an unrivaled mechanism acting on the S protein/ACE2 interaction and dampening membrane fusion in the viral envelope [17]. It mainly blocks both cell membranes and the fusion of viral endosomes through integration into cell membranes and intercession with the hydrogen bonding network of phospholipids [18]. Favipiravir (FPV) is a guanine analog with a pyrazine carboxamide structure, and competitively decreases purine nucleosides [19]. Through h phosphoribosylation and phosphorylation, FPV as a prodrug is transformed into active FPV ribofuranosyl phosphates as soon as it gets in the infected cells by endocytosis [19].

Oseltamivir (GS4104) is an ester prodrug, which is hydrolyzed by hepatic carboxylesterases to produce the active metabolite (GS4071), a potent, selective inhibitor of influenza virus neuraminidase. Viral neuraminidase disconnects the binding between the cell receptor and the virus during virus spreading from the cellular space to its periphery (budding). Thus, neuraminidase inhibitors (NAIs) inhibit neuraminidase. Renal filtration and tubular secretion are responsible for metabolite excretion [20]. Ribavirin acts by intracellular guanosine diminution inhibiting the inosine monophosphate dehydrogenase enzyme as an antiviral drug, interrupting guanosine synthesis. It can also affect the virus replication indirectly by accelerating IFN gene expression and modulating immune responses. Ribavirin is an inhibitor of both RNA synthesis and mRNA capping [21, 22]. Lopinavir (LPV) is a peptide-mimetic molecule augmenting the non-self-cleavage peptide linkage which is the main target of the HIV-1 protease enzyme, thus blocking the activity of that enzyme [23], while Ritonavir acts through an important step in the HIV life cycle through which protease enzyme cleaves polyproteins, afterward, immature proteins inside the virus aggregate into particles which bloom from the cell as infectious virions. Thereby, the main role of protease inhibitors is dedicated to compete for the active cleavage site on the protease enzyme to prevent the cleavage of these polyproteins and thus the formation of mature virions [24]. Given Baloxavir marboxil, it is an RNA polymerase inhibitor that hampers mRNA synthesis by hindering the cap-dependent endonuclease of PA, repressing virus propagation. PA, PB1, and PB2 are the components of the viral polymerase. Therefore, this antiviral agent limits the viral infection which takes place when hemagglutinin on the surface of the viral envelope ties up to receptors located on the cell surface of the airway in the human body. It is noteworthy that the virus ribonucleoprotein (RNP) complex is liberated in the intracellular space (shelling), and moves into the nucleus. Viral RNA transcription and viral genome RNA replication, which accounts for synthesizing mRNA, are independently spurred [25].

Regarding SARSCoV-2, Chloroquine can suppress the entrance of the virus and prohibit its cell-binding by impeding ACE2 receptor glycosylation and its fusion with spike protein, indicating earlier probable effectiveness of Chloroquine against COVID-19 infection, before reducing ACE2 expression and action [26 - 28].

Different Antiviral Drugs used in COVID-19 Treatment

Despite lacking definitive and specific treatment regimens, treating cases with SARS-CoV-2 infection is principally depending on those already well-known drugs and drawing on symptoms experienced by the infected patients. Antiviral medications are mainly used against COVID-19, especially in secondary infections triggered by ARDS [29]. However, the efficacy of these medications needs to be investigated by well-designed clinical experiments. Briefly, drugs targeting RNA respiratory viruses have guided some efficacious therapies, indicating obstacles for antivirals in COVID-19 infections treatment. Multiple antivirals are under study for symptomatic COVID-19 but no clear information boosting the usage of those agents. Remdesivir sounds promising *in vitro* against

SARS-CoV2 highlighting desirable results for inpatients in a compassionate use series with a short-term restoration and a mild decline in deaths. Presently, Remdesivir is under investigation in phase III clinical trials, the compassionate use series, and finally to approve its use in emergency cases. A randomized-controlled trial of Lopinavir/Ritonavir (LPV/r) showed no obvious clinical or virologic advantage, in addition, drug-drug interactions and adverse reactions restrict its usage. Antivirals such as Oseltamivir, which is commonly used in treating influenza, have restricted action against SARS-CoV-2, while those agents like FPV and Umifenovir target the virus through specific sites, and demand further examination. These antiviral drugs which have shown activity against the virus should be investigated to approve their usability as treatment and prophylaxis for those patients severely infected with COVID-19 [30].

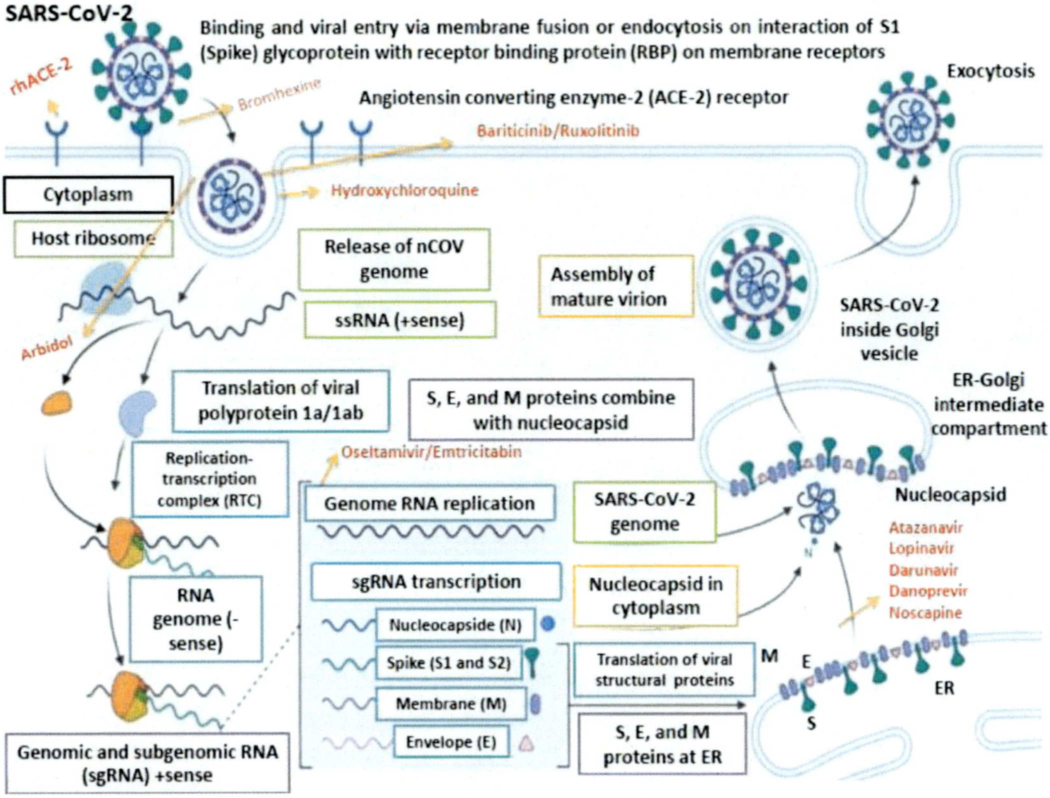

Fig. (1). Mechanism of action for medications used in the treatment of COVID-19 infection [10]. ACE2R: Angiotensin-converting Enzyme 2 receptor; TMPRSS2: Type II transmembrane serine protease; RdRp: RNA-dependent RNA polymerase.

Broad-spectrum Antiviral Agents (BSAA)

Remdesivir

Remdesivir is a phosphoramidite prodrug of an adenosine C nucleoside. In 2017, it was first synthesized, developed, and introduced by Gilead Sciences as a wide-spectrum antiviral drug against the Ebola virus, and used these days as a promising medication for COVID-19 treatment [31]. In mice infected with the virus MERS-CoV, it was found that Remdesivir can significantly improve lung function and alleviate pulmonary pathological damage *via* reducing the viral load in the lungs [32]. In another study, it was also revealed that low micromolar concentrations of Remdesivir can potently block SARS-CoV-2 infection with a high selectivity index (half-maximal effective concentration (EC50), 0.77 μM; half-cytotoxic concentration (CC50) > 100 μM; SI > 129.87) [26]. Holshue *et al.* revealed interesting findings of IV Remdesivir when has been utilized in a trial on a patient who had been cured of pneumonia but was infected with COVID-19 in the United States [33]. For evaluating its efficacy and safety COVID-19 infected cases, China has launched a randomized, placebo-controlled, double-blind, multicenter, phase III clinical trial on 308 and 452 cases, respectively, in February 2020. A 200 mg as an initial dose of Remdesivir has given to the patients in the case group followed by a subsequent IV infusion dose of 100 mg for 9 consecutive days accompanied by routine treatment, meanwhile, the same dose in placebo was given to patients in the control group. It was estimated that the trial results are going to be provided in mid-April but it has been suspended as no eligible patients can be recruited [34]. Currently, a 10-days regimen is recommended for Remdesivir including 200 mg loading dose on day 1, then 100 mg once-daily maintenance doses for 9 days. It is worthwhile that this experiment has been terminated as the epidemic has been controlled well in China [35]. Recently, case series in the USA investigating the compassionate use of Remdesivir on 61 inpatient adults infected with COVID-19 have shown an amelioration amongst 68% of those patients regarding oxygen therapy during an average of 18-day prosecution period, while the clinical status had worsened among 15% of the patients. Clinical amelioration was detected among 84% of ages less than 50 years old, but this was less noticed in patients aged 70 years old or more, and in patients who were on mechanical ventilation compared with patients on extubated ventilation. The mortality rate was 13% among old patients≥70 years old, and patients with higher baseline serum creatinine indicating a more elevated threat. The most common side effects observed in 60% of cases were; elevated liver enzymes (transaminases) (23%), diarrhea (9%), rash (8%), kidney dysfunction (8%), and hypotension (8%) [36]. Remdesivir exhibited changes in its characteristics depending on the abovementioned dose (linear pharmacokinetics), and an intracellular half-life when exceeds 35 hours.

Reversible aspartate aminotransferase and alanine transaminase elevations took place following multiple doses. Liver or kidney adjustments are not currently recommended, but at the start-up, the point might be necessary when the glomerular filtration rate is approximately lower than 30 mL/min [37, 38]. Accordingly, some other studies have supported the trials on Remdesivir against new COVID-19 based on its safety profile *in vivo* [16, 39]. It should be noted that the US Food and Drug Administration (FDA) authorized the use of Remdesivir for treating inpatients infected with COVID-19 in the emergency department, and this was in May 2020 [40]. It is noteworthy that Remdesivir has drawn a conditional marketing authorization from the European Commission for one year, due to the urgent need against the Covid-19 pandemic. The intravenous drug, manufactured by US pharma company Gilead Sciences, will be used for adults and children over the age of 12 who require supplemental oxygen. Subsequently, the authorization can be extended or became unconditional when further data is submitted. That encompasses data from presently ongoing phase III clinical trials [41].

Umifenovir (Arbidol)

Umifenovir (brand name, Arbidol), an indole carboxylic acids derivative, was firstly approved in Russia, then China as a prophylactic treatment in patients infected with influenza A and B, and some other arbovirus [42]. Subsequently, Umifenovir (brand name is Arbidol) has shown *in vitro* antiviral efficacy against multiple virus strains such as the Ebola, human herpesvirus 8 (HHV-8), hepatitis C virus (HCV), and Tacaribe arenavirus [43]. In the influenza virus, it acts on reducing the probability to reach the acidic media which is essential for the conversion of hemagglutinin (HA) into the fusogenic form [44]. Some studies have revealed the effectiveness of Umifenovir against both SARS-CoV-1 and SARS-CoV-2 *in vitro* [45, 46]. In China, an observational study has shown a decline in mortality rates in 67 COVID-19-infected patients, in addition to reduced length of hospital stay among 36 patients who used Umifenovir [47]. In contrast, in another Chinese retrospective study, Umifenovir failed to show negative tests for SARS-CoV-2 among 81 inpatients (not in the intensive care unit), nor in the length of stay when compared with the standard treatment [48]. Currently, there are two Chinese randomized and open-label trials aim at examining the efficacy and safety of Umifenovir while used in COVID-19 cases. One of these trials (NCT04252885) is for comparing the efficacy of the combination (Umifenovir and standard treatment) *versus* (LPV/r and standard treatment), whereas the other trial (NCT04260594) is for comparing (Umifenovir plus standard treatment) with standard treatment alone.

Favipiravir (T-705 or Avigan)

Favipiravir (FPV) (brand name, Avigan) was developed in 2014 by Fujifilm Toyama Chemical's Japanese company to treat avian influenza or other types of influenza resistant to neuraminidase inhibitors. FPV shows its broad-spectrum antiviral action *via* selective working on conservative catalytic RNA domain-dependent RNA polymerase (RdRp), interfering with the incorporation process of the nucleotide during RNA replication in the virus [19]. Those frequent transition mutations can be attributed to dysregulation occurring during RNA replication encompassing. For example, permutation of guanine (G) and cytosine (C) occurs due to adenine (A) and thymine (T), respectively. It leads to disables mutagenesis in RNA viruses [19]. Accordingly, FPV can play an important role in infections caused by RNA viruses such as influenza, Ebola, and norovirus [49]. One trial has concluded that FPV is needed in large doses for safe and efficacious clinical plans drawing on its activity in Vero E6 cells infected with SARS-CoV-2 with half-maximal effective concentration (EC50) of 61.88 μM and half-cytotoxic concentration (CC50) at over 400 μM [26]. In China, a randomized-controlled trial (ChiCTR200030254) has demonstrated that FPV was more effective than Umifenovir when both have been used to treat COVID-19 patients. This supremacy in terms of recovery rate was (71.43%) with FPV but (55.86%) with Umifenovir, moreover, and the time needed for relieving fever and cough also was profoundly shorter in the FPV group [50]. In a Chinese hospital, Jianjun Gao has carried out a study on 80 inpatients infected with COVID-19. It was found that FPV had a more potent antiviral activity than the LPV/r with no adverse effects [19]. The effective dose of FPV against COVID-19 is 600 mg Tid with 1,600 mg as a loading dose firstly for no more than 14 days, the half-life is approximately 5 hours [51]. However, FPV has exhibited teratogenic and embryotoxic effects in animals, therefore, it is contraindicated in pregnancy [51], [52]. FPV is used these days in Japan, but not in the United States, for clinical use. Up to Apr 15, 2020, eight clinical trials have been currently conducted in China and two in Japan to investigate the antiSARS-CoV-2 potential of FPV. These trials embrace non-randomized- and randomized-controlled trials to evaluate efficacy and safety of FPV as a single therapy (ChiCTR2000030113, JPRN-jRCTs031190226, JPRNjRCTs041190120), or when combined with IFN-α (ChiCTR2000029600), also with Baloxavir marboxil (ChiCTR2000029544, ChiCTR2000029548), with Tocilizumab (ChiCTR2000030894, NCT04310228), or with Chloroquine phosphate (ChiCTR2000030987, NCT04319900).

Oseltamivir (Tamiflu)

Oseltamivir (brand name is Tamiflu) is an antiviral medication approved to treat influenza A and B. Oseltamivir carboxylate is the active form of Oseltamivir, distinguished in a longer half-life, and formed by the hydrolysis of the prodrug, which is an ethyl ester in nature [53, 54]. The potential of Oseltamivir in decreasing death in cases infected with the H5N1 influenza virus was before the respiratory failure takes place and when the dose was 75 mg bid [55, 56]. Generally, patients require to take this drug for 5 days. Still, in influenza cases accompanied by acute respiratory distress syndrome (ARDS), pneumonia, or in immune-deficient patients, Oseltamivir should be used for 10 days [57]. Oseltamivir and Zanamivir are deemed as treatment and prophylactic first-line therapy in influenza, as shown in Table **1**. In Wuhan, China, a study has revealed that no positive results were detected after receiving Oseltamivir when treating COVID-19 [58]. Oseltamivir is in a clinical trial for Phase 3 to examine its efficacy against 2019-nCoV in COVID-19 therapy with an HIV protease inhibitor (ASC09F) as a 3CLpro inhibitor is in use individually in Phase 4 2019-nCoV [59].

Furthermore, Oseltamivir has been utilized per oral for treating 2019-nCoV and hospitalized cases in China, yet, its effectiveness in treating COVID-19 patients [59]. Oseltamivir has shown a wide safety margin while used in animals. In the clinical trials program, severe adverse reactions were documented at the same frequency as with placebo (1.3% with 75 mg bid, 0.7% with 150 mg bid, and 1.2% placebo) [20]. In addition, teratogenicity or fertility-related reactions were not evident. Oseltamivir has also been investigated as a prophylactic agent or even as a medication against influenza A and B. Transient gastrointestinal disturbances are the most prominent adverse effects that might appear with Oseltamivir. These disturbances can diminish when the drug is taken with a light meal [60].

Ribavirin

Ribavirin is a broad-spectrum antiviral drug, guanosine nucleoside analog in structure. It is used to treat several viral infections, such as respiratory syncytial virus (RSV), hepatitis C virus, bunyavirus, herpesvirus, adenovirus, poxvirus, and some viral hemorrhagic fevers. In studies on coronaviruses in animals, Ribavirin has shown a weak inhibitory effect. Nevertheless, it can minimize the release of pro-inflammatory cytokines from the macrophages through its immune-modulatory effect in mice and convert the Th-2 response to Th-1 response [61]. However, one of the adverse reactions of Ribavirin is the reduction in hemoglobin concentrations when given to ill-persons. It has limited use as an antiviral agent against SARS-CoV-2 [62, 63].

Lopinavir-Ritonavir

Lopinavir (LPV) is a highly specific inhibitor for HIV-1 protease; however, it is used exclusively in combination with Ritonavir. Kaletra was the brand name for this combination which was firstly produced by Abbott company in 2000 [64]. Ritonavir is responsible for enzyme inhibition and enhancing Lopinavir exposure by boosting oral bioavailability and reducing biotransformation [64]. In addition, Ritonavir results in increasing the area under curve related to LPV plasma concentration more than 100 folds in healthy volunteers [65]. In SARS, the protocol including lopinavir-ritonavir (LPV/r) (usually combined with corticosteroids) is effective in reducing deaths, lowering mechanical ventilation needs, decreasing rescue corticosteroid treatment, and minimizing the post-therapy load of the virus [66, 67]. According to these results, this combination was evaluated in patients with COVID-19. Early reports of LPV/r for COVID-19 treatment were mostly case reports of small-scale retrospective and non-randomized cohort studies. Hence, endorsing the role of this medication is not an easy task in this regard [67, 68]. Recently, in an open-label, individually randomized, controlled trial, LPV/r was investigated among patients with COVID-19 using a dose of 400mg/100 mg, orally twice daily plus standard of care, against others who were on the standard of care alone. No benefit was observed for LPV//r beyond standard care. The most frequent adverse effects related to LPV//r use were; diarrhea, nausea, and asthenia [69]. In a Korean report, LPV//r administration has significantly improved the clinical symptoms of coronavirus such as fever and cough.

Interestingly, also coronavirus titers were few or even undetected in the follow-up study. Nevertheless, the analysis encompassed only one infected person in the initial phase of the epidemic in Korea [70]. Another retrospective cohort study revealed a better effect of the combination of Umifenovir with LPV/r when compared with LPV/r alone when both groups have been applied containing 16 and 17 patients, respectively [71]. Undesirable reactions of LPV/r were abdominal disturbances such as nausea and diarrhea (up to 28%) and liver toxicity (2%-10%). Commonly, side effects of LPV/r might be escalated by using combination therapy. A percentage of patients may experience elevated transaminases [72]. Consequently, LPV/r-induced hepatotoxicity could limit the use of this combination [73].

Baloxavir Marboxil

Baloxavir marboxil is a new antiviral agent that can inhibit the process of RNA replication in influenza by acting on various parts of the proteins in the influenza polymerase complex. In short, the Baloxavir marboxil prohibits cap-dependent endonuclease [74]. As both are RNA viruses, Baloxavir marboxil seems to have a significant effect against SARS-CoV-2 by preventing its RNA synthesis. At the same time, it was revealed that the Baloxavir marboxil possesses antiviral activity against SARS-CoV-2 *in vitro*. Based on non-linear regression fitting, EC50 against SARS-CoV-2 was estimated to be 3.32, 5.48, and 10.4 μM for Umifenovir, Baloxavir acid, and LPV, respectively. In 24 patients (82.8%), the findings showed undetected viral RNA in two successive tests within 14 days post to the trial establishment. After 14 days, 70%, 77%, and 100% who have been treated with Baloxavir, FPV, and those in the control group, respectively, showed negative results according to the virus test. In this trial, the time needed for those patients for improvement was 14, 14, and 15 days in the cases treated with Baloxavir, FPV, and control group, respectively. In total, 7 days were sufficient for 15 patients (51.7%) to be free of the virus (60%, 44%, and 50% in Baloxavir, FPV, and control group, respectively. One and two patients in the Baloxavir marboxil, and FPV groups were admitted for intensive care within 7 days post to trial establishment based on the case aggravation, but no deaths have been reported. That patient in Baloxavir marboxil group needed to be treated with extracorporeal membrane oxygenation ten days after trial initiation. In short, it was concluded that adding Baloxavir or FPV in their usual dose to the existing standard treatment had not any contribution to clinical improvement in this study [75].

Chloroquine and Hydroxychloroquine

Chloroquine and Hydroxychloroquine are long-standing aminoquinolines, with similar structures. They are often clinically used in the treatment of various diseases such as malaria, amebiasis, rheumatoid arthritis (RA), and systemic lupus erythematosus (SLE) [76]. The hydroxyl group in Hydroxychloroquine, when compared with chloroquine, leads to a decrease in its toxicity while giving similar action. In humans, graft-*versus* -host disease can be controlled by targeting lysosomes which is one of these mechanisms of action of Chloroquine and Hydroxychloroquine [77]. These drugs accumulate in lysosomes and significantly change the entire pH. They are directly responsible for affecting lysosomal proteases' activity by influencing the disintegration of proteins and glycosaminoglycan [77, 78]. The effectiveness of Chloroquine is evident in mice models on viruses such as human coronavirus OC43, enterovirus EV-A71, Zika virus, and influenza A H5N1 virus, as well as *ex vivo* conditions on Ebola virus [47, 79, 80]. In both healthy and ill persons experiencing SLE and RA, Hydroxychloroquine has an anti-inflammatory effect on Th17-related cytokines (IL-6, IL-17, and IL-22) [81]. Based on one analysis, cytokine storm triggered by COVID-19 has a significant role in ARD, leading to death in infected patients. Interestingly, Chloroquine and Hydroxychloroquine can suppress cytokine storms in accordance with some evidence [82]. *In vitro*, it has been reported that Hydroxychloroquine has shown its effectiveness in repressing SARS-CoV-2 infection [28, 83, 84]. Wang *et al.* (2020) revealed that the EC50 of chloroquine against COVID-19 tested on VERO E6 was 1.13 μM and the EC90 was 6.90 μM.

It is noteworthy that after 24 hours of growth, Hydroxychloroquine demonstrated *in vitro* activity with a lower EC50 for SARS-CoV-2 when compared with Chloroquine (Hydroxychloroquine: EC50 = 6.14 μM and Chloroquine: EC50 = 23.90 μM) [85]. Nevertheless, the evidence on the safety and efficacy of these medications in the treatment of COVID-19, therefore, the risk/benefit relationship should be considered [86]. Accordingly, more clinical experiments to investigate the efficacy and safety of Hydroxychloroquine as a prophylactic and treatment agent against COVID-19 are underway. In the USA, Chloroquine and Hydroxychloroquine have been authorized for the emergency treatment of COVID-19 by the FDA. In one study, Chloroquine was not recommended for COVID-19 treatment (Table **1**) because of the high dosage utilized during the 10 days of needed for treatment plan (12 g) may result in serious cardiac effects [87]. Meanwhile, this was contrasted by another study in which Chloroquine was safely used in the treatment and resulted in radiologic findings improvement, viral clearance enhancement, and disease progression reduction [88]. Nevertheless, the design and outcomes data of this clinical trial have not yet been published for peer review which makes the validity of the results questionable. In France, a recent open-label non-randomized study recruited 36 patients have been divided into two groups, 20 in the Hydroxychloroquine group and 16 in the control group. The dose of Hydroxychloroquine was 200 mg bid per oral *versus* standard supportive care in the control group. By the sixth day, 70% of patients (14/20) in the Hydroxychloroquine group demonstrated virologic clearance using nasopharyngeal swabs, while this had happened in only 12% of patients (2/16) in the control group, the difference was statistically significant (p=0.001). In another Chinese prospective study in which 30 patients had been selected randomly. All were treated with 400 mg Hydroxychloroquine daily for 5 days combined with standard of care (*i.e.* supportive care, IFN, and other antivirals) *versus* standard care alone. The virologic outcomes were not different. On the seventh day, the difference in the virologic clearance between the two groups was not statistically significant (p> 0.05), this was 86.7% in the hydroxychloroquine plus standard of care group *versus* 93.3% in the standard care group, respectively [89]. Presently, there are numerous RCTs on both Chloroquine and Hydroxychloroquine evaluating their efficacy in COVID-19 treatment. Chloroquine prophylaxis was studied among health care employees (NCT04303507) and hydroxychloroquine for post-exposure prevention following risky exposures (NCT04308668) are planned or enrolled [90]. Chloroquine dose in COVID-19 is 500 mg per oral od or bid with scarceness of data about the maximum dose to assess its activity and safety profile [84]. Not withstanding the general indicated dose for hydroxychloroquine in most related diseases is 400 mg once a day per oral, but one study had probed the pharmacokinetics of the drug based on its physiological characteristics, and indicated that the optimal dose for hydroxychloroquine in

COVID-19 is a loading dose of 400 mg bid once for 1 day followed by 200 mg bid daily [85]. Conversely, another regimen for Whipple disease suggests the total daily dose of hydroxychloroquine 600 mg based on safety and clinical experience [84], hence, some more research is required to set out the optimal dose of hydroxychloroquine for COVID-19. Adverse reactions associated with chloroquine and hydroxychloroquine are rarely occurred as they relatively well-tolerated in SLE and malaria patients. However, serious side effects might appear in <10% of patients embracing QTc prolongation, hypoglycemia, neuropsychiatric effects, and retinopathy [91]. This necessitates baseline electrocardiography to check out heart status pre and post the use of these drugs in order to prevent arrhythmias, particularly in patients with a previous history, as well as to avoid drug-drug interaction with medications which prolong QT-interval such as azithromycin and fluoroquinolones [92]. Generally considered, chloroquine and hydroxychloroquine can be used safely in pregnancy [93], nevertheless, ocular toxicity has been reported as a side effect for these agents in one study had been conducted on 588 patients as a part of a review including 12 papers [94].

Other Antiviral Agents

Darunavir is one of the several antiretrovirals claimed to show *in vitro* activity when used against SARS-CoV-2. Clinically, still, there is no evidence on humans regarding the use of this medication in the treatment of COVID-19 [10]. Darunavir/Cobicistat (Prezcobix) and Darunavir /Cobicistat /Emtricitabine/ Tenofovir/ Alafenamide (Symtuza) are two Darunavir-based combinations produced by Johnson & Johnson, which has recently declared the lack of evidence to assure their usage as a therapy for SARS-CoV-2 [95]. Moreover, out of the three, one randomized, open-label clinical trial investigating Darunavir/Cobicistat for COVID-19 latterly indicated that this treatment was not efficient at clearing the virus on the seventh day after randomization when compared with the standard care [96].

BSAA Combination Therapy

Efficacious antiviral therapy is fundamental for combating the pandemic related to the novel coronavirus disease (COVID-19). One of these promising combinations in this regard is LPV/r, Ribavirin, and IFN beta-1b for treating COVID-19 infected patients. This combination was examined through a multicenter, prospective, open-label, randomized, phase 2 trial in adult patients infected with COVID-19. Those patients were admitted to six hospitals in Hong Kong, randomly selected (2:1), and divided into groups; combination and control.

The patients in the combination group have received a combination of LPV 400 mg and Ritonavir 100 mg bid, Ribavirin 400 mg bid, and three doses of 8 million international units of IFN beta-1b on reciprocal days for 14 days. In the control group, the patients were given LPV 400 mg and Ritonavir 100 mg every bid for 14 days. Nasopharyngeal swabs were obtained in the incipient final stage, and they were negative for SARS-CoV-2 RT-PCR and were carried out to treat the population deliberately. This trial was registered with (ClinicalTrials.gov: NCT04276688). In this trial, of the 127 recruited patients, 86 and 41 were randomly selected to the combination and control groups, respectively. Symptoms appearance and then starting the treatment was in the median duration, 5 days (IQR 3–7). Based on the negative nasopharyngeal swab, the time needed for getting this negative result in the combination group (7 days [IQR 5–11]) was significantly shorter than that required for the control group (12 days [8 - 15]; hazard ratio 4·37 [95% CI 1·86–10·24], p=0·0010). It should be noted that adverse reactions that accompanied the use of this combination were self-limited nausea and diarrhea in both groups. In the control group, only one patient paused LPV/r due to biochemical hepatitis. No deaths among patients have been reported during the study. Among those mild to moderate COVID-19 patients, this combination, triple antiviral therapy, was safe and more effective than LPV/r alone in mitigating symptoms and diminishing the duration of viral shedding, and reducing the length of hospital stay [97].

Umifenovir with LPV/r is another combination under investigation. However, this combination has demonstrated efficacy in one study [71]. Another prospective study (ChiCTR200030254) revealed the superiority of Favipiravir on Umifenovir concerning the clinical recuperation rate and alleviation of fever and cough [50]. Moreover, Darunavir with Umifenovir was a suggested combination to combat the SARS-CoV-2 outbreak reported in different recovering cases from the disease in China [98].

Many clinical experiments are currently investigating the effectiveness of Oseltamivir in the treatment of SARS-CoV-2 infection. In addition, Oseltamivir is also examined in clinical trials in numerous combinations, such as chloroquine and FPV [98].

Although the results of ribavirin and IFNα-2b in a MERS-CoV rhesus macaque model were promising, its results with IFN (either α2a or β1) on MERS-CoV infected patients were different. Mostly, Ribavirin exists in combinations with IFN but the findings vary from one type to another. It is noteworthy that the combination of IFNα-2b and Ribavirin for treating MERS-CoV demonstrated that their single-dose regimen had been decreased by 8 folds and 16 folds, respectively. They further activate cytokines, enhance immune system responses, reduce viral replication, host response modification, and clinical outcomes enhancement [63].

Table 1. Characteristics of the current treatments against COVID-19.

Class	Drug(s)	Rationale	Dosage Form	Dose	Comments
Broad-spectrum Antiviral agents	Remdesivir	Nucleotide analog prodrug, metabolized into Remdesivir triphosphate which acts as an analog of adenosine triphosphate.	Lyophilized injection powder (100mg/20ml/vial)	200 mg IV on day 1 then 100 mg daily 2-10 days	Initial FDA approval was for treatment of HIV1.
	Umifenovir (Arbidol)	Both direct-acting veridical and by viral life cycle stages inhibitor. A non-nucleoside antiviral and immune-modulating drug	Oral capsules 50mg – 100mg	Up to 200 mg four times daily for up to 14 days.	Initial approval was in Russia and China for prophylaxis and treatment of influenza and other respiratory viral infections [109]. As a monotherapy can be superior to LPV/r in treating COVID-19 [110].
	Favipiravir (Avigan)	Inhibits RNA polymerase. Metabolized into Favipiravir ribosyl triphosphate.	Oral tablet 200 mg	1600 mg twice daily for one day, then 600 mg twice a day for 4 days.	Initial approval was in Japan for the treatment of influenza (Fijifilm Co. leaflet).

(Table 1) cont.....

Class	Drug(s)	Rationale	Dosage Form	Dose	Comments
Antivirals	Oseltamivir (Tamiflu)	Neuraminidase inhibitor	Oral capsules and suspension	75 mg twice daily for five days	Initial FDA approval was for the treatment of influenza.
	Ribavirin	Nucleoside analog	Oral capsules or solution	800 mg – 1400 mg per day.	Initial approval was for the treatment of HCV (FDA).
	Baloxavir	RNA replication inhibitor	Oral	80 mg *orally* on day 1 and day 4, and another dose of 80 mg on day 7 (as needed); not to exceed 3 total doses [75], [111].	No data to date support use in the treatment of COVID-19.
Antivirals (combinations)	(Lopinavir/Ritonavir) (Kelatra)	Lopinavir is an HIV-1 protease inhibitor. Ritonavir increases the plasma levels of Lopinavir by inhibiting the CYP3A mediated metabolism of Lopinavir.	Oral combination capsules	400/100 mg twice daily	Initial FDA approval was for the treatment of HIV1 [96], [112].
	LPV/r combination with Umifenovir	-	-	Combination with Umifenovir 200mg/8h.	Combination therapy is superior to LPV/r monotherapy [71].
	-	-	-	-	-
Antivirals (combinations)	-	-	-	-	-
	-	-	-	-	-
	-	-	-	-	-

(Table 1) cont.....

Class	Drug(s)	Rationale	Dosage Form	Dose	Comments
Anti-malarial drugs	Hydroxychloroquine	-	Oral tablets	400 mg /12 h on day 1, then 200 mg /12h for 4 days	Reduced the risk of death in COVID-19 patients with ARDS.22 No significant effect [113].
	Chloroquine	-	Oral tablets	500 mg /12h for 7-10 days.	

Some other researches exhibited reduced ARDS and mortality among SARS patients when they are given a combination of Ribavirin plus LPV/r. Moreover, the reduction was significant by adding corticosteroids to treat patients with SARS-CoV [66, 99]. An *in vitro* study has been conducted recently and revealed that Ribavirin should be used in a high effective concentration (EC50= 109.50 μM) against SARS-CoV-2 [67]. There is no evidence on the benefit of inhaled Ribavirin over enteral or intravenous administration for nCoV or RSV treatment [100]. Four studies demonstrated possible undesirable reactions, including hematologic and hepatotoxicity [101]. In MERS therapy, the combination of Ribavirin with IFNs is generally showed no noticeable clinical outcomes or viral clearance [102, 103]. Ribavirin leads to severe dose-dependent hematologic toxicity. The large doses used in the SARS trials resulted in hemolytic anemia in more than 60% of cases. In addition, 75% of patients have experienced transaminase elevation [101]. Similarly, in the broadest MERS investigational experiment, around 40% of patients required blood transfusion after receiving a combination of Ribavirin plus IFN [103]. Ribavirin also has a known teratogenic effect, so it is contraindicated in pregnancy [104]. The combination therapy could be a good suggestion to overcome the indecisive efficacy data with Ribavirin for other nCoVs and its significant toxicity to treat COVID-19. In the present time, there is an experiment to evaluate the efficacy and safety of IFN-α. IFN-α combined with Ribavirin, LPV/r, or Ribavirin with LPV/r for SARS-CoV-2 cases in China (ChiCTR2000029387) work effectively.

Zinc inhibits SARS-CoV and retrovirus RNA polymerase *in vitro* models. It works as ionophores to prevent viral replication in cell culture. Zinc can act in combination withChloroquine or Hydroxychloroquine. This combination is currently under investigation [105]. Moreover, Zinc enhances Chloroquine intracellular uptake [106].

The combination of Azithromycin with Hydroxychloroquine has been reported in 6 patients led to viral clearance in all patients (100%) better than that of hydroxychloroquine monotherapy (57%) [107]. Notwithstanding these auspicious results, several major limitations had been reported, such as the small sample size and the exclusion of 6 patients in the hydroxychloroquine group from analysis due to early termination of treatment. These limitations might lead to critical illness or drug intolerance, variable baseline viral loads between Hydroxychloroquine alone and combination therapy groups, and no clinical or safety outcomes reported. Many clinical experiments areunder trial to assess the combined effect of Azithromycin plus Hydroxychloroquine in people infected with SARS-CoV-2. Three clinical studies are currently conducted in France using azithromycin (500 mg on the first day, then 250 mg od for four days) in combination with hydroxychloroquine (600 mg od for 10 days). One of these trials is in an open-label non-randomized study (6 patients) [107], the second is in an open-label uncontrolled study (11 patients) [108], and the third is an uncontrolled observational study (80 patients) [108]. Gautret *et al.* revealed a 100% viral clearance among their 6 patients by testing nasopharyngeal swabs [107]. Nonetheless, Molina *et al.* [106] have contrasted the results of another scientist after repeating the trials, thought the prompt and complete viral clearance was quite unpredictable as they revealed that 8 of 11 patients had serious comorbidities [108]. Depending on these findings, data exhibited so far are inadequate to weigh up possible clinical advantages of azithromycin in COVID-19 patients [108]. It is also worthwhile to take into account the cardiac toxicity resulting from the additive effect of hydroxychloroquine and azithromycin combination. Protraction of the QT interval is a common side effect for both agents and may potentiate the risk in people with cardiac-related comorbidities.

Clinical Trials on Treatments for COVID-19

COVID-19 has turned out to be one of the most severe challenges in medical history. Hence, the quick development and approval of effective and safe treatments are necessary for reducing the deaths resulting from this pandemic. Consequently, many companies seek to repurpose those current therapies of known efficacy and safety profiles that can act on COVID-19. Up to the date of writing, a search of ClinicalTrials.gov revealed almost 1,000 results for COVID-19 [114]. Here, some of the most promising clinical trials will be shown.

The first clinical trials on traditional antiviral drugs reported non-promising early results [69, 115]. To address the risk and weak evidence of multiple small trials, the WHO has established the international Solidarity study, which embraces more than 100 countries to compare the findings related to four treatments: Remdesivir, hydroxychloroquine, and Chloroquine, LPV/r, and LPV/r in combination with IFN β-1a [116]. Interestingly, the Solidarity Trial's International Steering Committee has recommended stalling the trials on both Hydroxychloroquine and LPV/r arms, and the WHO accepted this. These recommendations have been built in light of the temporal results and by reviewing the evidence of all trials presented in the WHO summit on COVID-19 research and innovation on 1-2 July 2020. These interim trial results indicated that Hydroxychloroquine and LPV/r as a combination have limited or with no effect in reducing mortality among inpatients infected with COVID-19 compared to standard care. For each of these medications, the tentative findings do not introduce robust evidence on the deadrise. However, the clinical lab results indicated the safety of this combination to some extent. This decision was only made concerning the conduct of the Solidarity trial in hospitalized patients, but will not affect the investigatory efforts to examine the use of Hydroxychloroquine or LPV/r in non-hospitalized patients or as pre- or post-exposure prophylaxis for COVID-19. The transitory solidarity findings are currently available for peer-reviewed publication [117].

Ribavirin (Virazole®, Bausch Health Companies Inc., Laval, Canada) is under investigation in an open-label, interventional trial to assess its safety and efficacy in inpatients adults who were COVID-19 positive and experienced severe respiratory distress [116]. A similar antiviral drug, Favipiravir (Avigan®, FUJIFILM Toyama Chemical Co., Ltd., Tokyo, Japan), is currently in phase II development (NCT04358549) [116]. Moreover, preclinical and clinical data imply the antiviral properties of Azithromycin (Zithromax®, Pfizer Inc., New York, NY, USA), and this is expected to be examined in COVID-19 patients soon [116].

Antibodies such as SLB (Kevzara®, Sanofi, New York, NY, USA, and Regeneron Pharmaceuticals, Inc., Tarrytown, NY, USA) and TZB (Actemra/RoActemra®, F. Hochmann-La Roche AG, Basel, Switzerland), which can effectively block IL-6 signal transduction. They are prioritized as the first agents to be examined in patients suffering complications from COVID-19 infection. Preliminary analysis of the phase II portion of Sanofi's trial investigating SLB (NCT04327388) manifested that it promptly decreased C-reactive protein, a key marker of inflammation. Nevertheless, SLB did not exhibit positive trends among severe cases that required oxygen supplementation but not mechanical, the results in critical cases that required mechanical ventilation were positive. Accordingly, the trial has been modified so that only critical patients are going to be enrolled to receive treatment. Evidence about TZB appears more auspicious, but the findings of the Roche global, randomized, double-blind, placebo-controlled phase II COVACTA trial (NCT04320615) will provide the pivotal answer about its profile [116]. Regarding Canakinumab, an IL-1β blocker, Novartis has also proclaimed a venture to launch a phase III clinical trial to investigate this treatment in patients with COVID-19 pneumonia, based on the reports of elevated levels of IL-1β in COVID-19-infected patients [116].

Evidence drawn from animal models on viral pneumonia indicates that complement inhibition may relieve lung injury, referred to as COVID-19 infection [118]. Complement is one of the innate immune response components to viruses that initiate pro-inflammatory responses. For the compassionate-use cases, Alexion is about initiating a global phase III trial to examine the use of Ravulizumab-cwvz (Ultomiris®, Alexion Pharmaceuticals, Boston, MA, USA) on mechanical ventilation term, hospitalization length of stay, and survival of patients with COVID-19 compared to best supportive care [119]. Eculizumab (Soliris®, Alexion Pharmaceuticals, Boston, MA, USA) is under investigation by Alexion in COVID-19 cases.

A preliminary study on 10 Chinese patients shows that immunotherapy using convalescent plasma-containing neutralizing antibodies improved clinical symptoms, raise blood oxygen levels and lymphocytes, decrease C-reactive protein levels and undetectable viral loads. Only two patients were detached from ventilators. It should be noted here that treatment with plasma was particularly successful when given within 14 days of symptoms appearance and with no detected adverse effects [120]. This result has to be assessed on a large scale.

Kiniksa Pharmaceuticals (Bermuda) recently has also declared evidence regarding Mavrilimumab treatment. This fully-human monoclonal antibody acts on granulocyte-macrophage colony-stimulating factor receptor alpha (GM-CSFRα) in 6 COVID-19-infected patients experiencing serious pneumonia and hyper-inflammation. All patients demonstrated an improvement in fever alleviation and oxygen levels within 1–3 days. There was no need for mechanical ventilation among those patients. However, further studies are still required [121].

Eli Lilly and Company has also established a phase II study (A study of LY3127804 in hospitalized COVID-19 participants with likely progressive ARDS or mechanical ventilation; NCT04342897) LY3127804, which is a selective monoclonal antibody against angiopoietin 2. Scientists hope that inhibition of angiopoetin 2 will reduce the advancement to ARDS or the demand for mechanical ventilation in COVID-19 patients [121]. With new trials being announced daily, many potential therapeutics will be in clinical development. Despite the accelerated rate of progress, wide gaps subsist in grasping the COVID-19 immunopathology. Collaborative efforts between pharmaceutical companies may embark and be reinforced to come up with effective therapies; however, this might need time for further investigation to be utilized in humans. Hopefully, these efforts will succeed sooner in possessing suitable and effective treatment and bringing people's life back to normal.

Only a few clinical trials have been undertaken these days to investigate Baloxavir for the treatment of COVID-19. In an exploratory, open-label, randomized controlled study at a single center in China (CHiCTR2000029544) was carried out. 29 COVID-19-infected inpatients on LPN/r, Darunavir/cobicistat, or Umifenovir, in combination with inhaled IFN-α, were randomized to treatment with Baloxavir marboxil (80 mg per oral on day 1 and day 4, and 80 mg per day on day 7 as required) (n=10), FPV (1600 or 2200 mg orally on day 1, followed by 600 mg Tid for up to 14 days) (n=9), or control (standard antiviral treatment) (n=10). After 14 days of treatment, 70, 77, and 100% of patients in the Baloxavir, FPV, and control groups, respectively, have shown negative viral RNA results according to 2 consecutive tests [75]. Another randomized controlled trial registered in China: (CHiCTR2000029548) [111].

FUTURE PERSPECTIVE

The COVID-19 pandemic is evident as a surpassing disastrous outbreak, particularly in the broadly influenced countries such as China, Italy, Iran, and the USA in enormous features, particularly health, social, and economic. However, it is too early to predict any *de facto* scenario, but definitely, it will significantly affect all countries around the world [122]. Special attention is paid to the future premises, which comprise identifying accurate and prompt diagnostic tools, proper control of disease transmission chain, manufacturing effective, safe, approved medications for the treatment of the infection. Meanwhile, efficacious prevention (vaccines) and treatment, especially for COVID-19 pneumonia, will be the time required for the real global threat to health attributed to SARS-CoV-2. Nevertheless, no official approval for any of COVID-19 drugs as they still represent a big problem for humans. Given the epidemiological aspects of SARS-CoV-2, it is substantial to interrupt the virus proliferation *via* some common methods such as quarantining the confirmed positive cases and controlling the spread of infection. Additionally, it is fundamental to benefit from the little evidence about medications these days to establish strategies to avoid and manage the SARS-CoV-2 transference. Based on the confirmation which stated that the genome sequence of SARS-CoV-2 is highly similar to both bat and human SARS-CoVs, some antiviral drugs for SARS-CoV infection have also been investigated for treating and preventing COVID-19 pneumonia. It seems that the most common concentration of ongoing clinical trials is on the repurposing of medications that has approval for other diseases into a COVID-19 disease treatment. Finally, among the literature, one novel perspective was recognized as an effective tool in the process of identifying new promising medications for the treatment of diseases generally. Furthermore, the need for designing and developing vaccines for SARS-CoV-2 cannot be ignored, moreover, developing new drugs and repurpose the previously used ones is of special concern. The establishment of animal models is one of the lessons extracted during the epidemics of SARS-CoV and MERS-CoV that should emphasize to retreat the various aspects of human disease as well as the safety and efficacy of the vaccine [123].

Interestingly, artificial intelligence is one of the fundamental suggestions that should be considered an effective method for early investigation of medications activity and safety in general and for COVID-19-related infections particularly. This technique can be used for both new medications design as well as for medication repurposing. Such applications are expected to introduce new medications with the adjusted estimation of safety and efficacy before any clinical trial. Through using different artificial intelligence techniques, several studies indicated mediations as potential treatments for COVID19 disease [124 - 126]. Within these studies, suggested medications include remdesivir, Atazanavir, Efavirenz, Grazoprevir, Ganciclovir, Daclatasvir, Simeprevir, Asunaprevir, Dolutegravir [126], while, other agents such as Carfilzomib, Valrubicin, LPV, Eravacycline, and Elbasvir as available medications for COVID19 disease based on computational drug repurposing study [125]. Some of the mentioned medications are involved in current clinical trials while others are still in the theoretical phase. In the literature, the most commonly promising COVID19 treatment based on clinical findings embraces Remdesivir [127], FPV [127], Chloroquine/Hydroxychloroquine, and Azithromycin combination [127]. Melatonin can also be considered as a promising treatment as adjuvant therapy [128]. Additionally, plasma from patients recovered from COVID-19 can be deemed as a potent medication as well [129].

CONCLUSION

Many studies have been published recently to address the possibilities of different antiviral drug repurposing and to develop new therapeutic agents to treat COVID-19. Every idea presented in these published studies revealed that two concepts are ideal, one is the repurposing of existing antiviral agents and the second is the design and development of multi-targeted drugs. This will provide a valid approach to the scientific community and hence will narrow the knowledge gap. The practical applications of such concepts will provide an opportunity to avail of new chemical entities that are most likely to be used in the fight against COVID-19.

CONSENT FOR PUBLICATION

Not Applicable.

CONFLICT OF INTEREST

The authors confirm that this chapter contents have no conflict of interest.

ACKNOWLEDGEMENT

Declared none.

REFERENCES

[1] Gorbalenya A, Baker S, Baric RS, Ziebuhr J. The species Severe acute respiratory syndrome- related coronavirus: classifying 2019-nCoV and naming it SARS-CoV-2 2019; (Box 1):

[2] Chen Y, Liu Q, Guo D. Emerging coronaviruses : Genome structure , replication , and pathogenesis 2020; (January): 23-418.

[3] Geier MR, Geier DA. Respiratory conditions in coronavirus disease 2019 (COVID-19): Important considerations regarding novel treatment strategies to reduce mortality. Med Hypotheses 2020; 140: 109760. [Internet]. [http://dx.doi.org/10.1016/j.mehy.2020.109760] [PMID: 32344310]

[4] WHO. https://www.who.int/ publications/i/item/clinical- management-of-severe-acute-respiratory-infection-when-novel-coronavirus-(ncov)- infection-is-suspected

[5] Centers for Disease Control and Prevention. https://www.cdc.gov/coronavirus/2019-ncov/hcp/clinica--guidance-management-patients.html

[6] Diagnosis and Treatment Protocol for COVID-19. https://www.chinadaily.com.cn/pdf/2020/1.Clinical.Protocols.for.the.Diagnosis.and.Treatment.of.COVID-19.V7.pdf

[7] Fragkou PC, Belhadi D, Moschopoulos CD, *et al.* Review of trials currently testing treatment and prevention of COVID-19. Clin Microbiol Infect 2020; 26(8): 988-98. [http://dx.doi.org/10.1016/j.cmi.2020.05.019]

[8] Vellingiri B, Jayaramayya K, Iyer M, *et al.* COVID-19: A promising cure for the global panic. Sci Total Environ 2020; 725: 138277. [Internet]. [http://dx.doi.org/10.1016/j.scitotenv.2020.138277] [PMID: 32278175]

[9] Scavone C, Brusco S, Bertini M, *et al.* Current pharmacological treatments for COVID-19: What's next? Br J Pharmacol 2020; 177(21): 4813-24.

[10] Sanders JM, Monogue ML, Jodlowski TZ, Cutrell JB. Pharmacologic Treatments for Coronavirus Disease 2019 (COVID-19): A Review. JAMA 2020; 323(18): 1824-36. [PMID: 32282022]

[11] Zhai P, Ding Y, Wu X, Long J, Zhong Y, Li Y. The epidemiology, diagnosis and treatment of COVID-19 2020. [http://dx.doi.org/10.1016/j.ijantimicag.2020.105955]

[12] Vijayvargiya P, Garrigos ZE, Almeida NEC, Gurram PR, Stevens RW, Razonable RR. Division of infectious diseases. Mayo Clin Proc 2020. [Internet]. [http://dx.doi.org/10.1016/j.mayocp.2020.04.027] [PMID: 32561148]

[13] Mehta N, Mazer-amirshahi M, Alkindi N, Pourmand A. Pharmacotherapy in COVID-19: A narrative review for emergency providers Am J Emerg Med 2020; 38(7): 1488-93.

[14] Neuman BW, Chamberlain P, Bowden F, Joseph J. Atlas of coronavirus replicase structure. Virus Res 2013; pp. 1-18. [http://dx.doi.org/10.1016/j.virusres.2013.12.004]

[15] Totura AL, Bavari S. Broad-spectrum coronavirus antiviral drug discovery. Expert Opin Drug Discov

2019; 14(4): 397-412.
[http://dx.doi.org/10.1080/17460441.2019.1581171] [PMID: 30849247]

[16] Brown AJ, Won JJ, Graham RL, *et al.* Broad spectrum antiviral remdesivir inhibits human endemic and zoonotic deltacoronaviruses with a highly divergent RNA dependent RNA polymerase. Antiviral Res 2019; 169(June): 104541.
[http://dx.doi.org/10.1016/j.antiviral.2019.104541] [PMID: 31233808]

[17] Kadam RU, Wilson IA. Structural basis of influenza virus fusion inhibition by the antiviral drug Arbidol. Proc Natl Acad Sci USA 2017; 114(2): 206-14.
[http://dx.doi.org/10.1073/pnas.1617020114] [PMID: 28003465]

[18] Villalaín J. Membranotropic effects of arbidol, a broad anti-viral molecule, on phospholipid model membranes. J Phys Chem B 2010; 114(25): 8544-54.
[http://dx.doi.org/10.1021/jp102619w] [PMID: 20527735]

[19] Furuta Y, Komeno T, Nakamura T. Favipiravir (T-705), a broad spectrum inhibitor of viral RNA polymerase. Proc Jpn Acad, Ser B, Phys Biol Sci 2017; 93(7): 449-63. https://www.ncbi.nlm.nih.gov/pmc/articles/PMC5713175/pdf/pjab-93-449
[http://dx.doi.org/10.2183/pjab.93.027] [PMID: 28769016]

[20] Aronson JK, Ed. Neuraminidase inhibitors.Meyler's Side Effects of Drugs: The International Encyclopedia of Adverse Drug Reactions and Interactions. 16th ed. Elsevier Science 2016; p. 7674.

[21] Martinez MA. Compounds with therapeutic potential against novel respiratory 2019 coronavirus. Antimicrob Agents Chemother 2020; 64(5): 1-7.
[http://dx.doi.org/10.1128/AAC.00399-20] [PMID: 32152082]

[22] Graci JD, Cameron CE. Mechanisms of action of ribavirin against distinct viruses. Rev Med Virol 2006; 16(1): 37-48.
[http://dx.doi.org/10.1002/rmv.483] [PMID: 16287208]

[23] De Clercq E. Anti-HIV drugs: 25 compounds approved within 25 years after the discovery of HIV. Int J Antimicrob Agents 2009; 33(4): 307-20.
[http://dx.doi.org/10.1016/j.ijantimicag.2008.10.010] [PMID: 19108994]

[24] 2020. Ritonavir (Norvir®) [Internet]. 2020 [cited 2020 Jul 8]. Available from: http://www.antimicrobe.org/drugpopup/ritonavir.htm

[25] Cap-dependent endonuclease inhibitor Baloxavir marboxil (Xofluza®) [Internet]. [cited 2020 Jul 8]. Available from: http://www.kansensho.or.jp/modules/en/index.php?content_id=2

[26] Wang M, Cao R, Zhang L, *et al.* Remdesivir and chloroquine effectively inhibit the recently emerged novel coronavirus (2019-nCoV) *in vitro*. Cell Res 2020; 30(3): 269-71.
[http://dx.doi.org/10.1038/s41422-020-0282-0] [PMID: 32020029]

[27] Savarino A, Di Trani L, Donatelli I, Cauda R, Cassone A. New insights into the antiviral effects of chloroquine. Lancet Infect Dis 2006; 6(2): 67-9.

[28] Liu J, Cao R, Xu M, Wang X, Zhang H, Hu H, *et al.* Hydroxychloroquine, a less toxic derivative of chloroquine, is effective in inhibiting SARS-CoV-2 infection *in vitro*. Cell Discov 2020; 6–9
[http://dx.doi.org/10.1038/s41421-020-0156-0]

[29] Lu H. Drug treatment options for the 2019-new coronavirus (2019-nCoV). Biosci Trends 2020; 14(1): 69-71.
[http://dx.doi.org/10.5582/bst.2020.01020] [PMID: 31996494]

[30] Hazafa A, Ur-Rahman K, Haq IU, *et al.* The broad-spectrum antiviral recommendations for drug discovery against COVID-19. Drug Metab Rev 2020; 52(3): 408-24.
[http://dx.doi.org/10.1080/03602532.2020.1770782] [PMID: 32546018]

[31] Siegel D, Hui HC, Doerffler E, *et al.* Discovery and synthesis of a phosphoramidate prodrug of a pyrrolo [2,1-f][triazin-4-amino] adenine C-nucleoside (GS-5734) for the treatment of ebola and

emerging viruses. J Med Chem 2017; 60(5): 1648-61.
[http://dx.doi.org/10.1021/acs.jmedchem.6b01594] [PMID: 28124907]

[32] Sheahan TP, Sims AC, Leist SR, *et al.* Comparative therapeutic efficacy of remdesivir and combination lopinavir, ritonavir, and interferon beta against MERS-CoV. Nat Commun 2020; 11(1): 222. [Internet].
[http://dx.doi.org/10.1038/s41467-019-13940-6] [PMID: 31924756]

[33] Holshue ML, DeBolt C, Lindquist S, *et al.* Washington State 2019-nCoV Case Investigation Team. First case of 2019 novel coronavirus in the United States. N Engl J Med 2020; 382(10): 929-36.
[http://dx.doi.org/10.1056/NEJMoa2001191] [PMID: 32004427]

[34] A trial of remdesivir in adults with mild and moderate COVID-19 [Internet]. Available from: https://clinicaltrials.gov/ct2/show/NCT04252664

[35] A trial of remdesivir in adults with severe COVID-19 [Internet]. Available from: https://clinicaltrials.gov/ct2/show/NCT04257656

[36] Grein J, Ohmagari N, Shin D, *et al.* Compassionate use of remdesivir for patients with severe COVID-19. N Engl J Med 2020; 382(24): 2327-36.
[http://dx.doi.org/10.1056/NEJMoa2007016] [PMID: 32275812]

[37] Jacobs M, Rodger A, Bell DJ, *et al.* Late Ebola virus relapse causing meningoencephalitis: a case report. Lancet 2016; 388(10043): 498-503. [Internet].
[http://dx.doi.org/10.1016/S0140-6736(16)30386-5] [PMID: 27209148]

[38] Kujawski S, Wong K, Collins J. First 12 patients with coronavirus disease 2019 (COVID-19) in the United States. J Chem Inf Model 2020; 53(9): 1689-99.

[39] de Wit E, Feldmann F, Cronin J, *et al.* Prophylactic and therapeutic remdesivir (GS-5734) treatment in the rhesus macaque model of MERS-CoV infection. Proc Natl Acad Sci USA 2020; 117(12): 6771-6.
[http://dx.doi.org/10.1073/pnas.1922083117] [PMID: 32054787]

[40] Srinivas P, Sacha GL, Koval C. Antivirals for COVID-19. Cleve Clin J Med 2020; 1-4.
[PMID: 32409433]

[41] Remdesivir becomes the first COVID-19 treatment approved in Europe. [Internet]. [cited 2020 Jul 11]. Available from: https://www.labiotech.eu/medical/covid-19-remdesivir-europe/

[42] Boriskin YS, Leneva IA, Pécheur E-I, Polyak SJ. Arbidol: a broad-spectrum antiviral compound that blocks viral fusion. Curr Med Chem 2008; 15(10): 997-1005.
[http://dx.doi.org/10.2174/092986708784049658] [PMID: 18393857]

[43] Pécheur E-I, Borisevich V, Halfmann P, *et al.* The synthetic antiviral drug arbidol inhibits globally prevalent pathogenic viruses. J Virol 2016; 90(6): 3086-92.
[http://dx.doi.org/10.1128/JVI.02077-15] [PMID: 26739045]

[44] Leneva IA, Russell RJ, Boriskin YS, Hay AJ. Characteristics of arbidol-resistant mutants of influenza virus: implications for the mechanism of anti-influenza action of arbidol. Antiviral Res 2009; 81(2): 132-40.
[http://dx.doi.org/10.1016/j.antiviral.2008.10.009] [PMID: 19028526]

[45] Blaising J, Polyak SJ, Pécheur EI. Arbidol as a broad-spectrum antiviral: an update. Antiviral Res 2014; 107(1): 84-94. [Internet].
[http://dx.doi.org/10.1016/j.antiviral.2014.04.006] [PMID: 24769245]

[46] Dong L, Hu S, Gao J. Discovering drugs to treat coronavirus disease 2019 (COVID-19). Drug Discov Ther 2020; 14(1): 58-60.
[http://dx.doi.org/10.5582/ddt.2020.01012] [PMID: 32147628]

[47] Wang Z, Yang B, Li Q, Wen L, Zhang R. Clinical Features of 69 Cases with Coronavirus Disease 2019 in Wuhan, China. Clin Infect Dis 2020; 71(215): 769-77.

[48] Lian N, Xie H, Lin S, Huang J, Zhao J, Lin Q. Umifenovir treatment is not associated with improved

outcomes in patients with coronavirus disease 2019: a retrospective study. Clin Microbiol Infect 2020; 26(7): 917-21. [Internet].
[http://dx.doi.org/10.1016/j.cmi.2020.04.026] [PMID: 32344167]

[49] De Clercq E. New nucleoside analogues for the treatment of hemorrhagic fever virus infections. Chem Asian J 2019; 14(22): 3962-8.
[http://dx.doi.org/10.1002/asia.201900841] [PMID: 31389664]

[50] Chen C, Huang J, Cheng Z, Wu J, Chen S, Zhang Y, *et al.* Favipiravir *versus* arbidol for COVID-19: a randomized clinical trial medRxiv 2020.
[http://dx.doi.org/10.1101/2020.03.17.20037432]

[51] Shiraki K, Daikoku T. Favipiravir, an anti-influenza drug against life-threatening RNA virus infections. Pharmacol Ther 2020; 209: 107512. [Internet].
[http://dx.doi.org/10.1016/j.pharmthera.2020.107512] [PMID: 32097670]

[52] Delang L, Abdelnabi R, Neyts J. Favipiravir as a potential countermeasure against neglected and emerging RNA viruses. Antiviral Res 2018; 153: 85-94.
[http://dx.doi.org/10.1016/j.antiviral.2018.03.003] [PMID: 29524445]

[53] McClellan K, Perry CM. Oseltamivir: a review of its use in influenza. Drugs 2001; 61(2): 263-83.
[http://dx.doi.org/10.2165/00003495-200161020-00011] [PMID: 11270942]

[54] Whitley RJ, Hayden FG, Reisinger KS, *et al.* Oral oseltamivir treatment of influenza in children. Pediatr Infect Dis J 2001; 20(2): 127-33.
[http://dx.doi.org/10.1097/00006454-200102000-00002] [PMID: 11224828]

[55] Adisasmito W, Chan PKS, Lee N, *et al.* Effectiveness of antiviral treatment in human influenza A(H5N1) infections: analysis of a global patient registry. J Infect Dis 2010; 202(8): 1154-60.
[http://dx.doi.org/10.1086/656316] [PMID: 20831384]

[56] Wang CB, Chiu ML, Lin PC, *et al.* Prompt oseltamivir therapy reduces medical care and mortality for patients with influenza infection. Medicine (Baltimore) 2015; 94(27): e1070.
[http://dx.doi.org/10.1097/MD.0000000000001070] [PMID: 26166080]

[57] Uyeki TM, Bernstein HH, Bradley JS, Englund JA, File T. Clinical practice guidelines by the infectious diseases society of America: 2018 update on diagnosis, treatment, chemoprophylaxis, and institutional outbreak management of seasonal influenzaa. Anesteziol a Intenziv Med 2019; 30(2): 97-8.

[58] Wang D, Hu B, Hu C, *et al.* Clinical characteristics of 138 hospitalized patients with 2019 novel coronavirus-infected pneumonia in Wuhan, China. JAMA 2020; 323(11): 1061-9.
[http://dx.doi.org/10.1001/jama.2020.1585] [PMID: 32031570]

[59] Li G, De Clercq E. Therapeutic options for the 2019 novel coronavirus (2019-nCoV). Nat Rev Drug Discov 2020; 19(3): 149-50. [Internet].
[http://dx.doi.org/10.1038/d41573-020-00016-0] [PMID: 32127666]

[60] Dutkowski R, Thakrar B, Froehlich E, Suter P, Oo C, Ward P. Safety and pharmacology of oseltamivir in clinical use 2003; 26(11): 787-801.

[61] Ning Q, Brown D, Parodo J, *et al.* Ribavirin inhibits viral-induced macrophage production of TNF, IL-1, the procoagulant fgl2 prothrombinase and preserves Th1 cytokine production but inhibits Th2 cytokine response. J Immunol 1998; 160(7): 3487-93.
[PMID: 9531310]

[62] Arabi YM, Mandourah Y, Al-Hameed F, *et al.* Saudi Critical Care Trial Group. Corticosteroid therapy for critically ill patients with middle east respiratory syndrome. Am J Respir Crit Care Med 2018; 197(6): 757-67.
[http://dx.doi.org/10.1164/rccm.201706-1172OC] [PMID: 29161116]

[63] Falzarano D, de Wit E, Rasmussen AL, *et al.* Treatment with interferon-α2b and ribavirin improves outcome in MERS-CoV-infected rhesus macaques. Nat Med 2013; 19(10): 1313-7.

[http://dx.doi.org/10.1038/nm.3362] [PMID: 24013700]

[64] KALETRA (lopinavir and ritonavir) tablet. 12/ 2019 [Internet]. Available from: https://www.accessdata.fda.gov/drugsatfda_docs/label/2019/%0A021251s058

[65] Hurst M, Faulds D. Lopinavir. Drugs 2000; 60(6): 1371-9. discussion 1380-1.

[66] Chu CM, Cheng VCC, Hung IFN, *et al.* Role of lopinavir/ritonavir in the treatment of SARS: initial virological and clinical findings. Thorax 2004; 59(3): 252-6. [http://dx.doi.org/10.1136/thorax.2003.012658] [PMID: 14985565]

[67] Chan KS, Lai ST, Chu CM, *et al.* Treatment of severe acute respiratory syndrome with lopinavir/ritonavir: a multicentre retrospective matched cohort study. Hong Kong Med J 2003; 9(6): 399-406. [PMID: 14660806]

[68] Yao TT, Qian JD, Zhu WY, Wang Y, Wang GQ. A systematic review of lopinavir therapy for SARS coronavirus and MERS coronavirus-A possible reference for coronavirus disease-19 treatment option. J Med Virol 2020; 92(6): 556-63. [http://dx.doi.org/10.1002/jmv.25729] [PMID: 32104907]

[69] Cao B, Wang Y, Wen D, *et al.* A trial of lopinavir-ritonavir in adults hospitalized with severe covid-19. N Engl J Med 2020; 382(19): 1787-99. [http://dx.doi.org/10.1056/NEJMoa2001282] [PMID: 32187464]

[70] Kim JY. Letter to the editor: Case of the index patient who caused tertiary transmission of coronavirus disease 2019 in Korea: The application of lopinavir/ritonavir for the treatment of COVID-19 pneumonia monitored by quantitative RT-PCR. J Korean Med Sci 2020; 35(7): 1-6.

[71] Deng L, Li C, Zeng Q, Liu X, Li X, Zhang H, *et al.* Arbidol combined with LPV/r *versus* LPV/r alone against corona virus disease 2019: A retrospective cohort study. J Infect 2020; 81(1): e1-5.

[72] Wu C, Chen X, Cai Y, *et al.* Risk factors associated with acute respiratory distress syndrome and death in patients with coronavirus disease 2019 pneumonia in Wuhan, China. JAMA Intern Med 2020; 180(7): 934-43. [http://dx.doi.org/10.1001/jamainternmed.2020.0994] [PMID: 32167524]

[73] ClinicalTrials.gov. [Internet]. [cited 2020 Jun 6]. Available from: https://clinicaltrials.gov/

[74] Chan JF, Yuan S, Kok KH, *et al.* A familial cluster of pneumonia associated with the 2019 novel coronavirus indicating person-to-person transmission: a study of a family cluster. Lancet 2020; 395(10223): 514-23. [http://dx.doi.org/10.1016/S0140-6736(20)30154-9] [PMID: 31986261]

[75] Lou Y, Liu L, Yao H, Hu X, Su J, Xu K, *et al.* Clinical Outcomes and Plasma Concentrations of Baloxavir Marboxil and Favipiravir in COVID-19 Patients: An Exploratory Randomized, Controlled Trial 2020.

[76] Rynes RI. Antimalarial drugs in the treatment of rheumatological diseases. 1996; 1997: 799-805.

[77] Schultz KR, Gilman AL. The lysosomotropic amines, chloroquine and hydroxychloroquine: a potentially novel therapy for graft-*versus*-host disease. 1997; 24(604): 10-201.

[78] Mauthe M, Orhon I, Rocchi C, *et al.* Chloroquine inhibits autophagic flux by decreasing autophagosome-lysosome fusion. Autophagy 2018; 14(8): 1435-55. [Internet]. [http://dx.doi.org/10.1080/15548627.2018.1474314] [PMID: 29940786]

[79] Sheahan TP, Sims AC, Graham RL, Menachery VD, Gralinski LE, Case JB, *et al.* Broad-spectrum antiviral GS-5734 inhibits both epidemic and zoonotic coronaviruses. Sci Transl Med 2017; 3(396): eaal3653. [http://dx.doi.org/10.1126/scitranslmed.aal3653]

[80] Tan YW, Yam WK, Sun J, Chu JJH. An evaluation of Chloroquine as a broad-acting antiviral against hand, foot and mouth disease. Antiviral Res 2018; 149(149): 143-9.

[http://dx.doi.org/10.1016/j.antiviral.2017.11.017] [PMID: 29175128]

[81] da Silva J, Mariz IHA, Junior L, de Oliveira P, Dantas A, Duarte A, *et al.* Hydroxychloroquine decreases Th17-related cyto- kines in systemic lupus erythematosus and rheuma- toid arthritis patients 2013; (8): 71-766.

[82] Cao X. COVID-19: immunopathology and its implications for therapy. Nat Rev Immunol 2019; 2019: 2019-20.
[http://dx.doi.org/10.1038/s41577-020-0308-3] [PMID: 32273594]

[83] Zhou P, Yang XL, Wang XG, *et al.* A pneumonia outbreak associated with a new coronavirus of probable bat origin. Nature 2020; 579(7798): 270-3.
[http://dx.doi.org/10.1038/s41586-020-2012-7] [PMID: 32015507]

[84] Colson P, Rolaine J-M, Lagier J-C, Brouqui P, Raoult D. Chloroquine and hydroxychloroquine as available weapons to fight COVID-19. Int J Antimicrob Agents 2020; 55(4): 105932.
[http://dx.doi.org/10.1016/j.ijantimicag.2020.105932]

[85] Yao X, Ye F, Zhang M, Cui C, Huang B, Niu P. *In Vitro* Antiviral Activity and Projection of Optimized Dosing Design of Hydroxychloroquine for the Treatment of Severe Acute Respiratory Syndrome Coronavirus 2 (SARS-CoV-2). Clin Infect Dis 2020; 71(15): 732-9.

[86] Juurlink D. Safety considerations with chloroquine, hydroxychloroquine and azithromycin in the management of SARS-CoV-2 infection. CMAJ 2020; 192(17): E450-3.
[http://dx.doi.org/10.1503/cmaj.200528]

[87] Borba M, Almeida Val F, Val A, Sampaio VS, Almeida M, Alexandre A, *et al.* Chloroquine diphosphate in two different dosages as adjunctive therapy of hospitalized patients with severe respiratory syndrome in the context of coronavirus (SARS-CoV-2) infection : Preliminary safety results of a randomized , double-blinded , phase I. 2020; 192(17): E450-3.

[88] Gao J, Tian Z, Yang X. Breakthrough: Chloroquine phosphate has shown apparent efficacy in treatment of COVID-19 associated pneumonia in clinical studies. Biosci Trends 2020; 14(1): 72-3.

[89] Chen Z, Hu J, Zhang Z, Jiang S, Han S, Yan D, *et al.* Efficacy of hydroxychloroquine in patients with COVID-19: results of a randomized clinical trial. 2020.
[http://dx.doi.org/10.1101/2020.03.22.20040758]

[90] Gotera C. Treatment and research lines for the patient with COVID-19. What do we have and where are we going? Int Braz J Uro 2020; 46(Suppl. 1): 125-32.

[91] Kalil AC. Treating COVID-19 — Off-Label Drug Use. Ther Adv Infect Dis. Compassionate Use, and Randomized Clinical Trials During Pandemics 2013; 1: pp. (5)155-65.

[92] Hancox JC, Hasnain M, Vieweg WVR, Crouse ELB, Baranchuk A. Azithromycin, cardiovascular risks, QTc interval prolongation, torsade de pointes, and regulatory issues: A narrative review based on the study of case reports. 2013; 66-155.

[93] Sperber K, Hom C, Chao CP, Shapiro D, Ash J. Systematic review of hydroxychloroquine use in pregnant patients with autoimmune diseases 2009.
[http://dx.doi.org/10.1186/1546-0096-7-9]

[94] Osadchy A, Ratnapalan T, Koren G, Osadchy A, Ratnapalan T, Koren G. Ocular toxicity in children exposed in utero to antimalarial drugs: review of the literature. J Rheumatol 2011; 38(12): 2504-8.
[http://dx.doi.org/10.3899/jrheum.110686] [PMID: 22002012]

[95] Johnson & Johnson Services I. Lack of evidence to support use of darunavir-based treatments for SARS-CoV-2. [cited 2020 May 6]. Available from: https://www.jnj.com/%0Alack-of-evidence-to-support-darunavir-based-hiv-treatments-forcoronavirus

[96] Bhimraj A, Morgan R, Shumaker A, Lavergne V, Baden L, Cheng VC, *et al.* Infectious Diseases Society of America Guidelines on the Treatment and Management of Patients with COVID-19. Clin Infect Dis 2020; ciaa478.

[97] Hung IF, Lung KC, Tso EY, *et al.* Triple combination of interferon beta-1b, lopinavir-ritonavir, and ribavirin in the treatment of patients admitted to hospital with COVID-19: an open-label, randomised, phase 2 trial. Lancet 2020; 395(10238): 1695-704. [Internet]. [http://dx.doi.org/10.1016/S0140-6736(20)31042-4] [PMID: 32401715]

[98] Rosa SGV, Santos WC. Clinical trials on drug repositioning for COVID-19 treatment. Rev Panam Salud Publica 2020; 44: e40. [http://dx.doi.org/10.26633/RPSP.2020.40] [PMID: 32256547]

[99] Zheng Y, Wang QY. Bioinformatics analysis on molecular mechanism of ribavirin and interferon-α in treating MERS-CoV. Zhonghua Liu Xing Bing Xue Za Zhi 2016; 37(2): 291-3. [PMID: 26917533]

[100] Foolad F, Aitken S, Shigle T, Prayag A, Ghantoji S, Ariza-Heredia E, *et al.* Oral *versus* aerosolized ribavirin for the treatment of respiratory syncytial virus infections in hematopoietic cell transplantation recipients. J Chem Inf Model 2018; 53(9): 1689-99.

[101] Stockman LJ, Bellamy R, Garner P. SARS: systematic review of treatment effects. PLoS Med 2006; 3(9): e343. [http://dx.doi.org/10.1371/journal.pmed.0030343] [PMID: 16968120]

[102] Morra ME, Van Thanh L, Kamel MG, *et al.* Clinical outcomes of current medical approaches for Middle East respiratory syndrome: A systematic review and meta-analysis. Rev Med Virol 2018; 28(3): e1977. [http://dx.doi.org/10.1002/rmv.1977] [PMID: 29664167]

[103] Arabi YM, Shalhoub S, Mandourah Y, *et al.* Ribavirin and interferon therapy for critically ill patients with middle east respiratory syndrome: a multicenter observational study. Clin Infect Dis 2020; 70(9): 1837-44. [http://dx.doi.org/10.1093/cid/ciz544] [PMID: 31925415]

[104] Altınbas S, Holmes JA, Altınbas A, Hepatitis C. Hepatitis c virus infection in pregnancy: an update. Gastroenterol Nurs 2020; 43(1): 12-21. [http://dx.doi.org/10.1097/SGA.0000000000000404] [PMID: 31990870]

[105] Velthuis AJW, Worm SHE, Van Den , *et al.* Zn2+ inhibits coronavirus and arterivirus RNA polymerase activity *In vitro* and zinc ionophores block the replication of these viruses in cell culture 2010; 6(11).

[106] Xue J, Moyer A, Peng B, Wu J, Hannafon BN, Ding W. Chloroquine is a zinc ionophore 2014; 9(10): 1-6.

[107] Gautret P, Lagier JC, Parola P, *et al.* Hydroxychloroquine and azithromycin as a treatment of COVID-19: results of an open-label non-randomized clinical trial. Int J Antimicrob Agents 2020; 56(1): 105949. [http://dx.doi.org/10.1016/j.ijantimicag.2020.105949] [PMID: 32205204]

[108] Molina JM, Delaugerre C, Le Goff J, *et al.* No evidence of rapid antiviral clearance or clinical benefit with the combination of hydroxychloroquine and azithromycin in patients with severe COVID-19 infection. Med Mal Infect 2020; 50(4): 384. [http://dx.doi.org/10.1016/j.medmal.2020.03.006] [PMID: 32240719]

[109] Huang L, Zhang L, Liu Y, Luo R, Zeng L, Telegina I, *et al.* Arbidol for preventing and treating influenza in adults and children (Protocol). 2017; (2): 2-5.

[110] Zhu Z, Lu Z, Xu T, Chen C, Yang G, Zha T, *et al.* Arbidol Monotherapy is Superior to Lopinavir/ritonavir in Treating COVID-19. J Infect 2020; 0-11. [http://dx.doi.org/10.1016/j.jinf.2020.03.060]

[111] Chinese Clinical Trial Registry. [cited 2020 May 11]. Available from: http://www.chictr.org.cn/enindex.aspx

[112] Li Y, Xie Z, Lin W, Cai W, Wen C, Guan Y, *et al.* Efficacy and safety of lopinavir/ritonavir or arbidol in adult patients with mild/moderate COVID-19: an exploratory randomized controlled trial. Med (N Y) 2020; 1(1): 105-13.
[http://dx.doi.org/10.1016/j.medj.2020.04.001]

[113] Rosenberg ES, Dufort EM, Udo T, Wilberschied LA, Kumar J, Tesoriero J, *et al.* Association of treatment with hydroxychloroquine or azithromycin with in-hospital mortality in patients with COVID-19 in New York State. 2020; 12203: 1-10.

[114] U.S. National Library of Medicine. http://ClinicalTrials.gov

[115] Mullard A. Flooded by the torrent: the COVID-19 drug pipeline. Lancet 2020; 395(10232): 1245-6. [Internet].
[http://dx.doi.org/10.1016/S0140-6736(20)30894-1] [PMID: 32305088]

[116] "Solidarity" clinical trial for COVID-19 treatments. [Internet]. [cited 2020 Apr 29]. Available from: www.who.int/emergencies/diseases/novel-coronavirus-2019/global-research-on-novel-coronavirus-2019-ncov/solidarity-clinical-trial-for-covid-19-treatments

[117] WHO. discontinues hydroxychloroquine and lopinavir/ritonavir treatment arms for COVID-19 [Internet]. [cited 2020 Jul 8]. Available from: https://www.who.int/news-room/detail/04-07-2020-who-discontinues-hydroxychloroquine-and-lopinavir -ritonavir-treatment-arms-for-covid-19mBio 2018; 9(5): e01753-18.

[118] Gralinski LE, Sheahan TP, Morrison TE, Menachery VD, Jensen K, Leist SR, *et al.* Complement activation contributes to severe acute respiratory syndrome coronavirus pathogenesis 2018; 9(5): 1-15.

[119] Alexion announces plans to initiate phase 3 study of ULTOMIRIS® (ravulizumab-cwvz) in hospitalized patients with severe COVID-19. [Internet]. [cited 2020 Apr 28]. Available from: https://ir.alexion.com/news-releases/news-release-details/alexion-announces-plans-initiate-phase-3-study-ultomirisr

[120] Duan K, Liu B, Li C, Zhang H, Yu T, Qu J, *et al.* Effectiveness of convalescent plasma therapy in severe COVID-19 patients. Proc Natl Acad Sci USA 2020; 117(17): 9490-6.
[http://dx.doi.org/10.1073/pnas.2004168117]

[121] Kiniksa announces early evidence of treatment response with mavrilimumab in 6 patients with severe COVID-19 pneumonia and hyperinflammation 2020.https://investors.kiniksa.com/news-releases/news-release-details/kiniksa-announces-early-evidence-treatment-response-mavrilimumab

[122] Gennaro F, Di , Pizzol D, *et al.* Coronavirus diseases (COVID-19) current status and future perspectives: a narrative review. Int J Environ Res Public Health 2012; 17(8): 2690.

[123] Li H, Liu S, Yu X, Tang S, Tang C. Coronavirus disease 2019 (COVID-19): current status and future perspectives 2020. January.

[124] Hu F, Jiang J, Yin P. Prediction of potential commercially inhibitors against SARS-CoV-2 by multi-task deep model. Data (Basel) 2020; 1-8.

[125] Wang J. Fast Identi fi cation of Possible Drug Treatment of Coronavirus Disease-19 (COVID-19) through Computational Drug Repurposing Study 2020.

[126] Beck BR, Shin B, Choi Y, Park S, Kang K. Predicting commercially available antiviral drugs that may act on the novel coronavirus (SARS-CoV-2) through a drug-target interaction deep learning model. Comput Struct Biotechnol J 2020; 18: 784-90. [Internet].
[http://dx.doi.org/10.1016/j.csbj.2020.03.025] [PMID: 32280433]

[127] Jean SS, Lee PI, Hsueh PR. Treatment options for COVID-19: The reality and challenges. J Microbiol Immunol Infect 2020; 53(3): 436-43.
[http://dx.doi.org/10.1016/j.jmii.2020.03.034] [PMID: 32307245]

[128] Zhang R, Wang X, Ni L, *et al.* COVID-19: Melatonin as a potential adjuvant treatment. Life Sci 2020; 250(February): 117583.

[http://dx.doi.org/10.1016/j.lfs.2020.117583] [PMID: 32217117]

[129] Saghazadeh A, Rezaei N. Towards treatment planning of COVID-19: Rationale and hypothesis for the use of multiple immunosuppressive agents: Anti-antibodies, immunoglobulins, and corticosteroids. Int Immunopharmacol 2020; 84(May): 106560. [http://dx.doi.org/10.1016/j.intimp.2020.106560] [PMID: 32413736]

CHAPTER 7

Phytochemicals Effective against COVID-19 and Future Perspective

Afshan Shafi[1], **Kashif Akram**[2], **Ismail Shah**[3] and **Fazlullah Khan**[4,*]

[1] *Department of Food Science and Technology, MNS University of Agriculture, Multan, Pakistan*

[2] *Department of Food Sciences, Faculty of Bio-Sciences, Cholistan University of Veterinary and Animal Sciences-Bahawalpur, Pakistan*

[3] *Department of Pharmacy, Garden Campus, Abdul Wali Khan University, Mardan, Pakistan*

[4] *Department of Allied Health Sciences, Bashir Institute of Health Sciences, Bharakahu, Islamabad, Pakistan*

Abstract: Novel coronavirus disease-19 (COVID-19) is the deadliest form of coronavirus, which has caused pandemics across the world. According to a recent survey of the World Health Organization (WHO), by August 8, 2020, shows around 19187943 cases and 716075 deaths from this virus globally. In addition to the shortage of effective drugs and vaccines, the outbreak of COVID-19 triggered by severe acute respiratory syndrome-coronavirus-2 (SARS-CoV-2) prompted the medical community to scramble for new antiviral formulations. Mankind utilizes the plants' origin medicines from ancient to treat and cure various diseases. They are the best possible tools to tackle the disease as they have the lowest possible side effects compared to other forms of drugs available and in use to treat the diseases. Several phytochemicals extracted from plants could provide a baseline for research into plant extracts in treating and preventing coronavirus. The present chapter aims to summarize phytochemicals' effectiveness against COVID-19.

Keywords: Antiviral, COVID-19, Inhibition mechanism, Phytochemicals, Phytoextracts activity.

INTRODUCTION

Novel coronavirus disease-19 (COVID-19) belongs to the family *Coronaviridae* and genus beta-coronavirus. An enveloped RNA virus has an average size from 60 nm to 140 nm in diameter and 79% identical to severe acute respiratory syndrome-coronavirus (SARS-CoV). Laboratory analysis of this virus showed that it is 88% identical to two SARS-like coronaviruses which are derived from

* **Corresponding author Fazlullah Khan:** Department of Allied Health Sciences, Bashir Institute of Health Sciences, Bharakahu, Islamabad, Pakistan; Tel: +92-3469433155; E-mail: fazlullahdr@gmail.com

Kamal Niaz & Muhammad Farrukh Nisar (Eds.)

the bat; (a) bat-SLCoVZXC21 and (b) bat-SL-CoVZC45, 50% identical to MERS-CoV (Middle East respiratory syndrome coronavirus) and 'its' similarity index to bat-CoV RaTG13 is 96.2% [1]. The novel coronavirus (nCoV-2019) or severe acute respiratory syndrome coronavirus-2 (SARS-CoV-2) was first reported in Wuhan (China), followed by a spread to other countries [2]. In December 2019, the first case was reported, then five patients were hospitalized with acute respiratory signs followed by the death of one of these patients [3]. The complete genome of a strain of SARS-CoV-2 (Wuhan-Hu-1-coronavirus WHCV) was first isolated and identified from a pneumonia patient in Wuhan. The size of the genome was 29.9 kb [4]. World Health Organization declared a public health emergency on January 30, 2020, of international concern for COVID-19 [5].

Novel COVID-19 has proved to be a highly deadly form of coronavirus that has special glycoprotein components on its surface that attach to the host body's immune complexes and leads to the arrest of the respiratory system of the host body. So far, there is no approved therapeutic drug or vaccine to combat coronavirus infection. As SARS-CoV-2 has created a global pandemic situation, the urgent discovery of novel antivirals is of utmost importance. Frequent mutations of the virus have made the discovery of vaccines a more challenging job for researchers [6]. Moreover, many vaccines are under trial, and researchers try their best to develop effective vaccines as soon as possible [7].

Globally, medicinal plants are used as alternative sources for the preparation of drugs. Several viral infections have long been treated using traditional medicinal plants that possess strong antiviral properties [8]. Secondary metabolites of medicinal plants (phytochemicals) pose beneficial health effects against viral infections. In many studies, the antiviral properties of phytochemicals such as glycosides, aliphatics, lactones, steroids, and alkaloids have been proved to cause beneficial health effects [9]. Plants have potential antiviral components, as found in flavonoids, coumarins, steroids, lignans, alkaloids, terpenes, and polyketides, *etc*[10]. Researchers have investigated luteolin-7-glucoside, kaempferol, catechin, quercetin, demethoxycurcumin, gingerol, apigenin-7-glucoside, naringenin, oleuropein, epicatechin gallate, zingerol, curcumin and allicin have inhibition activity against COVID-19 Table **1**. These phytochemicals ultimately lead to damage the cell membrane of this COVID-19, thus damaging its DNA components and composition and killing the virus. Another possibility is to develop phytocompounds which can damage the glycoprotein present on this COVID-19 coronavirus. Recent research on phytochemicals revealed that glycosides and flavonoids derived from garlic and Sena or *Salvia officinalis* could help develop specific phytochemicals that can damage the DNA gyrase SARS-CoV-2 [11]. From these all compounds such as catechin, kaempferol, epigallocatechin, quercetin, luteolin-7-glucoside, apigenin-7-glucoside, naringenin, demethoxycurcumin, curcumin, and oleuropein are the most suggested biological compounds extracted from medicinal plants that have inhibitory potential against COVID-19 Major protease (Mpro) [12], and their structure has been shown in Fig. (**1**). In the present chapter, the effectiveness of plant phytochemicals and possible antiviral therapies are highlighted, proving to be fruitful and effective to prevent and control this deadly disease.

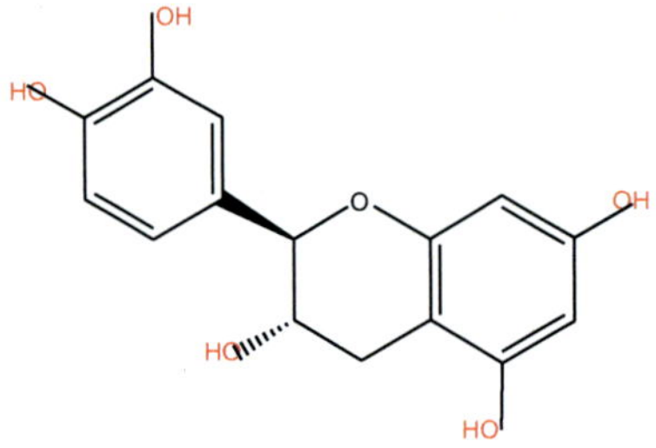

Catechin

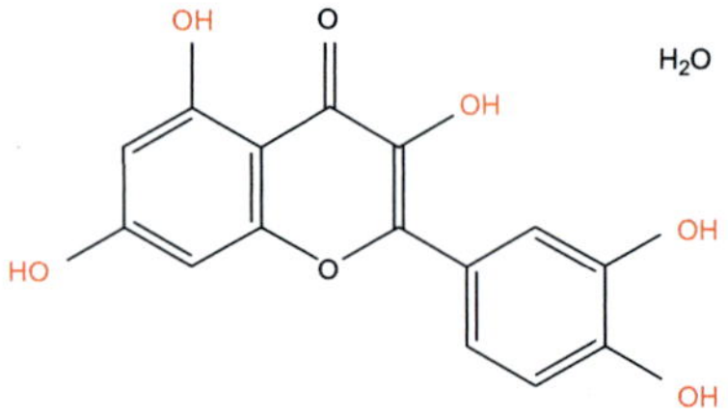

Quercetin

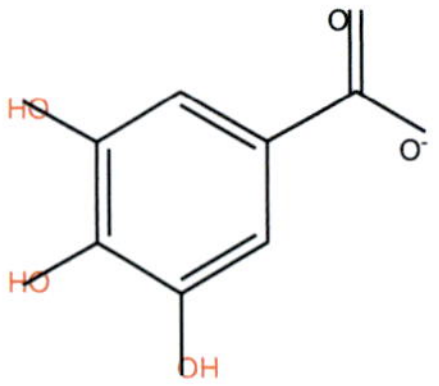

Gallate

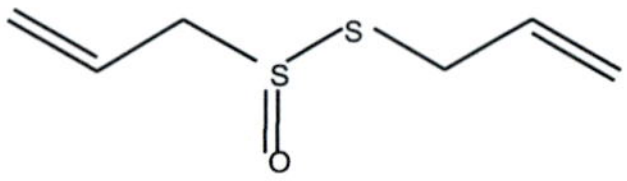

Allicin

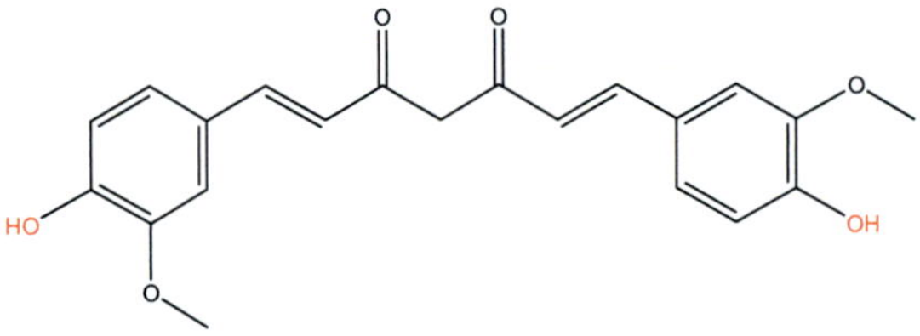

Curcumin

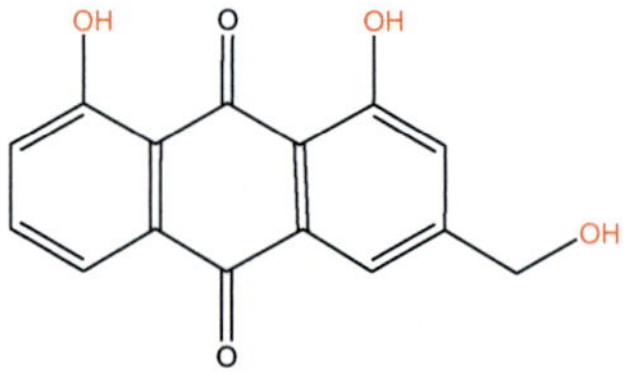

Aloe emodin

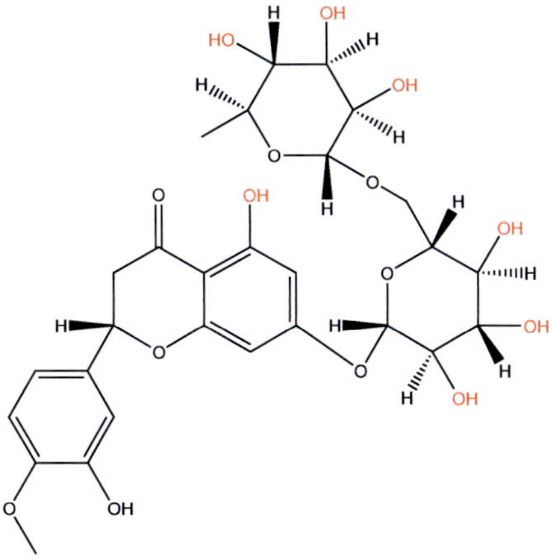

Hesperidin

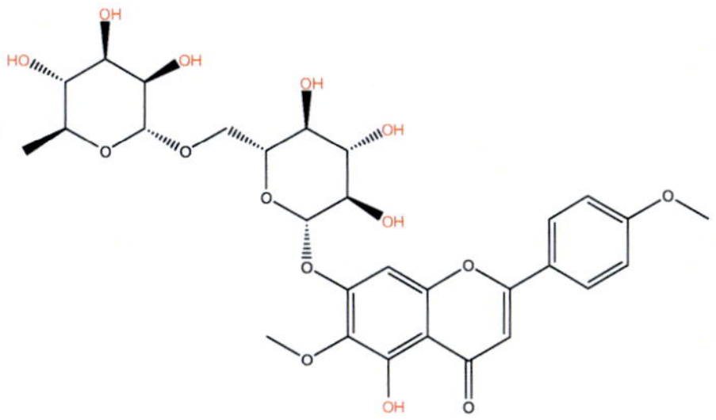

Pectolinarin

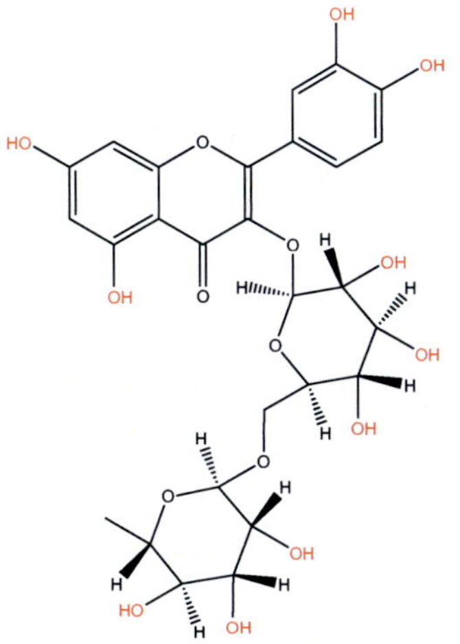

Rutin

Fig. (1). Structures of various compounds active in COVID-19.

Table 1. Active constituents, molecular formula, and mechanism of action in COVID-19.

Active Constituents	Molecular Formula	MOA	References
Epicatechin gallate	$C_{22}H_{18}O_{10}$	Interaction with Significant Protease catalytic residues	[13]
1,3,5-Trihydroxybenzene	$C_6H_6O_3$	Major protease (M^{pro}) inhibiters	[14]
Emodine	$C_{15}H_{10}O_5$	Spike protein and ACE2 inhibition	[15, 16]
Herbacetin	$C_{15}H_{10}O_7$	MERS -CoV protease inhibition	[17]
Catechin	$C_{15}H_{14}O_6$	inhibiting the cleavage of the viral polyprotein	[12]
Pectolinarin	$C_{29}H_{34}O_{15}$	SARS-CoV 3 carbon like protein inhibition	[17]

(Table 1) cont.....

Active Constituents	Molecular Formula	MOA	References
Curcumin	$C_{21}H_{20}O_6$	ACE 2 receptor inhibition	[10, 18]
Quercetin	$C_{15}H_{10}O_7$	Interaction with HA2	[19, 20]
Allicin	$C_6H_{10}OS_2$	ACE2 receptor inhibiter	[21]
Hesperidin	$C_{28}H_{34}O_{15}$	Major protein inhibiter	[22]

Various Phytochemicals Activities against COVID-19

Allicin (garlic compounds)

Most recent research on the antiviral potential of essential garlic oil against coronavirus demonstrated remarkable findings. The research also reported the inhibitory effect of garlic compounds against angiotensin-converting enzyme 2 (ACE2) proteins in the human body, leading to a crucial foundation for coronavirus resistance of individual compounds on the main protease (PDB6LU7) protein of SARS-CoV-2. The research outcomes demonstrated strong interaction with the amino acids of the ACE2 protein and the main protease PDB6LU7 of SARS-CoV-2. Study results concluded that garlic compounds' anti-coronavirus potential (allyl disulfide and allyl trisulfide) suggests that the essential garlic oil contributes to preventing the coronavirus's invasion into the human body [21]. The Anti-corona viral effect of garlic extract has been reported in research. The authors performed experimental trials on the chicken's embryonic stage. The study results expressed that garlic has a strong potential to inhibit the multiplication of coronavirus either through strengthening the immune responses or blocking the virus protein synthesis and genetic material [23].

Glycyrrhizin

The outbreak of SARS warrants the search for antiviral compounds to treat the disease. At present, no specific treatment has been identified for SARS-associated coronavirus infection. The antiviral potential of ribavirin, 6-azauridine, pyrazofurin, mycophenolic acid, and glycyrrhizin has been assessed against two clinical isolates of coronavirus (FFM-1 and FFM-2) from patients with SARS admitted to the clinical center of Frankfurt University, Germany. Of all the compounds, glycyrrhizin was the most active in inhibiting replication of the SARS-associated virus. The research findings suggest that glycyrrhizin should be assessed for the treatment of SARS [24].

Quercetin

The quercetin interferes with the dimer HA2 as well. The viral dimer HA2 is recognized as an antiviral vaccine base. In this way, quercetin interaction with

HA2 could present an antiviral effect. In addition, quercetin may inhibit virus entry [19]. Quercetin interferes with the S-protein S2 region with bonding energies of -8.5 kcal/mol. Quercetin creates hydrogen bonding with residues LEU 861, LYS 733, MET 731, PRO 1057, ALA 1056, SER 730, HIS 1058, and GLY 1059 and have hydrophobic interactions with ASP 867, ILE 870, PRO 863, MET 730, and VAL 860. Quercetin prevents the growth of tumor necrosis factor (TNF-) and IL-8 in cells [25].

Flavonoids

Catechin

Gallocatechin gallate and Catechin gallate are known as a type of catechin. Gallocatechin gallate and catechin gallates are the most abundant catechins, particularly in tea (especially green tea) and other plants, and they have antioxidant activity. This study revealed that the use of catechin and curcumin having significant antiviral properties (Table **2**). Infection of the virus may be treated with the use of catechin and curcumin. They are also known as inhibitory machinery because of blocking the entry of viral protein and receptors of the host cell to the virus [26].

Curcumin

Curcumin is a major constituent of turmeric, was already characterized to present increased anti-viral properties against a wide range of viruses, including Zika and chikungunya virus, dengue virus (serotype 2), HIV, herpes simplex virus. Curcumin attaches to the S1 region of the C-terminal of the S-protein through binding energy of -7.1 Kcal/mol in the prevention of coronavirus. This attachment quite likely inhibits the virus from bonding to ACE or internalizing throughout fusion. Reduced binding energy indicates a strong affinity of the ligand to the receptor. Curcumin forms H-bonding with amino acid residues like ASN 544, GLN 564, and ALA 520, and hydrophobic interactions exist with LEU 517, LEU 390, PHE 565, VAL 382, and THR 430 on the S1 domain [25]. Curcumin was shown to impede NF-B stimulation enhanced by numerous inflammatory impulses, including certain markers of inflammation (oxidized CD40 ligand, sCD40L), interleukin 6, solubilized vascular cell adhesion molecule 1 (sVCAM-1), and interleukin 1 beta [19].

Table 2. Phytochemicals with their antiviral effects.

Compound	Source/preparation Method	Effect	Reference
Catechin	Docking Method	inhibiting cleavage of the viral polyprotein	[12]

(Table 2) cont.....

Compound	Source/preparation Method	Effect	Reference
Catechin	Molecular docking analysis	blocking host cell receptor to virus	[27]

Miscellaneous Phytochemicals against COVID-19

Carvacrol, Oleanolic Acid and Ursolic Acid

The effect of natural polyphenols against COVID-19 while working on Potent COVID-19 Mpro Inhibitors from Natural Polyphenols: An *in-silico*f Strategy Unveils a Hope against CORONA has been studied. It has been found that phytochemicals hesperidin, rutin, diosmin, apiin, diacetyl curcumin, (E)-1--2-Hydroxy-4-methoxyphenyl)-3-[3-[(E)-3-(2-hydroxy-4- methoxyphenyl)---oxoprop-1-enyl]phenyl]prop-2 -en-1-one, and beta,beta'-(4-Methoxy-1,3-phenylene)bis(2'- hydroxy- 4',6'-dimethoxyac rylophenone have strong potential against COVID-19. The Mpro protein is seen to be an essential and fast-acting substrate for innovative COVID-19 inhibitors. The residues of amino acids have been involved in hydrophobic interactions between proteolytic enzymes and ligand molecules. Intermolecular interaction (hydrogen bonds and hydrophobic interactions) plays a crucial role in forming and sustaining the complexes at docking [22].

Gly143 amino acid was accused of developing a hydrogen bond with carvacrol (the major constituent of oregano and thyme) through Auto-Dock bonding energy 4.0 kcal/mol. Additionally, 6 more residues (Leu27, Met49, Met165, Asn142, His41, and Cys145) participated in hydrophobic interactions (d).

Oleanolic acid participated in docking with bonding energy of 6.0 kcal/mol. 2 amino acid residues exhibit (Cys145, His163) hydrophobic bonding whereas Gln189 forms hydrogen bonding (c) Bonding energy for ursolic acid was found to be 5.9 kcal/mol. The Ser46 makes hydrogen bonding at the active site of the protease. 9 amino acids (Thr24, Thr26, Asn142, Cys44, Thr25, Gly143, Glu166, Cys145, and Thr45) are involved in the van der Waals interactions (e) [28].

Catechin Quercetin
Gallate Allicin
Curcumin Aloe emodin
Hesperidin Pectolinarin
Rutin

Mechanism of Phytochemicals in Altering SARS-CoV-2 Infection

The treatment therapies against infection caused by SARS-CoV-2 can target and alter different pathways, including (a) Inhibition of structural proteins to bind with ACE2, which blocks its' entry into the host cell, and (b) Altering enzymes that are involved in RNA synthesis and viral replication. Advanced approaches in biology and bioinformatics help to estimate the treatment potential of phytochemicals against viral infections. These approaches also make drug development speedy, economical, safer, and reliable. Drug targets against viral infections are enzymes and receptors involved in the entry and development of SARS-CoV-2 in the host cells [29].

a. Inhibition of Spike Proteins to Bind with Angiotensin-converting Enzyme 2 (ACE2)

Four structural proteins of the coronavirus are; nucleocapsid protein (N), membrane protein (M), envelop protein (E), and spike protein (S) [30]. Spike proteins of SARS-CoV-2 play a crucial role in the entry of virus in host cells because these proteins attach with cell receptor ACE2 [31], diagrammatically showed in Fig. (**2**). In designing drugs against viral infections, both non-structural proteins and structural proteins play a crucial role. Recent studies have shown that ACE2 assists the entry of viruses into the host cells by viral binding spike (S) protein [32]. At the early stages of infection, the perfect drug target is spike protein involved in the entry of the virus into host cells. In RBD (Receptor binding domain), ACE2 binds with receptor binding motif (RBM) of spike protein and acts as a receptor of SARS-CoV-2 [33]. In host cells, the binding of ACE2 receptor with spike (S) protein of virus can be inhibited by different inhibitors. The drug nafamostat mesylate (Fusan) used against pancreatitis, has also shown inhibition properties that inhibit entry of MERS-SARS viruses in the host cells [34].

b. Inhibition of Viral Replication

In different viral infections such as Hepatitis C virus (HCV) and Human immunodeficiency virus (HIV), viral proteases have shown to be actual targets of antiviral therapies. Viral replication can be inhibited by targeting proteases that are involved in the replication. The main protease (M^{pro}, also called $3CL^{pro}$) is the best drug target to inhibit replication among coronaviruses [35]. There is a 96% similarity in the protein sequence of SARS-CoV-M^{pro} and SARS-CoV-2-M^{pro} [36]. In the life cycle of the virus, the functional significance of M^{pro} and the lack of similar homologs in humans make it an effective target in designing a drug against viral infection. Examples of protease inhibitors that are being used to treat COVID-19 infection are lopinavir-ritonavir combinations [37]. RNA replication is carried out by RdRp (RNA-dependent RNA-polymerase), which is another effective target in developing antiviral therapeutics.

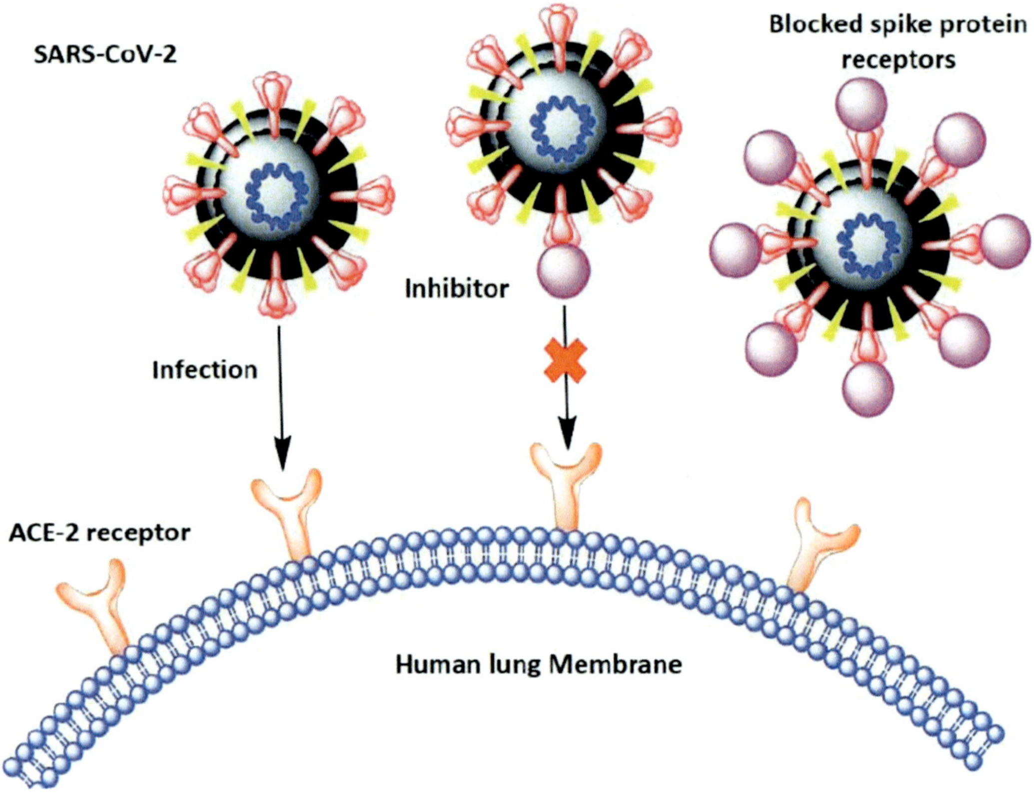

Fig. (2). Binding of Spike protein with ACE2 receptor. The figure illustrates that SARS-CoV-2 comprises four structural proteins, among which spike protein can bind with the ACE2 receptor on the host cell's surface. After binding with receptor hijacking of host cell machinery is carried out by the virus.

Plant Extracts and their Possible Anti-Viral Activities in COVID-19

Due to the lack of conventional therapeutic agents (vaccines, antibiotics) for COVID-19, broad-spectrum antibiotics along with antivirals and corticosteroids are in general use [13]. The WHO, US Food and Drug Administration (FDA), European Medicines Agency, and the Chinese Government and drug manufacturers are coordinating with scientists and industrials to speed up the development of new drugs for COVID-19 [38]. Natural products have high potentials in the treatment of viral infections [39]. Medicinal plants are used to be effective against SARS-CoV-2 with assorted secondary metabolites. Many can interrupt viral protein and enzymatic activities and stop viral penetration into host cells and (or) its replication [40]. Phytochemicals such as quercetin, catechin, and curcumin act to inhibit ACE2, demethylation of the gene, and histone modification (Fig. **3**).

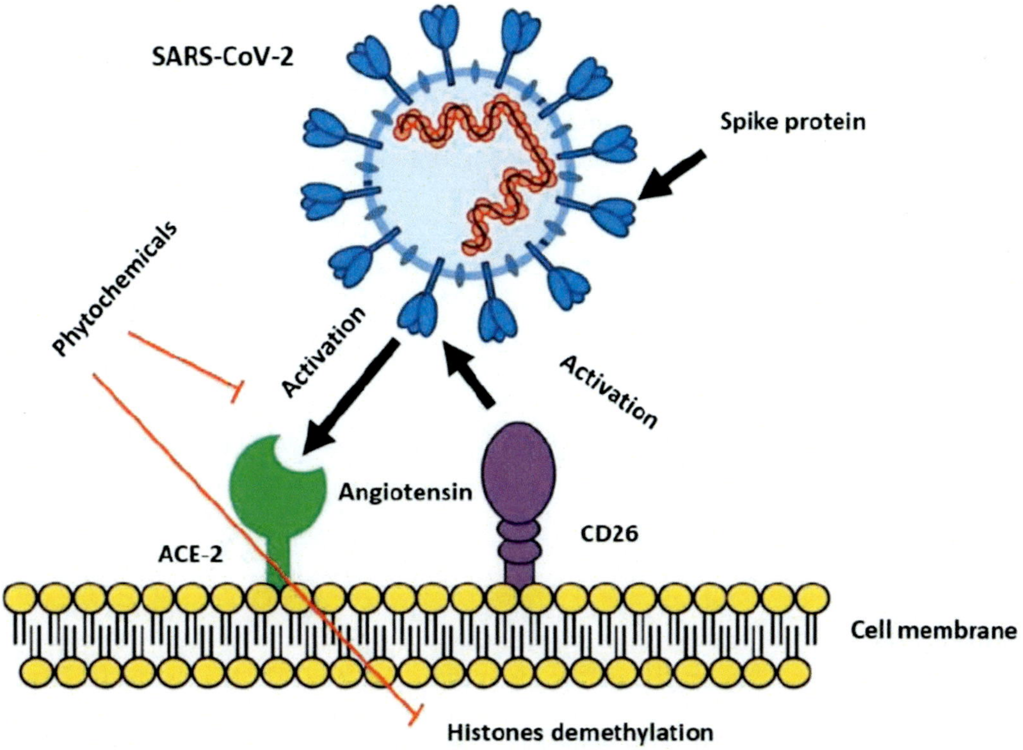

Fig. (3). Mechanism of action of phytochemicals against SARS-CoV-2.

Many medicinal plants have been testified to possess anti-coronaviral activity. *Platycodon grandiflorum*, a medicinal plant, has been tested scientifically on the PRRSV virus, and the result has been shown to inhibit viral replication and expression of pro-inflammatory cytokine [41]. *Reseda luteola,* another plant that has inhibited the entry of SARS-CoV, has a great attraction for S2 protein, thus interfering with the process of virus-cell fusion [42]. Medicinal plants can prevent replication of viruses are often preferred as favorable options against viral outbreaks. Thus, *Glycyrrhiza glabra* induces nitrous oxide synthase, which blocks viral replication in SARS-CoV [43]. *Clerodendrum inerme* Gaertn inactivates viral ribosome and protein translation of SARS-CoV 2 [44]. *Strobilanthes cusia* targets the HCoVs and inhibits RNA genome formation [45]. Similarly, *Anthemis hyaline* decreases gene expression of transient receptor potential proteins (TRP's) in coronavirus [46]. *Camellia japonica,* affects key structural protein synthesis in

PEDV coronavirus, thus blocking viral replication [47]. *Isatis indigotica*, inhibits viral cleavage activity in SARS-CoV [48]. *Vitis vinifera* reduces nucleocapsid (N) protein expression, also reduces MERS-CoV virus-induced apoptosis [49]. *Rosmarinus officinalis* blocks replication of the human respiratory syncytial (hRSV) virus [50]. Similarly, *Cedrela sinensis* inhibits SARS-CoV replication [51]. *Clerodendrum inerme* inactivates SARS-CoV-2 virus [52], and *Clitoria ternatea* inhibits metalloproteinase of SARS-CoV-2 [53]. *Coriandrum sativum* and *Embelia ribes* both inhibit ACE2 in SARS-CoV-2 [54]. Similarly, *Hyoscyamus niger* inhibits Ca2+ channels and acts as a bronchodilator in SARS-CoV-2 [55], and *Vitex trifolia* inhibits virus in SARS-CoV-2 [56]. Similarly, herbal extracts from *Dioscoreae rhizoma*, *Gentianae radix*, *Cassiae semen*, *Rhizoma cibotii*, and *Loranthi ramus* have a potential inhibitory effect SARS-CoV. Plant extracts (*Artemisia annua, Lycoris radiata, Lindera aggregate,* and *Pyrrosia lingua*) have resulted in the antiviral activity of SARS-CoV. Similarly, *Sanguisorbae radix, Sophorae radix,* and *Torilis fructus* extracts have antiviral effect and *Coptidis rhizome*, Meliae bark, Phellodendron bark extracts and Cimicifuga rhizomes have an effect on replication of coronavirus [57].

Many other plant extracts have an inhibitory role against HIV infections. They can also serve as favorable candidates in the development of the COVID-19 drug. *Eugenia jambolana* [58], *Acacia nilotica,* and *Euphorbia granulate* [59] are among these plants. Other plants like *Vitex negundo* [60] *Ocimum sanctum* [61], and *Solanum nigrum* [62] can target reverse transcriptase activity of HIV can also serve as favorable candidates in the development of COVID-19 drug. During pandemics, appropriateness is the basic requirement for developing any drug. Thus natural products can serve as proper and potential options as their safety is well-known. So it can be promptly assessed for combating patients.

FUTURE PERSPECTIVE OF PHYTOCHEMICALS IN COVID-19

Phytochemicals derived from plants such as *Allium sativum*, *Salvia officinalis,* and *Ficus racemose*, can help develop specific composition compounds that can ultimately damage DNA gyrase of SARS-CoV-2. Antiviral drug available which can kill the virus specifically are also the possible remedies for treating this deadly coronavirus. Plant medicines as antiviral therapy are also the best possible resources to arrest coronavirus spread from humans to humans. To stop the spread of this deadly coronavirus, using an alcoholic-based disinfectant would be beneficial to wipe out the risk of any possible infection chances.

Inside the body, the best way to stop the infection is to develop a medicine that will ultimately protect the host body's immune system from forming complexes with the SARS-CoV-2 glycoprotein, which further leads to the arrest of the respiratory system.

We need to develop a phytochemical component that makes the immune system flexible and strong to stop developing its complexes with viral glycoprotein. Using quantum computing technology, we can help develop unique components and compounds that make our immune system strong and have deadly environment development for the virus to survive inside the host body [63].

Phytochemicals can act as antioxidants, specific enzyme inhibitors, and protein receptors all over the virus's surface that blocks interactions. Specific medicinal plants with a broad range of biological activity can be used to source phytochemicals (polyphenols, sterols, and lipids). These substances offer hope that extracts from various plants described in this chapter may have antiviral effects, even against the family of coronaviruses. Awareness of their healing uses and application has been passed on from one generation to another. The new advances in biotechnology and medicine have made it possible to use substances of natural origin to a greater degree than in the preceding decades, often as nutritional supplements and nutraceuticals. A multidisciplinary approach (omics science-genomics, proteomics, metabolomics) has yet to examine their toxicity along with the processing period. New processing and formulating technologies may also help improve the solubility of bioactive antiviral compounds, their delivery strategies, and therapeutic activities, adapting these as useful antiviral foods and drugs. This way, the chances of developing better and speedy remedies to treat this deadly coronavirus will be possible, and we could stop this pandemic here itself.

CONCLUSION

COVID-19 is a severe respiratory infectious disease caused by a novel virus strain. The Coronavirus Study Group; taxonomists, working under the aegis of International Committee on Taxonomy of Viruses (ICTV), coined the nomenclature of SARS-COV-2 based on 82% identity to the SARS-CoV genome. This infectious disease has directed over 4,098,018 confirmed cases and 283,271 fatalities untill May 12, 2020. The number of cases across the globe is growing tersely. So far, no usual drug has proved to be effective for COVID-19 disease that has a high mortality rate, especially in immune-compromised patients. Nowadays, research and development programs are incessantly adopting methods focusing on plant-based products to develop drugs. There are several classes of phytochemicals, which are used as antiviral agents. These include phenolics, carotenoids, terpenoids, and alkaloids. The family of phenolics contains various subclasses, such as phenolic acids, flavonoids, stilbenes, coumarins, and tannins.

These viruses have either DNA or RNA as genetic material. Thus, phytochemicals exhibit a different mode of action against any infection or disease. Viral attachment can be inhibited by either blocking the viral binding sites or host receptors. The virus can be inhibited at various stages of its infection. Some of the strategies directly inhibit viral replication by targeting DNA/RNA polymerase, post-translation modification of viral proteins, or viral assembly. Phytochemicals have adopted several mechanisms to inhibit viral replication. For instance, epigallocatechin gallate (EGCG) inactivates the host enzyme or viral enzyme that promotes the virus's growth, such as RNA polymerase, protease, and reverse transcriptase. Another mechanism adopted by flavonoids is to inhibit phosphorylation of the protein, which restricts the replication of viruses.

CONSENT FOR PUBLICATION

Not Applicable.

CONFLICT OF INTEREST

The authors confirm that this chapter contents have no conflict of interest.

ACKNOWLEDGEMENT

Declared none.

REFERENCES

[1] Guo Y-R, Cao Q-D, Hong Z-S, *et al.* The origin, transmission and clinical therapies on coronavirus disease 2019 (COVID-19) outbreak–an update on the status. Mil Med Res 2020; 7(1): 1-10. [PMID: 31928528]

[2] Halaji M, Farahani A, Ranjbar R, Heiat M, Dehkordi FS. Emerging coronaviruses: first SARS, second MERS and third SARS-CoV-2: epidemiological updates of COVID-19. Infez Med 2020; 28 (Suppl. 1): 6-17. [PMID: 32532933]

[3] Singhal T. A review of coronavirus disease-2019 (COVID-19). Indian J Pediatr 2020; 87(4): 281-6. [PMID: 32166607]

[4] Wu F, Zhao S, Yu B, *et al.* A new coronavirus associated with human respiratory disease in China. Nature 2020; 579(7798): 265-9. [PMID: 32015508]

[5] Wu JT, Leung K, Leung GM. Nowcasting and forecasting the potential domestic and international spread of the 2019-nCoV outbreak originating in Wuhan, China: a modelling study. Lancet 2020; 395(10225): 689-97. [PMID: 32014114]

[6] Zhang L, Shen FM, Chen F, Lin Z. Origin and evolution of the 2019 novel coronavirus. Clin Infect Dis 2020; 71(15): 882-3. [PMID: 32011673]

[7] Amanat F, Krammer F. SARS-CoV-2 vaccines: status report. Immunity 2020; 52(4): 583-9. [PMID: 32259480]

[8] Dhama K, Karthik K, Khandia R, *et al.* Medicinal and therapeutic potential of herbs and plant metabolites/extracts countering viral pathogens-current knowledge and future prospects. Curr Drug Metab 2018; 19(3): 236-63.
[PMID: 29380697]

[9] Chikezie PC, Ibegbulem CO, Mbagwu FN. Bioactive principles from medicinal plants. Res J Phytochem 2015; 9(3): 88-115.

[10] Pandey P, Rane JS, Chatterjee A, *et al.* Targeting SARS-CoV-2 spike protein of COVID-19 with naturally occurring phytochemicals: an *in silico* study for drug development. J Biomol Struct Dyn 2020; 1-11.
[PMID: 32698689]

[11] Jo S, Kim S, Shin DH, Kim M-S. Inhibition of SARS-CoV 3CL protease by flavonoids. J Enzyme Inhib Med Chem 2020; 35(1): 145-51.
[PMID: 31724441]

[12] Khaerunnisa S, Kurniawan H, Awaluddin R, Suhartati S, Soetjipto S. Potential inhibitor of COVID-19 main protease (Mpro) from several medicinal plant compounds by molecular docking study. Prepr 2020; 20944: 1-14.

[13] Chojnacka K, Witek-Krowiak A, Skrzypczak D, Mikula K, Młynarz P. Phytochemicals containing biologically active polyphenols as an effective agent against Covid-19-inducing coronavirus. J Funct Foods 2020; 73: 104146.
[PMID: 32834835]

[14] Gentile D, Patamia V, Scala A, Sciortino MT, Piperno A, Rescifina A. Putative inhibitors of SARS-CoV-2 main protease from a library of marine natural products: A virtual screening and molecular modeling study. Mar Drugs 2020; 18(4): 225.
[PMID: 32340389]

[15] Ho T-Y, Wu S-L, Chen J-C, Li C-C, Hsiang C-Y. Emodin blocks the SARS coronavirus spike protein and angiotensin-converting enzyme 2 interaction. Antiviral Res 2007; 74(2): 92-101.
[PMID: 16730806]

[16] Schwarz S, Wang K, Yu W, Sun B, Schwarz W. Emodin inhibits current through SARS-associated coronavirus 3a protein. Antiviral Res 2011; 90(1): 64-9.
[PMID: 21356245]

[17] Jo S, Kim H, Kim S, Shin DH, Kim MS. Characteristics of flavonoids as potent MERS-CoV 3C-like protease inhibitors. Chem Biol Drug Des 2019; 94(6): 2023-30.
[PMID: 31436895]

[18] Azim KF, Ahmed SR, Banik A, Khan MMR, Deb A, Somana SR. Screening and druggability analysis of some plant metabolites against SARS-CoV-2: An integrative computational approach. Informatics in Medicine Unlocked 2020; p. 100367.

[19] Haslberger A, Jacob U, Hippe B, Karlic H. Mechanisms of selected functional foods against viral infections with a view on COVID-19: Mini review. Funct Food Health Dis 2020; 10(5): 195-209.

[20] Wu W, Li R, Li X, *et al.* Quercetin as an antiviral agent inhibits influenza A virus (IAV) entry. Viruses 2015; 8(1): 6.
[PMID: 26712783]

[21] Thuy BTP, My TTA, Hai NTT, *et al.* Investigation into SARS-CoV-2 resistance of compounds in garlic essential oil. ACS Omega 2020; 5(14): 8312-20.
[PMID: 32363255]

[22] Adem S, Eyupoglu V, Sarfraz I, Rasul A, Ali M. Identification of potent COVID-19 main protease (Mpro) inhibitors from natural polyphenols: An *in silico* strategy unveils a hope against CORONA. 2020.

[23] Mohajer Shojai T, Ghalyanchi Langeroudi A, Karimi V, Barin A, Sadri N. The effect of *Allium sativum* (Garlic) extract on infectious bronchitis virus in specific pathogen free embryonic egg. Avicenna J Phytomed 2016; 6(4): 458-267.
[PMID: 27516987]

[24] Cinatl J, Morgenstern B, Bauer G, Chandra P, Rabenau H, Doerr HW. Glycyrrhizin, an active component of liquorice roots, and replication of SARS-associated coronavirus. Lancet 2003; 361(9374): 2045-6.
[PMID: 12814717]

[25] Rane JS, Chatterjee A, Kumar A, Ray S. ChemRxiv 2020.

[26] Jena AB, Kanungo N, Nayak V, Chainy G, Dandapat J. Catechin and Curcumin interact with corona (2019-nCoV/SARS-CoV2) viral S protein and ACE2 of human cell membrane: insights from Computational study and implication for intervention 2020.

[27] Dandapat J, Jena A, Kanungo N, Nayak V, Chainy G. Catechin and Curcumin interact with corona (2019-nCoV/SARS-CoV2) viral S protein and ACE2 of human cell membrane: insights from Computational study and implication for intervention 2020.

[28] Kumar A, Choudhir G, Shukla SK, *et al.* Identification of phytochemical inhibitors against main protease of COVID-19 using molecular modeling approaches. J Biomol Structure and Dynamics 2020; (just-accepted): 1-21.

[29] Jin Z, Du X, Xu Y, *et al.* Structure-based drug design, virtual screening and high-throughput screening rapidly identify antiviral leads targeting COVID-19 BioRxiv 2020.

[30] Cui J, Li F, Shi Z-L. Origin and evolution of pathogenic coronaviruses. Nat Rev Microbiol 2019; 17(3): 181-92.
[PMID: 30531947]

[31] Wu A, Peng Y, Huang B, *et al.* Genome composition and divergence of the novel coronavirus (2019-nCoV) originating in China. Cell Host Microbe 2020; 27(3): 325-8.
[PMID: 32035028]

[32] Li W, Moore MJ, Vasilieva N, *et al.* Angiotensin-converting enzyme 2 is a functional receptor for the SARS coronavirus. Nature 2003; 426(6965): 450-4.
[PMID: 14647384]

[33] Tai W, He L, Zhang X, *et al.* Characterization of the receptor-binding domain (RBD) of 2019 novel coronavirus: implication for development of RBD protein as a viral attachment inhibitor and vaccine. Cell Mol Immunol 2020; 17(6): 613-20.
[PMID: 32203189]

[34] Elfiky AA. Zika viral polymerase inhibition using anti-HCV drugs both in market and under clinical trials. J Med Virol 2016; 88(12): 2044-51.
[PMID: 27604059]

[35] Anand K, Ziebuhr J, Wadhwani P, Mesters JR, Hilgenfeld R. Coronavirus main proteinase (3CLpro) structure: basis for design of anti-SARS drugs. Science 2003; 300(5626): 1763-7.
[PMID: 12746549]

[36] Liu X, Wang X-J. Potential inhibitors against 2019-nCoV coronavirus M protease from clinically approved medicines. J Genet Genomics 2020; 47(2): 119-21.
[PMID: 32173287]

[37] Lim J, Jeon S, Shin H-Y, *et al.* Case of the index patient who caused tertiary transmission of COVID-19 infection in Korea: the application of lopinavir/ritonavir for the treatment of COVID-19 infected pneumonia monitored by quantitative RT-PCR. J Korean Med Sci 2020; 35(6): e79.
[PMID: 32056407]

[38] Huang C, Wang Y, Li X, *et al.* Clinical features of patients infected with 2019 novel coronavirus in

Wuhan, China. Lancet 2020; 395(10223): 497-506.
[PMID: 31986264]

[39] Denaro M, Smeriglio A, Barreca D, *et al.* Antiviral activity of plants and their isolated bioactive compounds: An update. Phytother Res 2020; 34(4): 742-68.
[PMID: 31858645]

[40] Akram M, Tahir IM, Shah SMA, *et al.* Antiviral potential of medicinal plants against HIV, HSV, influenza, hepatitis, and coxsackievirus: A systematic review. Phytother Res 2018; 32(5): 811-22.
[PMID: 29356205]

[41] Nair R. HIV-1 reverse transcriptase inhibition by Vitex negundo L. leaf extract and quantification of flavonoids in relation to anti-HIV activity. Journal of Cell and Molecular Biology 2012; 10(2): 53-9.

[42] Zhang M, Du T, Long F, *et al.* Platycodin D suppresses type 2 porcine reproductive and respiratory syndrome virus in primary and established cell lines. Viruses 2018; 10(11): 657.
[PMID: 30469357]

[43] Yi L, Li Z, Yuan K, *et al.* Small molecules blocking the entry of severe acute respiratory syndrome coronavirus into host cells. J Virol 2004; 78(20): 11334-9.
[PMID: 15452254]

[44] Keyaerts E, Vijgen L, Pannecouque C, *et al.* Plant lectins are potent inhibitors of coronaviruses by interfering with two targets in the viral replication cycle. Antiviral Res 2007; 75(3): 179-87.
[PMID: 17428553]

[45] Olivieri F, Prasad V, Valbonesi P, *et al.* A systemic antiviral resistance-inducing protein isolated from Clerodendrum inerme Gaertn. is a polynucleotide:adenosine glycosidase (ribosome-inactivating protein). FEBS Lett 1996; 396(2-3): 132-4.
[PMID: 8914973]

[46] Lelešius R, Karpovaitė A, Mickienė R, *et al.* *In vitro* antiviral activity of fifteen plant extracts against avian infectious bronchitis virus. BMC Vet Res 2019; 15(1): 178.
[PMID: 31142304]

[47] Ulasli M, Gurses SA, Bayraktar R, *et al.* The effects of *Nigella sativa* (Ns), *Anthemis hyalina* (Ah) and *Citrus sinensis* (Cs) extracts on the replication of coronavirus and the expression of TRP genes family. Mol Biol Rep 2014; 41(3): 1703-11.
[PMID: 24413991]

[48] Rasool A, Khan MU, Ali MA, *et al.* Anti-avian influenza virus H9N2 activity of aqueous extracts of Zingiber officinalis (Ginger) and *Allium sativum* (Garlic) in chick embryos. Pak J Pharm Sci 2017; 30(4): 1341-4.
[PMID: 29039335]

[49] Lin C-W, Tsai F-J, Tsai C-H, *et al.* Anti-SARS coronavirus 3C-like protease effects of Isatis indigotica root and plant-derived phenolic compounds. Antiviral Res 2005; 68(1): 36-42.
[PMID: 16115693]

[50] Lin S-C, Ho C-T, Chuo W-H, Li S, Wang TT, Lin C-C. Effective inhibition of MERS-CoV infection by resveratrol. BMC Infect Dis 2017; 17(1): 144.
[PMID: 28193191]

[51] Younus I, Siddiq A, Ishaq H, Anwer L, Badar S, Ashraf M. Evaluation of antiviral activity of plant extracts against foot and mouth disease virus *in vitro*. Pak J Pharm Sci 2016; 29(4): 1263-8.
[PMID: 27393440]

[52] Mehrbod P, Amini E, Tavassoti-Kheiri M. Antiviral activity of garlic extract on influenza virus. Iran J Virol 2009; 3(1): 19-23.

[53] Shanthakumar B, Sathish M, Suresh A. *In vitro* antioxidant activity of extracts and stigmasterol from leaves of Clerodendrum inerme Linn. Res J Pharm Biol Chem Sci 2013; 4(4): 1411-8.

[54] Pandey A, Bigoniya P, Raj V, Patel KK. Pharmacological screening of *Coriandrum sativum* Linn. for hepatoprotective activity. J Pharm Bioallied Sci 2011; 3(3): 435-41.
[PMID: 21966166]

[55] Sood R, Swarup D, Bhatia S, *et al.* Antiviral activity of crude extracts of Eugenia jambolana Lam. against highly pathogenic avian influenza (H5N1) virus. Indian J Exp Biol 2012; 50(3): 179-86.

[56] Liou CJ, Cheng CY, Yeh KW, Wu YH, Huang WC. Protective effects of casticin from Vitex trifolia alleviate eosinophilic airway inflammation and oxidative stress in a murine asthma model. Front Pharmacol 2018; 9: 635.
[PMID: 29962952]

[57] Kim H-Y, Shin H-S, Park H, *et al. In vitro* inhibition of coronavirus replications by the traditionally used medicinal herbal extracts, Cimicifuga rhizoma, Meliae cortex, Coptidis rhizoma, and Phellodendron cortex. J Clin Virol 2008; 41(2): 122-8.
[PMID: 18036887]

[58] Liu Z, Xiao X, Wei X, *et al.* Composition and divergence of coronavirus spike proteins and host ACE2 receptors predict potential intermediate hosts of SARS-CoV-2. J Med Virol 2020; 92(6): 595-601.
[PMID: 32100877]

[59] Otake T, Mori H, Morimoto M, *et al.* Screening of Indonesian plant extracts for anti human immunodeficiency virus—type 1 (HIV 1) activity. Phytother Res 1995; 9(1): 6-10.

[60] Yu Y-B. The extracts of *Solanum nigrum* L. for inhibitory effects on HIV-1 and its essential enzymes. Korean J Orient Med 2004; 10(1): 119-26.

[61] Shanti B. Perspective of potential plants for medicine from Rajasthan, India. Int J Pharm Res 2016; 7(1): 1-6.

[62] Rege A, Chowdhary AS. Evaluation of *Ocimum sanctum* and *Tinospora cordifolia* as probable HIV protease inhibitors. Int J Pharm Sci Rev Res 2014; 25: 315.

[63] Ganjhu RK, Mudgal PP, Maity H, *et al.* Herbal plants and plant preparations as remedial approach for viral diseases. Virusdisease 2015; 26(4): 225-36.
[PMID: 26645032]

CHAPTER 8

Ultraviolet Radiation A (UVA): Modulates the Production of Nitric Oxide (NO) to Combat COVID-19

Muhammad Farrukh Nisar[1,*], Ahmad Uddin[2], Kamal Niaz[3], Shaukat Hussain Munawar[3], Qudratullulah[4], Faisal Siddique[5], Muhammad Yasir Waqas[1] and **Ahmad Farooq[6]**

[1] *Department of Physiology and Biochemistry, Faculty of Bio-Sciences, Cholistan University of Veterinary and Animal Sciences (CUVAS), Bahawalpur, 63100, Pakistan*

[2] *Drug Discovery Research Centre, Southwest Medical University, Luzhou 646000, China*

[3] *Department of Pharmacology and Toxicology, Faculty of Bio-Sciences, Cholistan University of Veterinary and Animal Sciences (CUVAS), Bahawalpur-63100, Pakistan*

[4] *Department of Surgery, Faculty of Veterinary Science, Cholistan University of Veterinary and Animal Sciences (CUVAS), Bahawalpur-63100, Pakistan*

[5] *Department of Microbiology, Faculty of Veterinary Science, Cholistan University of Veterinary and Animal Sciences (CUVAS), Bahawalpur-63100, Pakistan*

[6] *Department of Biological Sciences, International Islamic University, Islamabad, Pakistan*

Abstract: The ongoing outbreak of coronavirus-19 (COVID-19) has quickly become a daunting challenge to global health. The ultraviolet radiations (UVR) A wavebands fall in the region of 320-400 nm of the solar spectrum and comprise about 95% of overall ultraviolet (UVs) approaching the biosphere. The UVA is extensively used in phototherapy systems, as a disinfectant, and in various skin-related conditions. This chapter aimed to address the reduction of coronavirus replication by direct application of phototherapy (UVA) in lungs and modulation of nitric oxide (NO) in skin cells following UVA exposures. This NO influx inside the bloodstream to deliver into the lungs endothelial cells where it goes to incur cytoprotection to alveolar lung cells. Moreover, it is also proposed for direct application of therapeutic doses of UVA light inside the lungs. It uses a fiberoptic adapter to modulate the production of NO in lung endothelial cells, which will diffuse into the bronchi and lungs to leave bronchodilatory and vasodilatory effects. How NO reduces inflammatory burst and reactive oxygen species (ROS) in the lungs' alveolar cells is also discussed. Moreover, it is also

* **Corresponding author Muhammad Farrukh Nisar:** Department of Physiology and Biochemistry, Faculty of Bio-Sciences, Cholistan University of Veterinary and Animal Sciences (CUVAS), Bahawalpur, 63100, Pakistan. Tel.:+92 3457 1005 55; E-mail: mfarrukhnisar@cuvas.edu.pk

Kamal Niaz & Muhammad Farrukh Nisar (Eds.)

proposed that UVA radiation application should be limited to physiological doses and applied every 4-8 h, with at least 24 h of therapy before reassessment. The treating physician should determine discontinuation of this direct UVA treatment into the lungs following observation of the patient's condition and the safety and efficacy of the treatment. This study will highlight and emphasize the importance of utilizing UVA radiation to control this epidemic.

Keywords: Blood, COVID-19, Fiberoptic adapter, Lung endothelial cells, Nitric oxide, ROS, UVA.

INTRODUCTION

The coronavirus disease-2019 (COVID-19) pandemic has caused a momentous economic, healthcare, and social disorder worldwide since early 2020. This coronavirus disease is declared as a pandemic by the World Health Organization (WHO), and it exhibited human to human transmission with rapid spread across the globe [1]. However, it is still unknown to define proper measures to control or treat COVID-19. In December 2019, the COVID-19 epidemic was initially reported in Wuhan, China, responsible for 80904 confirmed cases as of August 31, 2020, China, with 24,854,140 cases reported worldwide 838924 mortalities. Upon the onset of this epidemic, the Chinese Government immediately has taken strict measures to control its transmission to other cities by completely lockdown Wuhan city, and many countries followed this practice. The number of COVID-19 cases is still increasing with few exceptions whatever the measures have been taken. A huge literature has been reported on the weather as an important factor in transmitting infectious diseases, especially influenza and severe acute respiratory syndrome (SARS). A remarked change in ambient temperature is linked with a higher risk of SARS [2], while influenza is linked with dry, hot, or cold air [3]. In Northern Europe, less temperature and low solar ultraviolet radiations (UVR) are examined to be linked with maximum activity and transmission of the influenza virus [4]. Based on the previous observations and reports, it is assumed that the COVID-19 epidemic can be reduced or even completely controlled as soon as the summer approaches. Seasonal variation (Temperature, humidity, and UVR) is important and is key to the spread of several infectious diseases [5 - 7]. Previously, the sunlight-driven nitric oxide (NO) mechanism was described as reducing blood pressure and a lower frequency of myocardial infarctions [8 - 10]. Most outcomes of COVID-19 are linked with dysfunctions of the vascular system, especially in the lungs.

Deadly infections are causing human morbidity and mortalities for centuries of known human history. Novel pathogenic conditions arise by the end of 2019, the novel severe acute respiratory syndrome coronavirus-2 (SARS-CoV-2) [11], and spread globally by early 2020. Certain secure, potent, and effective therapies are a dire need to minimize this SARS-CoV-2 pandemic unless a verified vaccine came into the market. Many studies indicate the shielding function of UVR in human health and for the disinfection of routine utensils. UVR is further divided into ultraviolet A (UVA) (320-400 nm), ultraviolet B (UVB) (280-320 nm), and ultraviolet C (UVC) (100-280 nm). UVR has long been recognized to pose strong anti-microbial effects. Among UVR, UVC is widely used to decontaminate and disinfect environmental objects and surfaces but is unsafe for human DNAs [12 - 15].

UVA radiation is a major environmental threat, but at the same time, certain therapeutic benefits have also been reported, and recently its potential use to minimize or reduce COVID-19. UVA (365 nm) is well known for inducing cellular signaling when irradiated in the physiological dose range. Solar UVR (UVA and UVB) is FDA-approved for various dermatological conditions such as skin lymphoma, psoriasis, and eczema [12, 16 - 18]. Still, we will elaborate on UVA light in the current draft only due to its least damaging effects for mammalian cells [13, 19]. Recent advancements in light-emitting diodes (LEDs) make it more versatile for the therapeutic application of lights for various internal organs [20]. FDA approves the only external application of the UVA light in therapeutic dosage range, but recently *in vivo* intraluminal UVA irradiations have produced no discernible endoscopic, histologic, or dysplastic changes in mice tissues [12]. Moreover, specific doses of UVA had strong inhibitory effects on coronavirus-229E and have proven a possible, safe, and quite effective treatment regimen for infectious diseases of internal viscera, but still demands clinical studies to define the safety, accuracy, and efficiency of UVA therapy in humans against COVID-19.

The current study aimed to propose the consideration of UVA therapy to control the cure for COVID-19 patients. The reduction of coronavirus replication in the lungs, modulation of NO in skin cells following UVA exposures, and this NO influx inside the bloodstream to deliver into lungs endothelial cells need to be evaluated. It incurs cytoprotection to lung alveolar cells shall be studied. Structural complexity, origin, classification, and molecular structure shall also be elucidated herein. Moreover, it is also proposed for direct application of therapeutic doses of UVA light inside the lungs to modulate the production of NO in lung endothelial cells, which will diffuse into the bronchi and lungs to leave bronchodilatory and vasodilatory effects. Moreover, how NO reduces inflammatory burst and ROS in the lungs' alveolar cells shall also be discussed.

Solar Light and Ultraviolet Radiation System

UV exposure is a key environmental factor that may affect skin functions significantly. Sunlight is an important environmental factor, which is further divided into various electromagnetic radiations, *e.g.,* UV light that spanned 100-400 nm of the solar spectrum. UVR can be classified into further sub-classes such as UV light with wavelengths of 100-280 nm is the UVC, which absorbs at the upper stratospheric layers and have no chance to get its entry into the biosphere. While wavelength between 280-320 nm are further split into two groups 280-311 nm (broadband), and 311-313 nm (narrowband) [21 - 23], and the longest wavebands in the UV region (320-400) is torn up to UVA2 (320-340 nm) and UVA1 (340-400 nm), which can make their way through the ozone layer and approach biosphere. Despite the various harmful effects of UVA and UVB, many different skin conditions, particularly psoriatic lesions and eczema, are being treated with these UV radiations [24]. A huge amount of literature claimed the differential effects/outcomes of both UVA and UVB in the human skin. Due to the deep penetration of UVA into the dermis and subcutaneous, but UVB affects the epidermal tissues. Hence the outcomes of both remained different [25, 26]. The exit has an inverse relationship with the energy and wavelength of UVs, *i.e.,* the longer the wavelength the less energy is, and vice versa. UVB radiations are five times more potent than UVA radiations. However, the former accounts for only 5% but later comprised 95% of the total UV light reaching the earth [3 - 7]' and both have differential penetration in the skin, but overall UVs effects are the same [27, 28]. Contemporary, UVR is also very useful to our skin in a way that, it synthesizes activated form of vitamin D3, immunomodulatory responses, reduces blood pressure, promotes healing of wounds, lessen pains, pigmentation of the skin, and production of NO [22, 24, 25, 29]. Short exposure to UVA light may protect the tissues from being irradiated [30].

Long term Environmental Exposure of Ambient Solar UVA Radiation and COVID-19

The sunlight is a source of energy in the biosphere in visible light, infrared radiation-producing heat, and invisible but harmful UVR. Fortunately, naturally, the ' 'Earth's atmosphere is shielding us from the harmful and damaging effects of UVR. Still, at the same time, our bodies need intermittent exposure to solar light to form skin vitamin D [31]. The ambient UVR in the biosphere is comprised of UVA (>95%) wavelengths, and the remaining is the UVB. This proportion of UVA to UVB may vary during different times of the day, season, latitude, and altitude. The peak proportion of UVB radiation is observed during midday time during summers at the low latitude and high altitude areas. Moreover, the cloud cover or haze may potentially act on the variation of the UVA to UVB proportion.

From 10 a.m. to 4:00 p.m, solar radiations have the maximum exposure for UVs. Still, it's more important for proper protective measures all year round because UVs are always strong even it's cloudy or haze, bright or sunny days, winter or summer, especially at altitudes [32]. In the invisible UVR, UVB (280-320 nm) parts are shorter but having more energy that easily enters through the outermost epidermis of the skin and produces burns, certain chemicals, inflammatory mediators, damage to the genetic materials in the cells leading to cancers even. Longer exposures affect the immune system by damaging the self-rebuild system of the tissue, activating melanocytes to provide melanin for filtration and protection of skin tissue under exposure [33].

UVA shows strong antiviral activity for positive sense, single-stranded RNA viruses such as coxsackievirus group B and coronavirus-229E [12]. It is assumed that UVA is involved in the alteration of the antiviral signaling mechanisms, especially the increased expression of mitochondrial antiviral signaling protein (MAVS), which is a major component of cellular antiviral immunity helping to suppress cellular viral invasion [34]. This suggests that UVA is involved in activating MAVS and later helps enter into an antiviral state without initiating antiviral apoptotic cell death.

On the other hand, UVA (320-400 nm) are longer waves, but less energetic than UVB may also have certain chronic damage [22]. UVA has far more penetration in the skin to dermal tissues, attacks cellular membranes, DNA damage, affects cellular signaling for transcriptional and translational levels mainly by the production of ROS and RNS [35]. UVR as a whole is linked with carcinogenesis, sagging of the skin, immune suppression, and sunburns, *etc.* Prolonged or chronic exposures to UVA may lead to dilated tiny blood vessels in the skin. Despite all the damaging effects of UVR, the therapeutic doses of UVA and UVB have useful effects on the human body. Specifically, a loose therapeutic dose of UVA may be used to boost immune response, regulate blood pressure, and adjust the redox balance of the cells [36]. Moreover, the UVA-mediated production of NO gets its entry to the blood vessels, and provides a protective and relaxing role in the lung tissues, and poses cytoprotective roles.

Sunlight has extensively been reported to inactivate SARS-CoV-2, a major cause of the COVID-19 under certain controlled studies. How increased aerosols help spread and transmit COVID-19 remained a big question for scientists. The aerosol is thought to be the possible way of transmitting COVID-19, and the whole phenomenon depends on multiple environmental conditions, especially the sunlight [37]. Moreover, simulated sunlight and matrix significantly affected the virus's decay rate, suggesting sunlight as a crucial factor that influences the risk of aerosol-mediated transmission of COVID-19 [37]. Sneezing, coughing, breathing, and talking can help generate aerosols in the respiratory tract [38, 39]. Coronaviruses HKU1, OC43, and NL63 genetic material have also been recovered from aerosols of exhaled breath of COVID-19 infected individuals. The genetic material of SARS-CoV-2 was also observed in upper respiratory tract specimens [10, 11].

The global impact of COVID-19 is numerous and uncountable. Still, precise forecasting of the coronavirus spread solely depends on historical data (total confirmed cases, number of deaths, and recoveries) may provide a chance to stop further spread. But at the same time, no forecast is certain as the future rarely repeats itself in the same way as the past because predictions rely on the source of the data, vested interests, and variables to be undertaken. Similarly, psychological factors significantly affect how people perceive and respond to the disease threats and internal fear that may affect badly [40].

Coronavirus

Coronaviruses (CoVs) are positive-sense, non-segmented single-stranded RNA-enveloped viruses that belong to the *Coronaviridae* family of the order Nidovirales [41]. Human CoVs (hCoV) were initially identified during the 1960s in patients with the common cold. Four known genera in this family are well recognized viz. *α-coronavirus* (*α*-CoV), *β-coronavirus* (*β*-CoV), *γ-coronavirus*(*γ* -CoV), and *Δ-coronavirus* (Δ-CoV). The *α*-CoV and *β*-CoV can only infect mammals, including bats, cats, pigs, and humans. The *γ*-CoV mostly infects birds while Δ-CoV infects both mammals and birds. Six CoVs are known to be responsible for causing fatal infections in humans viz. human-CoVNL63 (hCoV-NL63) and human-CoV229E (hCoV-229E) of the genera *α*-CoV; human-CoVHKU1 (hCoV HKU1) and human-CoV OC43 (hCoV-OC43) in *β*-CoV lineage A are frequently involved in common cold symptoms in immunocompetent people. SARSr-CoV of *β*-CoV lineage B, and MERS-CoV belonging to *β*-CoV lineage C [42]. These are also known as zoonotic viruses due to their capacity for movement across the *trans*-species and well adaptation in various animals. CoVs involved in human diseases includes SARS, MERS, other respiratory infections, or gastrointestinal infections to attack birds and mammals [43]. SARS-CoV was initially identified during SARS outbreaks in 2002-03 in Guangdong province, China [44, 45]. MERS-CoV is responsible for causing severe respiratory disease outbreaks during 2012 in the Middle East [46]. These viruses are turned into a pandemic, and SARS caused over 8096 infections in 26 countries with almost 800 deaths, while MERS was identified in 2500 confirmed cases of infection in 27 different countries, which leads to 860 mortalities [47, 48].

The emergence potential of CoVs is mainly linked with its mutation and recombination, allowing the generation of new viral strains with higher susceptibility for new hosts [49 - 55]. The novel SARS-CoV-2 causing 2019 novel COVID-19 first appeared in Wuhan, Hubei province, China, in December 2019. COVID-19 causes severe respiratory infections, including pneumonia. Initially, unidentified sources of pneumonia was later found associated with the seafood and wet animal wholesale market in Wuhan, Hubei Province of China [56]. Later on, deep sequencing analysis of lower respiratory tract pathological samples from infected individuals indicated a novel coronavirus strain that was later designated as SARS-CoV-2. However, SARS-COV-2 spread in over 185 countries around the globe, including countries in almost every continent, caused around 19,462,112 infections and 722,285 deaths [58]. Initially, the mortality rate of COVID-19 in China was 2.3% compared with other viruses, viz. MERS (34.4%) and SARS (9.6%) announced by WHO [57]. Due to the daily increase in cases and death globally, make it hard to conclude about the exact fatality rate of the disease. But the latest data showed a sudden increase in Italy, the Islamic Republic of Iran, and the Republic of Korea during March 2020 [58]. Initial clinical studies reported the laboratory, clinical, radiological characteristics, and possible epidemiological features of such viruses [59].

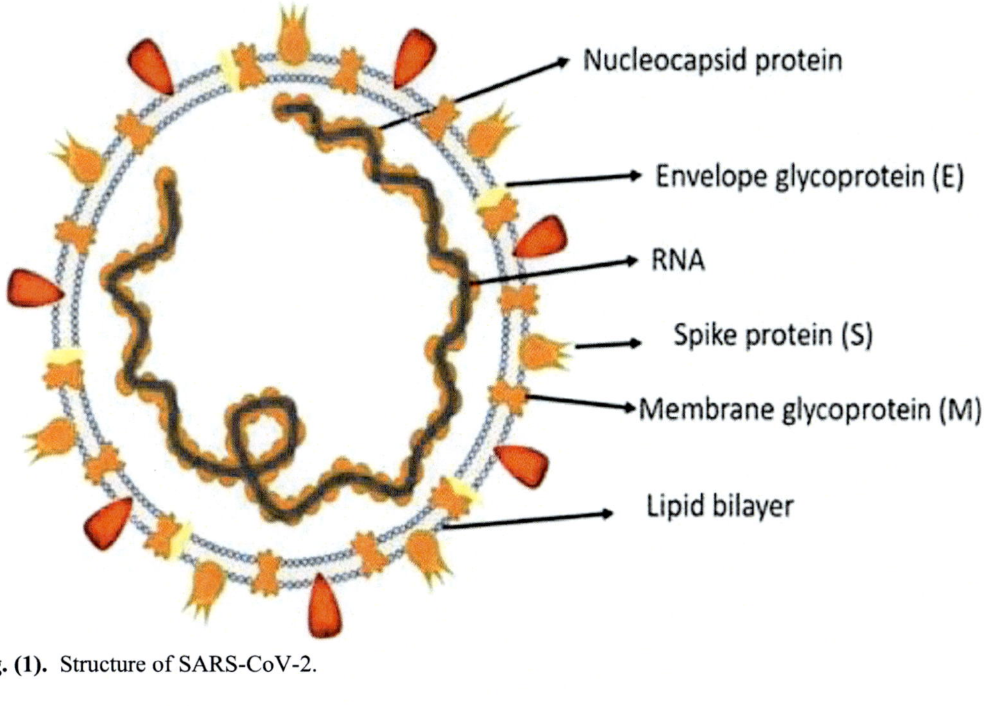

Fig. (1). Structure of SARS-CoV-2.

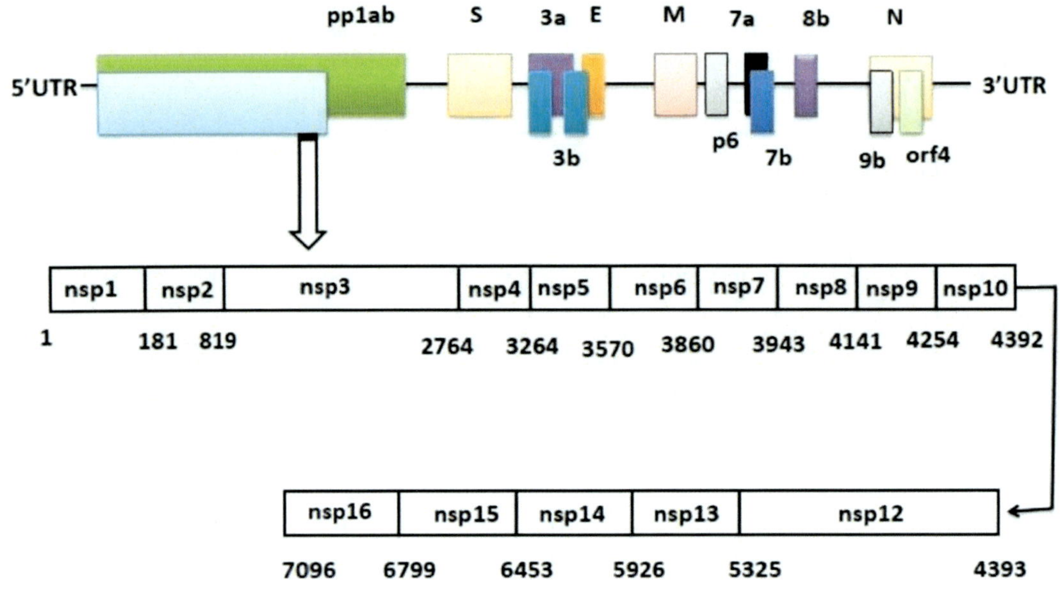

Fig. (2). Details of the genome of SARS-CoV-2 that comprised of approximately ~30 kb, which encodes both structural and non-structural proteins.

What is SARS-CoV-2?

SARS-CoV-2 (Fig. **1**) is a single-stranded RNA enveloped β-CoV and efficiently causes acute respiratory syndrome named COVID-19. SARS-CoV-2 genome is comprised of approximately ~30 kilobases, which encodes both structural and non-structural proteins (Fig. **2**). The later proteins such as 3-chymotrypsin-like protease, papain-like protease, RNA-dependent RNA polymerase, and helicases are vital enzymes in maintaining the virus particle life cycle within the cell. The pairwise protein sequence analysis of these seven protein conserved non-structural proteins demonstrate that the virus belongs to the species of SARSr-CoV [60]. On the contrary, the structural proteins include spike glycoprotein and its accessory proteins required for the virus to cell receptor interactions during viral entry into the host cell [61]. Therefore, these proteins are documented as potential targets to develop antiviral drugs against SARS and MERS [62], and probably almost mimicking in the case of COVID-19 as revealed by recent genomic data of this novel virus from Wuhan [63]. This on-time identification of receptors and binding proteins will be helpful in vaccine developments and using therapies of the past

SARS and MERS outbreak to cure current COVID-19 patients. The evolutionary history of SARS-CoV-2 and those of other CoVs genomes to track its origin. The full-length genome phylogenetic analyses suggested that COVID-19 shares about 79.5% sequence identify SARS-CoV (Fig. **3**) [64 - 66]. This data suggests SARS-CoV-2 as a novel β-CoV from the subgenus Sarbecovirus [64 - 67].

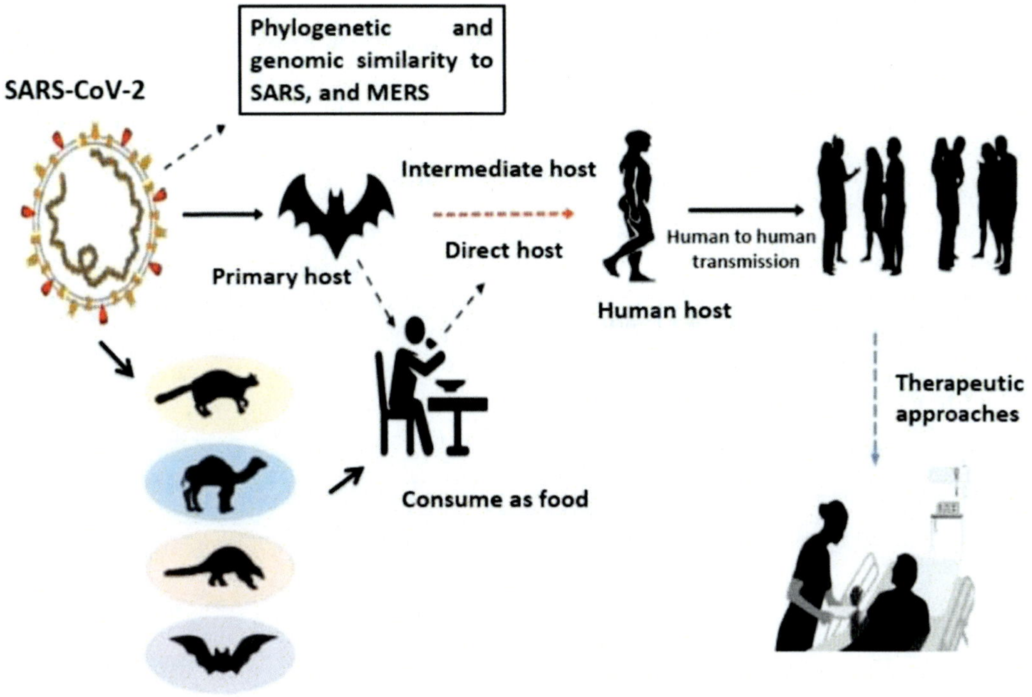

Fig. (3). A comparative evolutionary history of SARS-CoV-2 with other CoVs genomes to track its origin.

The 21st century has witnessed two pandemics by coronaviruses, MERS-CoV and SARS-CoV [68, 69], which were highly pathogenic. Starting during December 2019, in Wuhan, China [56], a cluster of people with pneumonia from unknown sources and epidemiology was linked to a seafood and wild animal wholesale market. SARS-CoV-2 can infect humans through the mouth and nose mucous membranes and use mucous membranes in the eyes, boosting regional circulation and large-scale spread [70]. Remarkable scientific advancements and united global efforts enable rapid identification of the novel coronavirus as SARS-CoV-2 and help its epidemic prevention. Notably, SARS-CoV-2 was closely related with 88% sequence similarity to two Zhoushan, Eastern China, bat-derived SARS-like coronaviruses, *i.e.,* bat-SL-CoVZXC21 and bat-SL-CoVZC45, but was more distant from MERS-CoV (50% sequence similarity) and SARS-CoV (79% sequence similarity) [63]. Phylogenetically, the 2019 novel CoV originated from the genus β-CoV, which includes coronaviruses (SARS/SARS-like -CoV and others) identified in bats, humans, and few wild animals [71]. The spike (S) proteins, crucial for host tropism and transmission capacity, mediates receptor binding through its domain S1 and plasma membrane fusion through S2. S protein of SARS-CoV-2 shared high sequence similarity (88%) with SARS-CoV suggesting its possible utilization of Angiotensin-Converting Enzyme 2 (ACE2) as a cell receptor [72]. However, several key residues required for the binding of the ACE2 receptor to the coronavirus receptor-binding domain displayed similarly between the receptor-binding domains of SARS-CoV and SARS-CoV-2.

Unlike MERS-CoV and SARS-CoV receptor-binding domain, the SARS-CoV-2 receptor binding domain contains several mutations but still employs the ACE2 binding receptor. This mutation was introduced at Furin protease, which may enhance the transmissibility and significantly improve the efficiency of infecting cells by SARS-CoV-2 than SARS-CoV. The lessons learned through experiences resulted from the outbreaks of CoVs prevalence over the last two decades, tremendous advances, and valuable insight toward unraveling the physiognomies of SARS-CoV-2 have been achieved at an unprecedented speed. It is still might be able to use this binding receptor. Whether mutations in ACE2 affect its binding or change receptor tropism need to explore in detail [63].

Mode of Transmission of SARS-CoV-2

Since the outbreak of SARS-CoV-2, the level of infections and severity, mode of transmission, and mortality rate appear unclear and controversial till now. In the emergence of the SARS-CoV-2 outbreak, health officials and administrations mostly rely on prevention to use face masks in public places. Whole cities were in quarantine to reduce surge capacity [73]. Emerging evidence supported asymptomatic transmission [74] while numerous ways of transmission are adding up. In the current scenario, a health official Guangfa Wang, with a protective face mask N95 complained about eye redness before the onset of pneumonia was infected with the novel virus in Wuhan [75]. Lu and colleagues [76] confirmed the ocular transmission of this deadly virus almost similar to 2003 SARS-CoV, the primary way it transmits through the mucus membrane [77]. Thus, the ocular transmission of SARS-CoV-19 should not be underestimated. The current study suggests the better protection of health workers is a more effective way to prevent disease amplification.

Additionally, the Government has already warned and instructed the general public about SARS-CoV-19 ocular transmission. More recently, the appalling human-to-human hospitalized transmission was 44 cases (29%) [78]. This makes it more amiable to speculate that there would be more unknown ways of transmission of COVID-19 [79]. Hence certain robust and serious precautions are needed to prevent or check transmissions. Urine and stool samples should be tested to prevent a possible alternative transmission route at this stage [79].

Moreover, researchers speculated sewage transmission in Hongkong and Guangzhou, China, as a viral infection has had been demonstrated in Caco-2 cell lines when co-cultured with samples from infected individuals in Germany [80, 81]. This suggested that, like SARS and MERS, COVID-19 shares a similar transmission mode [82]. This evidence adding up anxiety in the SARS-CoV-2 outbreak and require further in-depth studies of contact patterns on epidemic dynamics, hence certain robust and serious precautions needed to prevent or check transmissions.

Prevention Strategies Adopted

Although SARS-like outbreaks have not been reported over a decade, modeling SARS transmission and control in the healthcare systems can be applied to control COVID-19 outbreaks [83 - 85]. MERS, SARS, and COVID-19 share certain common features that could be implemented in healthcare systems and display transmission heterogeneity [86]. The lack of an appropriate animal model that mimics the natural history of the disease has slowed down the development of effective pharmaceutical interventions against MERS-CoV [87] and SARS and now for COVID-19. The CDC recommends a set of preventive measures to help check the amplification of respiratory viruses [83, 84].

Like the SARS outbreak, reducing close contact by quarantine people to their houses and a travel ban would be an effective measure to limit the spread of SARS-CoV-2 [88]. Furthermore, due to persons to person, asymptomatic transmissions and incubation period [74, 89] make their way far more vigilant for control measures of the epidemic which seems to be pandemic. One such measure taken by the Chinese Government was the quick isolation of suspected, infected, and close contact individuals. In addition, SARS-CoV and MERS-CoV super spreading events [90] cannot be completely ignored in the current SARS-CoV-2 outbreak. So far, the transmission of COVID-19 occurs either through close contact or aerosol, which seems controversial along with fecal transmission [91]. Health workers should follow SARS and MERS type infection standard procedures while handling infected patients and during sample collection [92].

UVA Mediates Production of NO

The increasing literature ever portrays the positive effects of solar radiation;

especially UVA radiation reduces blood pressure mainly by producing NO in the skin keratinocytes and microvascular endothelial cells [29]. NO is well known for killing or inhibiting the replication of intracellular pathogens, specifically viruses, where NO targets viral proteases necessary for virulence and the life cycle of many viruses [93 - 98]. NO mainly targets Coxsackievirus proteases 3C, torn the virus polyproteins into individual polypeptides, and S-nitrosylate cysteine residues present in the active-site of protease 3C to inhibit protease activity [93]. COVID-19 pandemic is not finished yet, though some signs of the second phase are striking ears for days, *e.g.*, Hongkong's recent COVID-19 outbreak in the last July 2020, according to WHO. Keeping in view the continuous and vigorous spread of COVID-19, certain risk factors (temperature, humidity, and solar UVR) are seriously considered while attempting to minimize the SARS-CoV-2 [99]. The human skin gets exposed to solar light, UVA light induces the discharge of NO from skin cells making its way to enter the bloodstream (Fig. **4**), which dilates blood vessels and minimizes blood pressure, promoting cardiovascular disease and metabolic health [99]. This produces a reduction in the risk of death from COVID19 since heart disease, vascular conditions, and metabolic syndrome are high-risk factors [99].

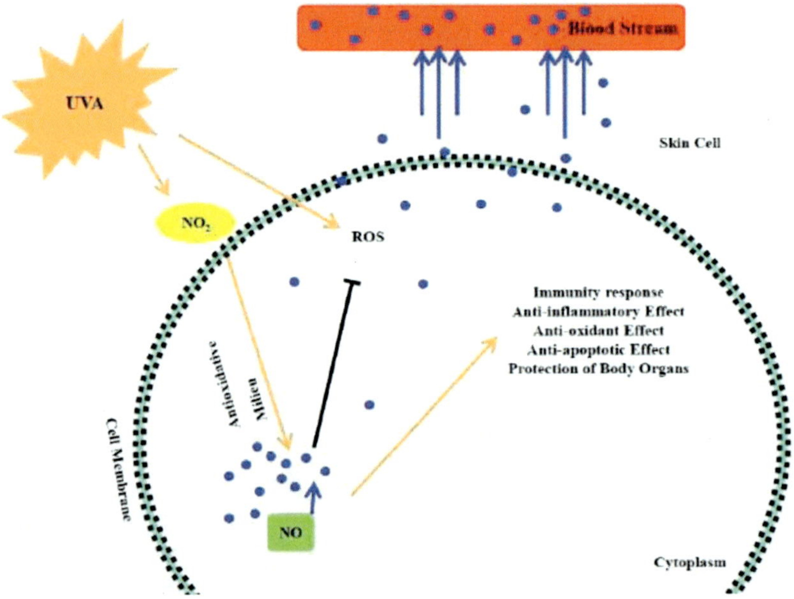

Fig. (4). Possible molecular mechanisms involved in mediating the beneficial effects of solar ultraviolet radiation.

Moreover, UVA irradiation is also suggested to inactivate the virus in airborne droplets and fomites. The spread rate reduction and the size of the inoculating dose in those coming into contact with infectious material, hence reducing infection levels [99]. It is also said that NO may modulate the expression of proteins of the Bcl-2 family, which appears as the molecular mechanism underlying this cellular protection [100].

Effect of NO on SARS-CoV-2

NO a key signaling molecule between cells, shows an inhibitory effect on some virus infections [101]. Infection caused by SARS-CoV-2 may lead to a diversity of cardiopulmonary and vascular complications, specifically upper respiratory tract issues, severe acute respiratory distress syndrome (ARDS), shock, acute kidney injury, and thromboembolic complications [102, 103]. Various reactive oxygen and nitrogen species play important roles in human physiology, but gaseous NO is quite an important signaling molecule.

In vascular smooth muscle cells showed high expression levels of the canonical receptor (guanylate cyclase) that gets activated after the NO attaches to heme moiety and remarkably increases its enzymatic conversion guanosine-5--triphosphate to cyclic guanosine monophosphate, which subsequently promotes vasorelaxation. The gaseous NO has distinctive pharmacological properties, especially import into well-ventilated lung units promoting local vasodilatation. The extremely short half-life NO after getting entered into the blood quickly forms a complex with intraerythrocytic Hb and inactivated. It will lead to a strong check on its systemic effects [104]. Gaseous NO preferentially vasodilates pulmonary arterioles in well-ventilated lung units. It decreases the relative blood flow to poorly ventilated lung units and enhances V/Q matching to increase blood oxygenation [105].

Moreover, NO is also said to induce mild bronchodilation and check neutrophil-mediated oxidative burst [105 - 108]. In SARS patients, inhaled nitric oxide (iNO) is linked with enhanced oxygenation in a severity-matched observational cohort [109]. Both endogenous and exogenous NO showed to inhibit SARS-CoV virus replication [101] (Fig. **5**). On the other hand, iNO has significant effects on oxygenation in ARDS patients and hence reduces pulmonary vascular resistance [105]. Such therapeutic activities give an idea that iNO may be used as an early cure during CoVID-19 infection to minimize the demand for invasive mechanical ventilation [104]. Certain recent cases reported the superiority of iNO delivery systems to facilitate patients even at their homes. At the same time, GENOSYL DS (VERO Biotech) has designed a tankless system to deliver at homes [110]. Still, many other systems such as Nu-Med Plus (UT), INOpulse (Bellerophon Therapeutics), and an iridium electric NO generator have also been introduced due to easy portability. Still, all these iNO therapy systems have certain limitations for their universality.

In a randomized and placebo-controlled trial of ambulatory patients with fibrotic lung disease requiring long-term oxygen. INOpulse therapy was associated with greater physical activity than placebo. In an acute dose-escalation study of patients with pulmonary hypertension associated with pulmonary fibrosis, iNO delivered through the INOpulse system lead to a 30% reduction in pulmonary vascular resistance, with improvements in Q and pulmonary artery compliance.

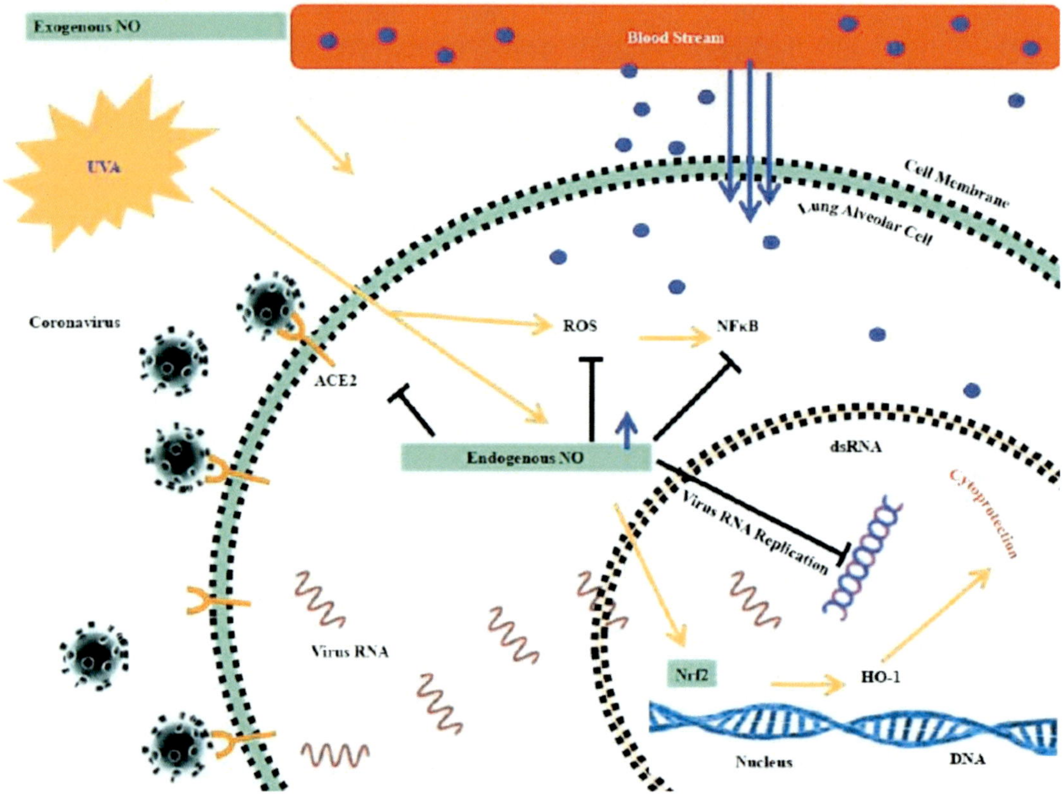

Fig. (5). Role of UVA and exogenous NO in lung alveolar cell to inhibit SARS-CoV-2.

NO: A Key Player in the Airways

Various biological and pathological outcomes of NO are due to some deleterious or cytoprotective effects primarily depends on the immediate micro-environment [111, 112] (Fig. **5**). For decades, NO remained a major atmospheric pollutant and cause of acid rains [113]. Still, late in the 20th century, NO appeared as a mimicking factor of endothelium-derived relaxing factor (EDRF) [114], performing multiple functions in the human body, especially the respiratory tract.

Nitric oxide synthase (NOS) exists in two isoforms, namely inducible (iNOS) and constitutive (cNOS), which help to release endogenous NO into the airways. The constitutive NOS poses protective effects on airways against excessive bronchoconstriction. It inducible NOS modulates airways inflammatory conditions, particularly in asthma [115], platelet aggregation [116], and neurotransmission [117]. A higher NO level is suggested in asthmatic conditions due to overexpression of NOS [118, 119]. Moreover, endothelial and epithelial cells of the lung airways and inflammatory cells are capable of producing NO.

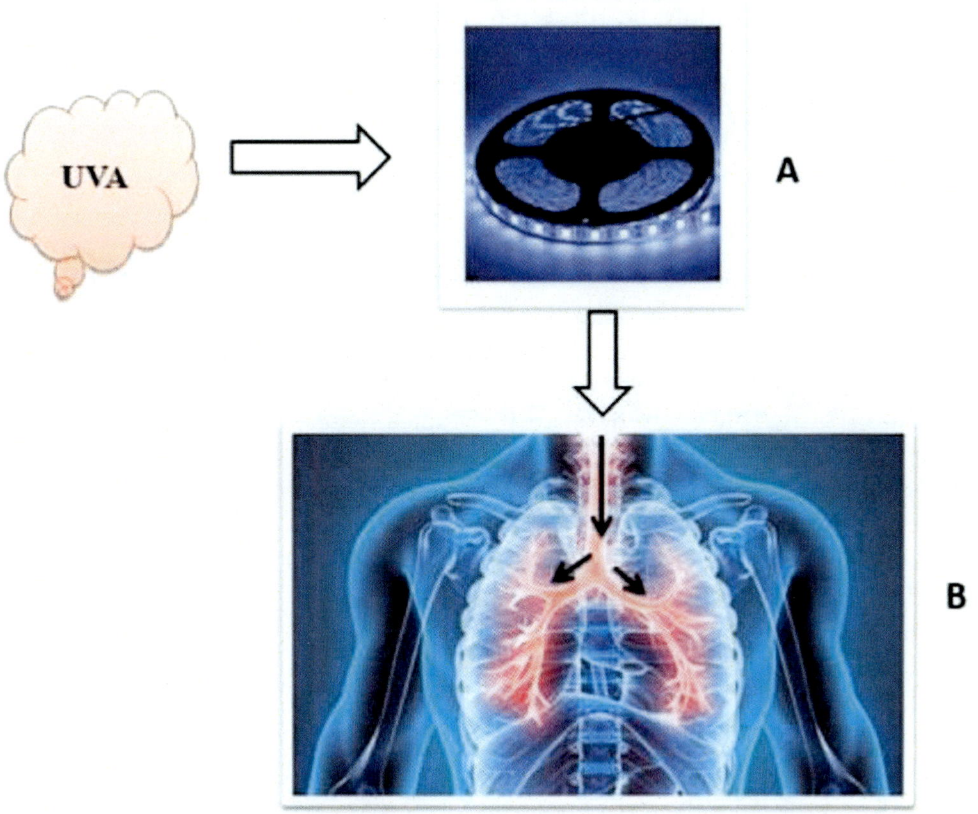

Fig. (6). Schematic representation of UVA-based direct tracheobronchial UVR applications: (A) Appropriate UVA (365 nm) source with a fiberoptic adapter; (B) direct bronchoscopic application of UVA. Note that radiation intensity should be limited to physiological doses and that treatments should be applied every 4-8 h, with at least 24 h of therapy before reassessment. Discontinuation of treatment should be determined by the treating physician after considering: (a) the status of the patient's condition and (b) the safety and efficacy of the treatment.

Many studies reported the negative role of NO in health. Still, minor oxidative stress leads to releasing the redox-active chelate iron pool (CIP) of the cell, which potentially and actively amplifies the cellular ROS led to oxidative stress later to pose multiple pathologies. In macrophages exposed to NO, the CIP gets complexed with NO to form di-nitrosyl iron with thiol-containing ligands (DNICs) [120]. At the cellular level, NO slowed or check H_2O_2 metabolism that suggests some H_2O_2 is consumed during cellular iron metabolism to pose cytoprotection against iron toxicity [120]. In severe lung issues specifically, asthmatic individuals, increased levels of NO have been observed. Keeping this fact in mind, we proposed a UVA-based direct tracheobronchial UVR application shown in Fig. (**6**). It needs an appropriate UVA (365 nm) source with a fiberoptic adapter for the direct bronchoscopic application of UVA. Moreover, UVA radiation application should be limited to physiological doses and applied every 4-8 h, with at least 24 h of therapy before reassessment. The treating physician should determine discontinuation of treatment following observation of the patient's condition and the safety and efficacy of the treatment.

NO Blocks Virus Replication Inside Host Cells

NO is an important signaling molecule between cells that have been shown to have an inhibitory effect on some virus infections. For a long time, NO has been considered a physiological mediator of endothelial cell relaxation, especially in hypertension. Previously, NO was studied extensively as an intracellular messenger and reported as a potent mediator of endothelial cell relaxation that plays a significant role in hypotension. Macrophages, natural killer cells, and neutrophils comprise the innate immune system. It mainly use pattern recognition receptors to identify molecular patterns linked with inhibition of various pathogens, mainly by checking replication and release of numerous effector molecules, particularly NO [121]. iNOS mediated NO potentially inhibits the SARS-CoV replication cycle at some early stages of infection [101, 122]. The diffusion of NO through the cell membrane to reach the virus should be significantly more effective at the very high NO concentration [122]. NO plays certain key roles in pulmonary vascular functions during viral infections and many pulmonary conditions [123]. The lung cells are reported to have higher levels of iNOS when there is a viral attack, and NO checks the replication of the SARS-CoV-1 virus mainly through certain cytotoxic intermediate reactions such as the formation of peroxynitrite [101]. Nitrosation of various surface thiols of red blood cells (RBC) and β-chains of the hemoglobin tetramer help stabilize for hemolysis and oxidative damage, respectively. It depicts the potential of NO to stop SARS-CoV-2 RBC-linked pathogenic processes [124, 125]. SARS-CoV-2 primarily attack to infect lung endothelial cells, which are the main resource for NO production. Hence naturally, NO is holding a better position to respond against virus attacks quickly [123].

iNOS mediated NO being an important inter/intracellular molecule, has shown an increased level in various microbial infections with appreciable effects for the protozoans and pathogenic bacterial strains, but also shows inhibitory effects on certain virus infections well [101]. An *in vitro* study, where NO donor S-nitros--N-acetylepenicillamine checks the replication of the SARS CoV in a concentration-dependent fashion both at translational and transcriptional levels [101]. Some studies reported the suppression of virus replication, where the infected murine macrophages start releasing iNOS-mediated NO without an accessory protein C (4C(-)) from the Sendai virus (SeV). The underlying mechanism in the virus replication is an increased expression of IFN-β and activation of NFκB, and the former modulates the induction of iNOS *via* the JAK-STAT pathway [126]. NF-κB is a key regulator of transcription of the iNOS gene modulate by 4C(–) infection. It plays a vital role in inducing NO production, and iNOS expression significantly decreased in the cells that express influenza virus NS1 protein constitutively. So, it sequesters double-stranded (ds)RNA, which is an essential factor to trigger signaling pathways leading to activation of NF-κB and IRF3. C protein is marked as suppressing NF-κB activation to inhibit iNOS expression leading to NO production, possibly by limiting dsRNA generation in the context of viral infection [126].

NO Reduces the Inflammatory Influx and Oxidative Stress

The available reports showed that severe patients of COVID-19 had been found with higher levels of pro-inflammatory cytokines such as interleukin (IL)-6 [127]. Higher IL-6 levels show poor prognosis in COVID-19, moreover, excessive infiltration of pro-inflammatory cells viz. T-helper 17 cells and macrophages have been observed in lung tissues of COVID-19 patients. It is assumed that "cytokine burst" may aid in the mortality of COVID-19. SARS-Cov-2 selectively induces a high level of IL-6 and results in the exhaustion of lymphocytes [127].

Both neutrophils and the following monocytes get involved during the inflammations where the former helps to kill pathogenic microbes and ultimately undergoes apoptosis. Monocytes turned to macrophages at the inflammatory tissue, other phagocytes help clear the apoptotic neutrophils and reduce the inflammation.

NO is recently reported to be involved in regulating the inflammatory burst, immune responses and retards the growth of the microorganisms [128]. Moreover, NO has a pivotal role in alleviating oxidative stress by neutralizing ROS (Fig. **5**). In certain lungs, asthma and some viral infections, higher levels of NO are examined. Alveolar macrophages (AM) and bronchoalveolar lavage fluid (BALF) in patients with asthma showed a higher level of inflammatory cytokines are being modulated by the presence of NO [129]. Paranasal sinuses continuously generate NO as a ROS agent. It gets diffused into the bronchi and lungs to leave bronchodilatory and vasodilatory effects [130]. NO may lead to initiate an array of reactive nitrogen oxide species [131]. Still, it goes to react with different targets [3], either some free radicals (dioxygen, superoxide, *etc.*) or free cellular iron (Fe^{2+}) [132] to stabilize the unpaired electron on NO [133], and hence the free radicals get neutralized. It is well established that iNOS-mediated NO modulates the production of various chemokines, which are involved in the neutrophils and monocytes infiltration during inflammations [134]. The levels of NO are the key players in identifying the balanced production of such chemokines. Moreover, the production of pro-inflammatory cytokines appears to be actively suppressed by TGF-β and NO. Phagocytes produce them upon interaction with apoptotic cells [134]. NO is playing a key role in inflammations and, therefore, is considered a potent candidate for developing therapeutics for inflammatory diseases, particularly in COVID-19.

CONCLUSION

The outbreak of COVID-19 is still a big challenge for global health. It is obvious after discussion of the bi-phasic mechanism of UVA radiations that can trigger vasodilatory effects. The UVA as a potential therapeutic source could be used in various conditions. NO production can evidence that nitrites in skin cells are the major source of UV-mediated NO release. The reduction of coronavirus replication can be made by directly applying therapeutic doses of UVA in lungs using a fiberoptic adapter through the modulation of NO. Similar effects can be achieved by exposing the skin cells to UVA radiations that produce the influx of NO inside the bloodstream to deliver into lung endothelial cells to incur cytoprotection to alveolar lung cells. Moreover, it is also being proposed that UVA-mediated production of NO in lung endothelial cells can easily diffuse into the bronchi. It leaves the lungs with bronchodilatory and vasodilatory effects that reduce inflammation to burst and produce ROS. The application of physiological doses of UVA (365 nm) every 4-8 hours for 24 hours before reassessment, while discontinuation of direct UVA application can be done following physician's observations about the status of the patient's condition and the safety and efficacy of the treatment.

CONSENT FOR PUBLICATION

Not Applicable.

CONFLICT OF INTEREST

The author confirms that this chapter contents have no conflict of interest.

ACKNOWLEDGEMENT

Declared none.

REFERENCES

[1] Bai Y, Yao L, Wei T, *et al.* Presumed asymptomatic carrier transmission of COVID-19. JAMA 2020; 323(14): 1406-7.
[http://dx.doi.org/10.1001/jama.2020.2565] [PMID: 32083643]

[2] Tan J, Mu L, Huang J, Yu S, Chen B, Yin J. An initial investigation of the association between the SARS outbreak and weather: with the view of the environmental temperature and its variation. J Epidemiol Community Health 2005; 59(3): 186-92.
[http://dx.doi.org/10.1136/jech.2004.020180] [PMID: 15709076]

[3] Xu Z, Hu W, Williams G, Clements AC, Kan H, Tong S. Air pollution, temperature and pediatric influenza in Brisbane, Australia. Environ Int 2013; 59: 384-8.
[http://dx.doi.org/10.1016/j.envint.2013.06.022] [PMID: 23911338]

[4] Ianevski A, Zusinaite E, Shtaida N, *et al.* Low temperature and low UV indexes correlated with peaks of influenza virus activity in Northern Europe during 2010–2018. Viruses 2019; 11(3): 207.
[http://dx.doi.org/10.3390/v11030207] [PMID: 30832226]

[5] Fisman D. Seasonality of viral infections: mechanisms and unknowns. Clin Microbiol Infect 2012; 18(10): 946-54.
[http://dx.doi.org/10.1111/j.1469-0691.2012.03968.x] [PMID: 22817528]

[6] Shaman J, Pitzer VE, Viboud C, Grenfell BT, Lipsitch M. Absolute humidity and the seasonal onset of influenza in the continental United States. PLoS Biol 2010; 8(2): e1000316.
[http://dx.doi.org/10.1371/journal.pbio.1000316] [PMID: 20186267]

[7] Charland KM, Buckeridge DL, Sturtevant JL, *et al.* Effect of environmental factors on the spatio-temporal patterns of influenza spread. Epidemiol Infect 2009; 137(10): 1377-87.
[http://dx.doi.org/10.1017/S0950268809002283] [PMID: 19296868]

[8] Liu D, Fernandez BO, Hamilton A, *et al.* UVA irradiation of human skin vasodilates arterial vasculature and lowers blood pressure independently of nitric oxide synthase. J Invest Dermatol 2014; 134(7): 1839-46.
[http://dx.doi.org/10.1038/jid.2014.27] [PMID: 24445737]

[9] Weller RB, Wang Y, He J, *et al.* Does incident solar ultraviolet radiation lower blood pressure? J Am Heart Assoc 2020; 9(5): e013837.
[http://dx.doi.org/10.1161/JAHA.119.013837] [PMID: 32106744]

[10] Mackay DF, Clemens TL, Hastie CE, Cherrie MPC, Dibben C, Pell JP. UVA and Seasonal Patterning of 56 370 Myocardial Infarctions Across Scotland, 2000-2011. J Am Heart Assoc 2019; 8(23): e012551.
[http://dx.doi.org/10.1161/JAHA.119.012551] [PMID: 31747863]

[11] Huang C, Wang Y, Li X, *et al.* Clinical features of patients infected with 2019 novel coronavirus in Wuhan, China. Lancet 2020; 395(10223): 497-506.
[http://dx.doi.org/10.1016/S0140-6736(20)30183-5] [PMID: 31986264]

[12] Rezaie A, Leite GGS, Melmed GY, *et al.* Ultraviolet A light effectively reduces bacteria and viruses including coronavirus. PLoS One 2020; 15(7): e0236199.
[http://dx.doi.org/10.1371/journal.pone.0236199] [PMID: 32673355]

[13] Vecchia P, Hietanen M, Stuck BE, van Deventer E, Niu S. Protecting workers from ultraviolet radiation. Citeseer 2007.

[14] Reed NG. The history of ultraviolet germicidal irradiation for air disinfection. Public Health Rep 2010;

125(1): 15-27.
[http://dx.doi.org/10.1177/003335491012500105] [PMID: 20402193]

[15] Roy S. In Ultraviolet Light in Human Health, Diseases and Environment. Springer 2017; pp. 207-19.
[http://dx.doi.org/10.1007/978-3-319-56017-5_17]

[16] Bhutani T, Liao W. A practical approach to home UVB phototherapy for the treatment of generalized psoriasis. Pract Dermatol 2010; 7(2): 31-5.
[PMID: 25191138]

[17] Patrizi A. Raone, B.; Ravaioli, G.M.Ultraviolet Light in Human Health, Diseases and Environment. Springer 2017; pp. 319-31.
[http://dx.doi.org/10.1007/978-3-319-56017-5_27]

[18] Tarabadkar ES, Shinohara MM. Skin directed therapy in cutaneous T-cell lymphoma. Front Oncol 2019; 9: 260.
[http://dx.doi.org/10.3389/fonc.2019.00260] [PMID: 31032224]

[19] Reichrath J. Rass, K.Sunlight, Vitamin D and Skin Cancer. Springer 2014; pp. 208-33.
[http://dx.doi.org/10.1007/978-1-4939-0437-2_12]

[20] Robatto M, Pavie MC, Garcia I, *et al.* Ultraviolet A/blue light-emitting diode therapy for vulvovaginal candidiasis: a case presentation. Lasers Med Sci 2019; 34(9): 1819-27.
[http://dx.doi.org/10.1007/s10103-019-02782-9] [PMID: 30945022]

[21] Diffey BL. What is light? Photodermatol Photoimmunol Photomed 2002; 18(2): 68-74.
[http://dx.doi.org/10.1034/j.1600-0781.2002.180203.x] [PMID: 12147039]

[22] Nisar MF, Parsons KSG, Bian CX, Zhong JL. UVA irradiation induced heme oxygenase-1: a novel phototherapy for morphea. Photochem Photobiol 2015; 91(1): 210-20.
[http://dx.doi.org/10.1111/php.12342] [PMID: 25207998]

[23] Sklar LR, Almutawa F, Lim HW, Hamzavi I. Effects of ultraviolet radiation, visible light, and infrared radiation on erythema and pigmentation: a review. Photochem Photobiol Sci 2013; 12(1): 54-64.
[http://dx.doi.org/10.1039/C2PP25152C] [PMID: 23111621]

[24] Tyrrell RM. Activation of mammalian gene expression by the UV component of sunlight--from models to reality. BioEssays 1996; 18(2): 139-48.
[http://dx.doi.org/10.1002/bies.950180210] [PMID: 8851047]

[25] de Gruijl FR. In Methods in enzymology. Elsevier 2000; Vol. 319: pp. 359-66.

[26] York NR, Jacobe HT. UVA1 phototherapy: a review of mechanism and therapeutic application. Int J Dermatol 2010; 49(6): 623-30.
[http://dx.doi.org/10.1111/j.1365-4632.2009.04427.x] [PMID: 20618465]

[27] de Gruijl FR, Van der Leun JC. Estimate of the wavelength dependency of ultraviolet carcinogenesis in humans and its relevance to the risk assessment of a stratospheric ozone depletion. Health Phys 1994; 67(4): 319-25.
[http://dx.doi.org/10.1097/00004032-199410000-00001] [PMID: 8083043]

[28] Fisher GJ, Datta SC, Talwar HS, *et al.* Molecular basis of sun-induced premature skin ageing and retinoid antagonism. Nature 1996; 379(6563): 335-9.
[http://dx.doi.org/10.1038/379335a0] [PMID: 8552187]

[29] Holliman G, Lowe D, Cohen H, Felton S, Raj K. Ultraviolet radiation-induced production of nitric oxide: a multi-cell and multi-donor analysis. Sci Rep 2017; 7(1): 11105.
[http://dx.doi.org/10.1038/s41598-017-11567-5] [PMID: 28894213]

[30] Reeve V, Tyrrell RM. UVA and inducible protection. Biophysical and Physiological Effects of Solar Radiation on Human Skin 2007; 10: 293.
[http://dx.doi.org/10.1039/9781847557957-00293]

[31] Trummer C, Pandis M, Verheyen N, *et al.* Beneficial effects of UV-radiation: vitamin D and beyond.

Int J Environ Res Public Health 2016; 13(10): 1028.
[http://dx.doi.org/10.3390/ijerph13101028] [PMID: 27775585]

[32] Sam S, Lim J, Liau M, Toh M, Aw D. Knowledge, attitude and practices of adults in relation to sun exposure and photodamage. notice to authors. 2018.

[33] Brenner M, Hearing VJ. The protective role of melanin against UV damage in human skin. Photochem Photobiol 2008; 84(3): 539-49.
[http://dx.doi.org/10.1111/j.1751-1097.2007.00226.x] [PMID: 18435612]

[34] Biacchesi S, LeBerre M, Lamoureux A, *et al.* Mitochondrial antiviral signaling protein plays a major role in induction of the fish innate immune response against RNA and DNA viruses. J Virol 2009; 83(16): 7815-27.
[http://dx.doi.org/10.1128/JVI.00404-09] [PMID: 19474100]

[35] Dunaway S, Odin R, Zhou L, Ji L, Zhang Y, Kadekaro AL. Natural antioxidants: multiple mechanisms to protect skin from solar radiation. Front Pharmacol 2018; 9: 392.
[http://dx.doi.org/10.3389/fphar.2018.00392] [PMID: 29740318]

[36] Juzeniene A, Moan J. Beneficial effects of UV radiation other than *via* vitamin D production. Dermatoendocrinol 2012; 4(2): 109-17.
[http://dx.doi.org/10.4161/derm.20013] [PMID: 22928066]

[37] Schuit M, Ratnesar-Shumate S, Yolitz J, *et al.* Airborne SARS-CoV-2 is rapidly inactivated by simulated sunlight. J Infect Dis 2020; 222(4): 564-71.
[http://dx.doi.org/10.1093/infdis/jiaa334] [PMID: 32525979]

[38] Lindsley WG, Pearce TA, Hudnall JB, *et al.* Quantity and size distribution of cough-generated aerosol particles produced by influenza patients during and after illness. J Occup Environ Hyg 2012; 9(7): 443-9.
[http://dx.doi.org/10.1080/15459624.2012.684582] [PMID: 22651099]

[39] Morawska L, Johnson G, Ristovski Z, *et al.* Size distribution and sites of origin of droplets expelled from the human respiratory tract during expiratory activities. J Aerosol Sci 2009; 40(3): 256-69.
[http://dx.doi.org/10.1016/j.jaerosci.2008.11.002]

[40] Petropoulos F, Makridakis S. Forecasting the novel coronavirus COVID-19. PLoS One 2020; 15(3): e0231236.
[http://dx.doi.org/10.1371/journal.pone.0231236] [PMID: 32231392]

[41] Huang C, Wang Y, Li X, *et al.* Clinical features of patients infected with 2019 novel coronavirus in Wuhan, China. Lancet 2020; 395(10223): 497-506.
[http://dx.doi.org/10.1016/S0140-6736(20)30183-5] [PMID: 31986264]

[42] Su S, Wong G, Shi W, *et al.* Epidemiology, genetic recombination, and pathogenesis of coronaviruses. Trends Microbiol 2016; 24(6): 490-502.
[http://dx.doi.org/10.1016/j.tim.2016.03.003] [PMID: 27012512]

[43] Denison MR, Graham RL, Donaldson EF, Eckerle LD, Baric RS. Coronaviruses: an RNA proofreading machine regulates replication fidelity and diversity. RNA Biol 2011; 8(2): 270-9.
[http://dx.doi.org/10.4161/rna.8.2.15013] [PMID: 21593585]

[44] Zhong NS, Zheng BJ, Li YM, *et al.* Epidemiology and cause of severe acute respiratory syndrome (SARS) in Guangdong, People's Republic of China, in February, 2003. Lancet 2003; 362(9393): 1353-8.
[http://dx.doi.org/10.1016/S0140-6736(03)14630-2] [PMID: 14585636]

[45] Ksiazek TG, Erdman D, Goldsmith CS, *et al.* SARS Working Group. A novel coronavirus associated with severe acute respiratory syndrome. N Engl J Med 2003; 348(20): 1953-66.
[http://dx.doi.org/10.1056/NEJMoa030781] [PMID: 12690092]

[46] Zaki AM, van Boheemen S, Bestebroer TM, Osterhaus AD, Fouchier RA. Isolation of a novel coronavirus from a man with pneumonia in Saudi Arabia. N Engl J Med 2012; 367(19): 1814-20.

[http://dx.doi.org/10.1056/NEJMoa1211721] [PMID: 23075143]

[47] WHO Summary of probable SARS cases with onset of illness from November 01 2002 to July 31 2003.

[48] WHO. Middle East respiratory syndrome coronavirus. MERS-CoV 2019.

[49] Woo PC, Wang M, Lau SK, *et al.* Comparative analysis of twelve genomes of three novel group 2c and group 2d coronaviruses reveals unique group and subgroup features. J Virol 2007; 81(4): 1574-85. [http://dx.doi.org/10.1128/JVI.02182-06] [PMID: 17121802]

[50] Woo PC, Lau SK, Yip CC, *et al.* Comparative analysis of 22 coronavirus HKU1 genomes reveals a novel genotype and evidence of natural recombination in coronavirus HKU1. J Virol 2006; 80(14): 7136-45.
[http://dx.doi.org/10.1128/JVI.00509-06] [PMID: 16809319]

[51] Kottier SA, Cavanagh D, Britton P. Experimental evidence of recombination in coronavirus infectious bronchitis virus. Virology 1995; 213(2): 569-80.
[http://dx.doi.org/10.1006/viro.1995.0029] [PMID: 7491781]

[52] Lau SK, Woo PC, Yip CC, *et al.* Isolation and characterization of a novel Betacoronavirus subgroup A coronavirus, rabbit coronavirus HKU14, from domestic rabbits. J Virol 2012; 86(10): 5481-96.
[http://dx.doi.org/10.1128/JVI.06927-11] [PMID: 22398294]

[53] Lau SK, Li KS, Huang Y, *et al.* Ecoepidemiology and complete genome comparison of different strains of severe acute respiratory syndrome-related Rhinolophus bat coronavirus in China reveal bats as a reservoir for acute, self-limiting infection that allows recombination events. J Virol 2010; 84(6): 2808-19.
[http://dx.doi.org/10.1128/JVI.02219-09] [PMID: 20071579]

[54] Lau SK, Lee P, Tsang AK, *et al.* Molecular epidemiology of human coronavirus OC43 reveals evolution of different genotypes over time and recent emergence of a novel genotype due to natural recombination. J Virol 2011; 85(21): 11325-37.
[http://dx.doi.org/10.1128/JVI.05512-11] [PMID: 21849456]

[55] Lau SK, Poon RW, Wong BH, *et al.* Coexistence of different genotypes in the same bat and serological characterization of Rousettus bat coronavirus HKU9 belonging to a novel Betacoronavirus subgroup. J Virol 2010; 84(21): 11385-94.
[http://dx.doi.org/10.1128/JVI.01121-10] [PMID: 20702646]

[56] Wuhan; Commission, MH, Report of clustering pneumonia of unknown etiology in Wuhan City. Wuhan Municipal Health Commission 2019.

[57] CDC. Coronavirus Disease 2019 (COVID-19). Situation Summary 2020.

[58] WHO. SARS-CoV-2 Report 202, August 09, 20202020.

[59] Stadler K, Masignani V, Eickmann M, *et al.* SARS--beginning to understand a new virus. Nat Rev Microbiol 2003; 1(3): 209-18.
[http://dx.doi.org/10.1038/nrmicro775] [PMID: 15035025]

[60] Zhou P, Yang X-L, Wang X-G, *et al.* A pneumonia outbreak associated with a new coronavirus of probable bat origin. Nature 2020; 579(7798): 270-3.
[http://dx.doi.org/10.1038/s41586-020-2951-z]

[61] Li G. Erik De Clercq, therapeutic options for the 2019 novel coronavirus (2019-nCoV). Nat Rev Drug Discov 2020; 19(3): 149-50.

[62] Zumla A, Chan JF, Azhar EI, Hui DS, Yuen KY. Coronaviruses - drug discovery and therapeutic options. Nat Rev Drug Discov 2016; 15(5): 327-47.
[http://dx.doi.org/10.1038/nrd.2015.37] [PMID: 26868298]

[63] Lu R, Zhao X, Li J, *et al.* Genomic characterisation and epidemiology of 2019 novel coronavirus: implications for virus origins and receptor binding. Lancet 2020; 395(10224): 565-74.

[http://dx.doi.org/10.1016/S0140-6736(20)30251-8] [PMID: 32007145]

[64] Ahmed SF, Quadeer AA, McKay MR. Preliminary identification of potential vaccine targets for the COVID-19 coronavirus (SARS-CoV-2) based on SARS-CoV immunological studies bioRxiv 2020.

[65] Zhou P, Yang XL, Wang XG, *et al.* A pneumonia outbreak associated with a new coronavirus of probable bat origin. Nature 2020; 579(7798): 270-3.
[http://dx.doi.org/10.1038/s41586-020-2951-z]

[66] Lu R, Zhao X, Li J, *et al.* Genomic characterisation and epidemiology of 2019 novel coronavirus: implications for virus origins and receptor binding. Lancet 2020; 395(10224): 565-74.
[http://dx.doi.org/10.1016/S0140-6736(20)30251-8]

[67] Lu R, Zhao X, Li J, *et al.* Genomic characterisation and epidemiology of 2019 novel coronavirus: implications for virus origins and receptor binding. Lancet 2020; 395(10224): 565-74.
[http://dx.doi.org/10.1016/S0140-6736(20)30251-8] [PMID: 32007145]

[68] Zhong NS, Zheng BJ, Li YM, *et al.* Epidemiology and cause of severe acute respiratory syndrome (SARS) in Guangdong, People's Republic of China, in February, 2003. Lancet 2003; 362(9393): 1353-8.
[http://dx.doi.org/10.1016/S0140-6736(03)14630-2] [PMID: 14585636]

[69] Rota PA, Oberste MS, Monroe SS, *et al.* Characterization of a novel coronavirus associated with severe acute respiratory syndrome. Science 2003; 300(5624): 1394-9.
[http://dx.doi.org/10.1126/science.1085952] [PMID: 12730500]

[70] Lu CW, Liu XF, Jia ZF. -nCoV transmission through the ocular surface must not be ignored. Lancet 2019; 395(10224): e39.
[PMID: 32035510]

[71] Zhu N, Zhang D, Wang W, *et al.* China Novel Coronavirus Investigating and Research Team. A Novel Coronavirus from Patients with Pneumonia in China, 2019. N Engl J Med 2020; 382(8): 727-33.
[http://dx.doi.org/10.1056/NEJMoa2001017] [PMID: 31978945]

[72] Bao L, Deng W, Huang B, *et al.* The pathogenicity of SARS-CoV-2 in hACE2 transgenic mice. bioRxiv 2020.
[http://dx.doi.org/10.1101/2020.02.07.939389]

[73] Editorial. Stop the Wuhan virus. Nature Editorial 2020.

[74] Rothe C, Schunk M, Sothmann P, *et al.* Transmission of 2019-nCoV infection from an asymptomatic contact in Germany. N Engl J Med 2020; 382(10): 970-1.
[http://dx.doi.org/10.1056/NEJMc2001468] [PMID: 32003551]

[75] Xing D. Peking University Hospital Wang Guangfa disclosed treatment status on Weibo and suspected infection without wearing goggles. 2020.

[76] Borah A, Paul R, Choudhury S, *et al.* Neuroprotective potential of silymarin against CNS disorders: insight into the pathways and molecular mechanisms of action. CNS Neurosci Ther 2013; 19(11): 847-53.
[http://dx.doi.org/10.1111/cns.12175] [PMID: 24118806]

[77] Belser JA, Rota PA, Tumpey TM. Ocular tropism of respiratory viruses. Microbiol Mol Biol Rev 2013; 77(1): 144-56.
[http://dx.doi.org/10.1128/MMBR.00058-12] [PMID: 23471620]

[78] Wang D, Hu B, Hu C, *et al.* Clinical characteristics of 138 hospitalized patients with. Novel coronavirus-infected pneumonia in Wuhan, China. JAMA 2020; 323(11): 1061-9.
[http://dx.doi.org/10.1001/jama.2020.1585] [PMID: 32031570]

[79] Lucey D. 2019-nCoV: Fecal-oral transmission of the new coronavirus? More research urgently needed 2020.

[80] Gander K. Coronavirus Could Spread Through Pipes in Buildings, Officials Fear. Newsweek 2020.

[81] Hoehl S, Rabenau H, Berger A, *et al.* Evidence of sars-cov-2 infection in returning travelers from Wuhan, China. N Engl J Med 2020; 382(13): 1278-80. [http://dx.doi.org/10.1056/NEJMc2001899] [PMID: 32069388]

[82] WHO Inadequate plumbing systems likely contributed to SARS transmission. https://www.who.int/news-room/detail/26-09-2003-inadequate-plumbing-systems-likely- contributed-to-sars-transmission

[83] World health organization: middle east respiratory syndrome coronavirus (MERS-CoV)-factsheet. 2017.

[84] Gañán-Gómez I, Wei Y, Yang H, Boyano-Adánez MC, García-Manero G. Oncogenic functions of the transcription factor Nrf2. Free Radic Biol Med 2013; 65: 750-64. [http://dx.doi.org/10.1016/j.freeradbiomed.2013.06.041] [PMID: 23820265]

[85] Chen N, Zhou M, Dong X, *et al.* Epidemiological and clinical characteristics of 99 cases of 2019 novel coronavirus pneumonia in Wuhan, China: a descriptive study. Lancet 2020; 395(10223): 507-13. [http://dx.doi.org/10.1016/S0140-6736(20)30211-7] [PMID: 32007143]

[86] Chowell G, Abdirizak F, Lee S, *et al.* Transmission characteristics of MERS and SARS in the healthcare setting: a comparative study. BMC Med 2015; 13: 210. [http://dx.doi.org/10.1186/s12916-015-0450-0] [PMID: 26336062]

[87] Modjarrad K. MERS-CoV vaccine candidates in development: The current landscape. Vaccine 2016; 34(26): 2982-7. [http://dx.doi.org/10.1016/j.vaccine.2016.03.104] [PMID: 27083424]

[88] Munster VJ, Koopmans M, van Doremalen N, van Riel D, de Wit E. A novel coronavirus emerging in China-key questions for impact assessment. N Engl J Med 2020; 382(8): 692-4. [http://dx.doi.org/10.1056/NEJMp2000929] [PMID: 31978293]

[89] Chan JF-W, Yuan S, Kok K-H, *et al.* A familial cluster of pneumonia associated with the 2019 novel coronavirus indicating person-to-person transmission: a study of a family cluster. Lancet 2020; 395(10223): 514-23. [http://dx.doi.org/10.1016/S0140-6736(20)30154-9] [PMID: 31986261]

[90] Wong G, Liu W, Liu Y, Zhou B, Bi Y, Gao GF. MERS, SARS, and Ebola: the role of super-spreaders in infectious disease. Cell Host Microbe 2015; 18(4): 398-401. [http://dx.doi.org/10.1016/j.chom.2015.09.013] [PMID: 26468744]

[91] Holshue ML, DeBolt C, Lindquist S, *et al.* Washington state 2019-nCoV case investigation team. First case of 2019 novel coronavirus in the United States. N Engl J Med 2020; 382(10): 929-36. [http://dx.doi.org/10.1056/NEJMoa2001191] [PMID: 32004427]

[92] PG Sick. Interim laboratory biosafety guidelines for handling and processing specimens associated with coronavirus disease 2019 (COVID-19). Atlanta, GA: Centers for Disease Control and Prevention 2020 Mar.

[93] Saura M, Zaragoza C, McMillan A, *et al.* An antiviral mechanism of nitric oxide: inhibition of a viral protease. Immunity 1999; 10(1): 21-8. [http://dx.doi.org/10.1016/S1074-7613(00)80003-5] [PMID: 10023767]

[94] Perrone LA, Belser JA, Wadford DA, Katz JM, Tumpey TM. Inducible nitric oxide contributes to viral pathogenesis following highly pathogenic influenza virus infection in mice. J Infect Dis 2013; 207(10): 1576-84. [http://dx.doi.org/10.1093/infdis/jit062] [PMID: 23420903]

[95] Pertile TL, Karaca K, Sharma JM, Walser MM. An antiviral effect of nitric oxide: inhibition of reovirus replication. Avian Dis 1996; 40(2): 342-8. [http://dx.doi.org/10.2307/1592230] [PMID: 8790884]

[96] Bi Z, Reiss CS. Inhibition of vesicular stomatitis virus infection by nitric oxide. J Virol 1995; 69(4):

2208-13.
[http://dx.doi.org/10.1128/jvi.69.4.2208-2213.1995] [PMID: 7533852]

[97] Komatsu T, Bi Z, Reiss CS. Interferon-γ induced type I nitric oxide synthase activity inhibits viral replication in neurons. J Neuroimmunol 1996; 68(1-2): 101-8.
[http://dx.doi.org/10.1016/0165-5728(96)00083-5] [PMID: 8784266]

[98] Karupiah G, Xie QW, Buller RM, Nathan C, Duarte C, MacMicking JD. Inhibition of viral replication by interferon-gamma-induced nitric oxide synthase. Science 1993; 261(5127): 1445-8.
[http://dx.doi.org/10.1126/science.7690156] [PMID: 7690156]

[99] Cherrie M, Clemens T, Colandrea C, *et al.* Radiation and COVID-19 deaths: a multi country study. medRxiv 2020.

[100] Suschek CV, Krischel V, Bruch-Gerharz D, *et al.* Nitric oxide fully protects against UVA-induced apoptosis in tight correlation with Bcl-2 up-regulation. J Biol Chem 1999; 274(10): 6130-7.
[http://dx.doi.org/10.1074/jbc.274.10.6130] [PMID: 10037696]

[101] Akerström S, Mousavi-Jazi M, Klingström J, Leijon M, Lundkvist A, Mirazimi A. Nitric oxide inhibits the replication cycle of severe acute respiratory syndrome coronavirus. J Virol 2005; 79(3): 1966-9.
[http://dx.doi.org/10.1128/JVI.79.3.1966-1969.2005] [PMID: 15650225]

[102] Oxley TJ, Mocco J, Majidi S, *et al.* Large-vessel stroke as a presenting feature of COVID-19 in the young. N Engl J Med 2020; 382(20): e60.
[http://dx.doi.org/10.1056/NEJMc2009787] [PMID: 32343504]

[103] Ye Z, Zhang Y, Wang Y, Huang Z, Song B. Chest CT manifestations of new coronavirus disease 2019 (COVID-19): a pictorial review. Eur Radiol 2020; 30(8): 4381-9.
[http://dx.doi.org/10.1007/s00330-020-06801-0] [PMID: 32193638]

[104] Alvarez RA, Berra L, Gladwin MT. Home nitric oxide therapy for COVID-19. Am J Respir Crit Care Med 2020; 202(1): 16-20.
[http://dx.doi.org/10.1164/rccm.202005-1906ED] [PMID: 32437250]

[105] Griffiths MJ, Evans TW. Inhaled nitric oxide therapy in adults. N Engl J Med 2005; 353(25): 2683-95.
[http://dx.doi.org/10.1056/NEJMra051884] [PMID: 16371634]

[106] Brown RH, Mitzner W. Airway response to deep inspiration: role of nitric oxide. Eur Respir J 2003; 22(1): 57-61.
[http://dx.doi.org/10.1183/09031936.03.00090403] [PMID: 12882451]

[107] Kacmarek RM, Ripple R, Cockrill BA, Bloch KJ, Zapol WM, Johnson DC. Inhaled nitric oxide. A bronchodilator in mild asthmatics with methacholine-induced bronchospasm. Am J Respir Crit Care Med 1996; 153(1): 128-35.
[http://dx.doi.org/10.1164/ajrccm.153.1.8542105] [PMID: 8542105]

[108] Prado CM, Martins MA, Tibério IF. Nitric oxide in asthma physiopathology ISRN allergy, 2011 2011.
[http://dx.doi.org/10.5402/2011/832560]

[109] Chen L, Liu P, Gao H, *et al.* Inhalation of nitric oxide in the treatment of severe acute respiratory syndrome: a rescue trial in Beijing. Clin Infect Dis 2004; 39(10): 1531-5.
[http://dx.doi.org/10.1086/425357] [PMID: 15546092]

[110] Zamanian RT, Pollack Jr CV, Gentile MA, *et al.* Outpatient inhaled nitric oxide in a patient with vasoreactive IPAH and COVID-19 infection. American Journal of Respiratory and Critical Care Medicine 2020. ja

[111] Wink DA, Miranda KM, Espey MG, *et al.* Mechanisms of the antioxidant effects of nitric oxide. Antioxid Redox Signal 2001; 3(2): 203-13.
[http://dx.doi.org/10.1089/152308601300185179] [PMID: 11396476]

[112] Thomas DD, Heinecke JL, Ridnour LA, *et al.* Signaling and stress: The redox landscape in NOS2

biology. Free Radic Biol Med 2015; 87: 204-25.
[http://dx.doi.org/10.1016/j.freeradbiomed.2015.06.002] [PMID: 26117324]

[113] Culotta E, Koshland DE Jr. NO news is good news. Science 1992; 258(5090): 1862-5.
[http://dx.doi.org/10.1126/science.1361684] [PMID: 1361684]

[114] Palmer RM, Ferrige AG, Moncada S. Nitric oxide release accounts for the biological activity of endothelium-derived relaxing factor. Nature 1987; 327(6122): 524-6.
[http://dx.doi.org/10.1038/327524a0] [PMID: 3495737]

[115] Ricciardolo FLM. Multiple roles of nitric oxide in the airways. Thorax 2003; 58(2): 175-82.
[http://dx.doi.org/10.1136/thorax.58.2.175] [PMID: 12554905]

[116] Radomski MW, Palmer RM, Moncada S. An L-arginine/nitric oxide pathway present in human platelets regulates aggregation. Proc Natl Acad Sci USA 1990; 87(13): 5193-7.
[http://dx.doi.org/10.1073/pnas.87.13.5193] [PMID: 1695013]

[117] Bredt DS, Snyder SH. Nitric oxide mediates glutamate-linked enhancement of cGMP levels in the cerebellum. Proc Natl Acad Sci USA 1989; 86(22): 9030-3.
[http://dx.doi.org/10.1073/pnas.86.22.9030] [PMID: 2573074]

[118] Hamid Q, Springall DR, Riveros-Moreno V, *et al.* Induction of nitric oxide synthase in asthma. Lancet 1993; 342(8886-8887): 1510-3.
[http://dx.doi.org/10.1016/S0140-6736(05)80083-2] [PMID: 7504773]

[119] Kobzik L, Bredt DS, Lowenstein CJ, *et al.* Nitric oxide synthase in human and rat lung: immunocytochemical and histochemical localization. Am J Respir Cell Mol Biol 1993; 9(4): 371-7.
[http://dx.doi.org/10.1165/ajrcmb/9.4.371] [PMID: 7691109]

[120] Sahni S, Hickok JR, Thomas DD. Nitric oxide reduces oxidative stress in cancer cells by forming dinitrosyliron complexes. Nitric Oxide 2018; 76: 37-44.
[http://dx.doi.org/10.1016/j.niox.2018.03.003] [PMID: 29522907]

[121] Tripathi P. Nitric oxide and immune response. Indian J Biochem Biophys 2007; 44(5): 310-9.

[122] Hedenstierna G, Chen L, Hedenstierna M, Lieberman R, Fine DH. Nitric oxide dosed in short bursts at high concentrations may protect against Covid 19. Nitric Oxide 2020; 103: 1-3.
[http://dx.doi.org/10.1016/j.niox.2020.06.005] [PMID: 32590117]

[123] Adusumilli NC, Zhang D, Friedman JM, Friedman AJ. Harnessing nitric oxide for preventing, limiting and treating the severe pulmonary consequences of COVID-19. Nitric Oxide 2020; 103: 4-8.
[http://dx.doi.org/10.1016/j.niox.2020.07.003] [PMID: 32681986]

[124] Zhang R, Hess DT, Qian Z, *et al.* Hemoglobin βCys93 is essential for cardiovascular function and integrated response to hypoxia. Proc Natl Acad Sci USA 2015; 112(20): 6425-30.
[http://dx.doi.org/10.1073/pnas.1502285112] [PMID: 25810253]

[125] Cabrales P. Examining and mitigating acellular hemoglobin vasoactivity. Antioxid Redox Signal 2013; 18(17): 2329-41.
[http://dx.doi.org/10.1089/ars.2012.4922] [PMID: 22938394]

[126] Odkhuu E, Komatsu T, Koide N, *et al.* Sendai virus C protein limits NO production in infected RAW264.7 macrophages. Innate Immun 2018; 24(7): 430-8.
[http://dx.doi.org/10.1177/1753425918796619] [PMID: 30189760]

[127] Tang Y, Liu J, Zhang D, Xu Z, Ji J, Wen C. Cytokine storm in COVID-19: the current evidence and treatment strategies. Front Immunol 2020; 11: 1708.
[http://dx.doi.org/10.3389/fimmu.2020.01708] [PMID: 32754163]

[128] Moilanen E, Vapaatalo H. Nitric oxide in inflammation and immune response. Ann Med 1995; 27(3): 359-67.
[http://dx.doi.org/10.3109/07853899509002589] [PMID: 7546626]

[129] Thomassen MJ, Buhrow LT, Connors MJ, Kaneko FT, Erzurum SC, Kavuru MS. Nitric oxide inhibits

inflammatory cytokine production by human alveolar macrophages. Am J Respir Cell Mol Biol 1997; 17(3): 279-83.
[http://dx.doi.org/10.1165/ajrcmb.17.3.2998m] [PMID: 9308913]

[130] Martel J, Ko Y-F, Young JD, Ojcius DM. Could nasal nitric oxide help to mitigate the severity of COVID-19? Microbes Infect 2020; 22(4-5): 168-71.

[131] Lancaster JR Jr. Nitroxidative, nitrosative, and nitrative stress: kinetic predictions of reactive nitrogen species chemistry under biological conditions. Chem Res Toxicol 2006; 19(9): 1160-74.
[http://dx.doi.org/10.1021/tx060061w] [PMID: 16978020]

[132] Toledo JC Jr, Bosworth CA, Hennon SW, Mahtani HA, Bergonia HA, Lancaster JR Jr. Nitric oxide-induced conversion of cellular chelatable iron into macromolecule-bound paramagnetic dinitrosyliron complexes. J Biol Chem 2008; 283(43): 28926-33.
[http://dx.doi.org/10.1074/jbc.M707862200] [PMID: 18480062]

[133] Ford PC, Lorkovic IM. Mechanistic aspects of the reactions of nitric oxide with transition-metal complexes. Chem Rev 2002; 102(4): 993-1018.
[http://dx.doi.org/10.1021/cr0000271] [PMID: 11942785]

[134] Kobayashi Y. The regulatory role of nitric oxide in proinflammatory cytokine expression during the induction and resolution of inflammation. J Leukoc Biol 2010; 88(6): 1157-62.
[http://dx.doi.org/10.1189/jlb.0310149] [PMID: 20807706]

CHAPTER 9

Herbal Remedies Effective against COVID-19

Laiba Hassan[1], Muhammad Ali Syed[1,*] and **Mohammad Ejaz[1]**

[1] *Department of Microbiology, The University of Haripur, Haripur, Pakistan*

Abstract: Coronavirus disease-2019 (COVID-19) first originated from China, named Wuhan, and now becomes a pandemic disease. The COVID-19 infections range from asymptomatic to mild and severe conditions. Medicinal plants have potential therapeutic effects for different infectious diseases and have long been used to treat many diseases. Wild plants are well-known for their anti-viral activities and are also used in herbal treatment for COVID-19 infection. Various traditional medicine systems use plants for the treatment of COVID-19. The considerable therapeutic effect was achieved by using traditional Chinese medicine (TCM) during the 2003 outbreak of severe acute respiratory syndrome (SARS), which brought new hope preventing and treating COVID-19. The Ministry of Ayurveda, Yoga & Naturopathy, Unani, Siddha, and Homoeopathy (AYUSH) focuses on prophylactic treatment, dietary management, and simple traditional remedies for the treatment of symptoms of COVID-19 by using medicinal plants. Telemedicine was focused on a new health care model to prevent transmission of COVID-19 by avoiding person-to-person contact. The purpose of this chapter is to identify the effective herbal treatment for COVID-19.

Keywords: AYUSH, COVID-19, TCM, Telemedicine, Wild plants.

INTRODUCTION

Coronaviruses belong to the family of *Coronaviridae*, which include viruses that commonly cause respiratory tract diseases ranging from the common cold to severe conditions. It has Middle East respiratory syndrome-coronavirus (MERS-CoV) or severe acute respiratory syndrome-coronavirus (SARS- CoV) [1]. A new strain of the corona virus was identified in the city of China, named Wuhan, at the end of 2019 [2] and was initially named the 2019-novel Corona Virus (2019-nCoV) [3]. The International Committee on Taxonomy of Viruses (ICTV) named this novel coronavirus as "severe acute respiratory syndrome coronavirus 2" (SARS-CoV2) on February 11, 2020, by picking its name from the causative virus of the 2003 outbreak of severe acute respiratory syndrome (SARS). It is genetically similar to the SARS virus [4]. After that, the World Health Organizat-

* **Corresponding author Muhammad Ali Syed:** Infectious Diseases Research Group, Department of Microbiology University of Haripur; Pakistan; Tel: +92 3325 256 722; E-mail: mirwah2000@yahoo.de

Kamal Niaz & Muhammad Farrukh Nisar (Eds.)

ion (WHO) officially declared the disease name caused by this virus as COVID-19 (coronavirus disease-2019) [5]. After identifying the first case of the novel coronavirus in late December 2019 in China, it rapidly spread to other countries such as Germany, the USA, France, Iran, Spain, Italy, India, and now spread worldwide [6]. COVID-19 has over 1 million cases across the globe, almost 50,000 deaths are caused, and 203 countries are affected by this novel coronavirus decalred by WHO. Emergency Committee of WHO declared the SARS-CoV-2 a global pandemic on March 11, 2020 [7].

The period from exposure of the virus to the appearance of symptoms ranges from 2 to 14 days, but the average incubation period is 5 days [3]. Initial symptoms of COVID-19 are commonly non-specific such as dry cough, fever, and fatigue, *etc*. It may involve multiple systems such as the respiratory system causing sore throat, shortness of breath, cough, chest pain, hemoptysis and rhinorrhea, musculoskeletal causing muscle ache, gastrointestinal causing nausea, vomiting, diarrhea, and neurologic causing confusion and headache [8]. In severe cases, COVID-19 causes multiple organ failure and lead to death [9].

Currently, there is no specific vaccine or treatment available for COVID-19 [10]. Some studies have investigated anti-viral drugs, including protease inhibitors such as Ritonavir/Lopinavir, neuraminidase inhibitors, nucleoside analogs, Lamivudine, Tenofovir Disoproxil, Umifenovir, and Remdesivir for the treatment of patients of COVID-19 [11]. The results of these studies for therapeutic use are clinically not approved for the treatment of infected patients of COVID-19 [12]. Supportive therapies and preventive measures are implemented to avoid further complications of COVID-19 and prevent organ damage [13].

Symptomatic Comparison of SARS-CoV, MERS-CoV, and COVID-19

For the last two decades, the world has suffered from a few of the most devastating outbreaks of viral diseases. It includes the epidemics of coronaviruses like SARS-CoV that emerged in Guangdong, China, MERS-CoV emergence in Saudi Arabia, and newly emerged SARS-CoV-2 in Wuhan, China causing several causalities. HCoV-OC43, HCoV-229E, HCoV-NL63, and HCoV-HKU1 are among the other viruses belonging to the same family causing outbreaks in different regions [14, 15]. The viruses are closely related to each other as several studies reported the sequence homology of SARS-CoV-2 with other viruses belonging to β-*coronaviridae*. The studies conducted by Wu *et al.* [16] and Zhou *et al.* [8] in 2020 reported the sequence homology of 79.5% between SARS-Co--2 and SARS-CoV. However, Chan *et al.* (2020) reported the sequence homology of 89% and 82% with bat SARS-like CoVZXC21 and human SARS-CoV [17]. The previous epidemic of SARS-CoV and MERS-CoV reported being zoonotically originated from bats and transmitted to humans *via* intermediate hosts of civet cats and camel, respectively. For SARS-CoV-2, bats were considered as native hosts as the virus has 96% similarity with SARS-like coronaviruses, including bat- SL-CoVZX21 and bat-SL-CoVZX45 [18, 19]. The potential route of transmission from person to person is through inhalation of infectious aerosol. The potential of COVID-19 spreading is higher compared to other phylogenetically related viruses. This may be due to mutations like longer 8b segments, shorter 3b segments, absence of 8a, the difference in open reading frame 8 (ORF8), and open reading frame 10 (ORF10), and the difference in nsp2 and nsp3 proteins [20 - 23]. Besides these mutations, the changes in the nsp2 protein of SARS-CoV-2 lead to an increased potential to become more contagious than other related viruses [24].

After incubation of about 5-7 days, SARS-CoV leads to the onset of the disease typically associated with symptoms like fever, headache, myalgia, malaise, dyspnea, and dry cough, in which 25% of the patients develop watery diarrhea. In some severe cases, the disease progresses to severe pneumonia and respiratory distress [25 - 28]. A similar disease goes in the MERS-CoV infected individuals who may develop an asymptomatic or mild infection, including fever, chills, myalgia, and dyspnea, followed by a nonproductive cough. Abdominal pain, diarrhea, and vomiting are reported in 25% of infected individuals. The severity of the progression of the disease may result in acute renal failure along with respiratory distress and pneumonia [29, 30]. The case fatality rate in MERS-CoV infected individuals is 34.4% compared to SARS-CoV with a fatality rate of 9.6%, and SARS-CoV-2, with a mortality rate of >3.4% [31 - 33].

The mean incubation period of SARS-CoV-2 is 5.2 days and 14 days of median duration from onset of symptom to death, and the mortality rate is alarming in the patients with age more than 70 years as they have a median duration of 11.5 days from the initial onset of the symptoms to the death [34]. Human coronaviruses are mostly associated with the upper respiratory tract causing mild to moderate illness. Still, in some moderate to severe cases, the lower respiratory tract can be infected and result in severe complications [35]. The COVID-19 infection ranges from asymptomatic to mild and severe infection as similar to SARS-CoV and MERS-CoV. The symptoms include fever, myalgia, dry cough, fatigue, chest pain, anorexia, nausea, vomiting, dyspnea, arrhythmia, and diarrhea. Complications related to coronaviruses infection involve acute respiratory distress syndrome, multiple organ failure, various degrees of liver infection [36], testicular tissue damage [37], kidney infections, RNAemia, cardiac injury, and metabolic acidosis [38]. Moreover, the infected individual can be observed with ground-glass opacities and peripheral consolidation in the lungs. The bilateral finding seems to be higher in SARS-CoV-2 infected patients [39].

The symptomatic comparison of SARS-CoV, MERS-CoV, and SARS-CoV-2 is shown in Table **1**. In COVID-19 disease, the viral load is higher compared to SARS-CoV and MERS-CoV infections, even in asymptomatic or mild infections [40]. The laboratory findings of these coronaviruses (SARS-CoV, MERS-CoV, and SARS-CoV-2) are also similar, indicating the lymphopenia, thrombocytopenia, elevated LDH level, elevated cytokines level (IL-1, IL-2, IL-6, and IL-10 INFγ), and elevated C-reactive protein [30, 41 - 43].

Table 1. Comparison of symptoms associated with SARS-CoV, MERS-CoV, and COVID-19 infections.

Disease	Emergence	Transmission	Incubation Period	Symptoms	Complications	Recovery Period	Treatment
SARS-CoV	2002, China	Human to Human *via* respiratory droplets, Inhalation of aerosol, Nosocomial transmission, Zoonotic transmission	2-7 days post-exposure	Fever, dry cough, breathing difficulties, myalgia, diarrhea, and loss of appetite	Acute respiratory distress syndrome (ADRS), Severe pneumonia	5-6 weeks	Oxygen therapy, Anti-viral drugs, Corticosteroids to reduce inflammation in the lungs
MERS-CoV	2012, Saudi Arabia	Human to Human *via* respiratory droplets, Inhalation of aerosol, Nosocomial transmission, Zoonotic transmission	5-6 days post-exposure	Fever, dry cough, nasal congestion, sore throat, chills, nausea, and vomiting	Acute renal failure, Pneumonia, Multiple organ failure ARDS,	6-8 weeks	No proper treatment, Only symptoms are treated
SARS-CoV-2	2019, China	Human to Human *via* respiratory droplets, Inhalation of aerosol, Nosocomial transmission, Zoonotic transmission, Oral-fecal transmission	2-14 days post-exposure	Fever, sore throat, myalgia, nasal congestion, shortness of breath, vomiting, diarrhea, and dry cough	Severe pneumonia, Septic shock, Pulmonary edema, ARDS and organ failure	2-8 weeks	No vaccine and No treatment, Symptoms are treated, Breathing ventilator for oxygen therapy

Medicinal Plants against Coronaviruses

Medicinal plants have potential therapeutic effects for different infectious diseases and have long been used to treat the diseases in the past. Medicinal plants can be used as a whole, as an extract of the plant or phytochemicals isolated from plants [44] and endophytes isolated to extract secondary metabolites that have therapeutic effects [45]. More than 60,000 plant species have been used for medicinal purposes worldwide, in which 3,000 species are traded internationally, and 28,000 species are well documented, with one-third are known to be cultivated commercially [46]. There is a wide range of medicinal plants and treatment applications based on the plants that have been practiced in the Indian subcontinent and China for a long time. Traditional medicinal practices in India use medicinal plants that directly include Unani, Homeopathy, Ayurveda, Naturopathy, and Siddha. AYUSH system of medicine focuses on the prophylactic treatment, dietary management, and simple traditional remedies for the treatment of symptoms by using medicinal plants [47]

Ni *et al.* [48] reported the case study for the treatment of COVID-19 using TCM called Shuanghuanglian. Shuanghuanglian (SHL) is a TCM that contains the extract from three medicinal plants, namely *Forsythia, Scutellaria baicalensis,* and *Honeysuckle.* It is usually used to treat the common cold with fever, cough, and sore throat. The case study reported the effectiveness of this medicine with no adverse side effects. Thus a clinical trial is needed to be used in the future for treating the COVID-19 patients.

Andrographis paniculata is a medicinal plant that has shown the therapeutic ability for viral respiratory infections in Ayurveda and other natural remedies-based treatment systems [49]. It was reported that *Andrographis paniculata* suppressed the increase in caspase-1, interleukin-1β, and NOD-like receptor protein involved in SARS-CoV's pathogenesis and more likely of SARS-CoV-2 infection [50]. The plants like *Allium sativum* [51] and *Glycyrrhiza glabra* [52] are known to target SARS-CoV replication; thus, they can be promising candidates against the COVID-19 causative agent SARS-CoV-2. Similarly, the herbal medicinal plant is called *Clerodendrum inerme* (L.) *Gaertn* has the potential to neutralize the viral infection by inactivating the virus, thus can be investigated as potential candidate for the drug that targets SARS-CoV-2 proteins translation [53]. *Hyoscyamus niger*, the medicinal plant, has inhibitory effects on the Ca^2+ channel and has bronchodilation ability, thus targeting the Ca^{2+} channels of orf3a that trigger various downstream pathways after the infection of the virus [54].

Moreover, *Sambucus ebulus* is found to inhibit the activity of enveloped viruses and can be a potential target for treating COVID-19 individuals [55]. Some of the medicinal plants produce bioactive molecules like flavonoids that have anti-viral activities. The medicinal plants including *Spinacia oleracea*, *Brassica oleracea*, *Anethum graveolens*, *Sauropus androgynous*, *Foeniculum vulgare*, *Allium cepa,* and *Oregano vulgare* are reported to produce the secondary metabolite like Kaempferol and Quercetin that can be used as anti-viral agents [56, 57].

TCM system is also in practice to find its effectiveness in treating COVID-19 infections. These TCM use medicinal plants to extract the phytochemicals or secondary metabolites for the treatment of COVID-19. Some studies have reported that TCM plants can modulate T-cells to enhance the host defense system [58, 59]. Another Chinese herb, Liquorice root, contains an active compound called glycyrrhizin, which can potentially inhibit the replication of the SARS-CoV virus in clinical isolates [60]. Furthermore, the TCM extracts from *Houttuynia cordata* [61], *a* flavonoid extracted from seeds of litchi [62], beta-sitosterol extracted from the roots of *Isatis indigotica* [63], and *Rhubarb* extracts have shown the enzymatic activity against the SARS 3CLpro (3-chymotrypsi--like protease). The compound is important for replicating viral particles and can thus be a promising drug target for SARS-CoV-2 and other coronaviruses [64].

Western medicines in practice cannot effectively treat COVID-19 infected patients. The main strategy for treating the infectious individual of COVID-19 is supportive care, supplemented by a combination of anti-virals, broad-spectrum antibiotics, convalescent plasma therapy, and corticosteroids. Therefore, herbal medicines have become an important area of interest for preventing and treating COVID-19 [61].

Traditional Chinese Medicine (TCM) against Coronaviruses

TCM is a system of medical field based on principles of herbal pharmacology, theories, pathogenesis, symptoms, diagnosis, and treatment of disease. It differs from Western naturopathy and orthodox medicine. The application of TCM has evolved over millennia from knowledge gained through observation of clinical diseases and treatment. TCM has quickly expanded in recent years, and its users account for 3.2% of overall medicines [65].

There has been a long history of TCM, which played an important role in preventing and treating many epidemic diseases [66]. TCM has been used since 2003 to fight against several viral diseases such as SARS, MERS, H7N9, H1N1, and EBOV [67]. A considerable therapeutic effect was achieved by using TCM during the outbreak of SARS that occurred in 2003 [68].

Results of many clinical practices revealed that TCM plays a vital role in treating infection of COVID-19, which brings a new hope to control and prevent COVID-19 [66]. "New Coronavirus Pneumonia Diagnosis and Treatment Plan" also recommended TCM to treat symptoms caused by COVID-19 [69].

TCM Prescription for COVID 19

Many TCM have been described in the publications of medical institutions and local government [70]. The Chinese medicinal herbs used to treat COVID-19 patients mainly include *Trichosanthes*, *Ephedra*, *Glycyrrhiza*, *Amomum*, bitter almond, reed root, and gypsum. The main functions of these herbal medicines include toxicity clearance and heat removal from the lungs, improve immunity, and relieving cough [71]. The patent medicines used to treat COVID-19 patients mainly include the Suhuang Zhike capsule, *Reduning* injection, and Xuebijing [69].

The combined study of the Virology Institute in Wuhan, the Chinese Academy of Sciences, and Materia Medica institute in Shanghai reported that the oral liquid of Shuanghuanglian could inhibit COVID-19 [48]. Shuanghuanglian is composed of a Chinese skullcap, honeysuckle flowers, and forsythia. Previous studies reported that components such as forsythin, chlorogenic acid, and baicalin could inhibit many bacteria and viruses [72]. The mechanism of therapeutic effect might be achieved by decreasing the inflammatory response caused by bacteria and viruses in the body through these components [73]. Shuanghuanglian is effective for the treatment of cough, fever, and sore throat [74].

Based on the overall symptoms of pneumonia caused by COVID-19, TCM has suggested prescriptions that might be effective, such as qingfei touxie fuzheng recipe, sheganmahuang decoction, gancaoganjiang decoction, and qingfei paidu decoction (QPD), *etc*., [66]. QPD consists of *Zingiberis Rhizoma Recens, Zingibere et Alumine, Asteris Radix et Rhizoma, Pinelliae Rhizoma Praepratum cum, Farfarae Flos, Scutellariae Radix, Belamcandae Rhizoma, Bupleuri Radix, Asari Radix et Rhizoma, Poria, Atractylodis Macrocephalae Rhizoma, Dioscoreae Rhizoma, Pogostemonis Herba, Ephedrae Herba, Citri Reticulatae Pericarpium, Glycyrrhizae, Aurantii Fructus Immaturus, Radix et Rhizoma Praeprata cum Melle, Polyporus, Armeniacae Semen Amarum, Alismatis Rhizoma, Cinnamomi Ramulus* and *Cinnamomi Ramulus.* In China, QPD is promoted to be included in the general prescription plan for the diagnosis and treatment of COVID-19 [75]. The QPD effective rate to cure COVID-19 is more than 90%. This decoction is primarily specific for the treatment of lung diseases. It can act on various ribosomal proteins of COVID-19, as a result, block viral replication. It removes inflammation by regulating immune response and related pathways of cytokine action [76]. Molecular docking predicts that shionone, ergosterol, and patchouli alcohol found in the formula of QPD is highly effective against COVID-19, which can provide a molecular structure for the development of new drugs [66].

Treatment measures of COVID-19 patients revealed that early involvement of TCM plays a vital role in reducing the disease course, enhance the cure rate, delay the progression of the disease, and low the mortality rate. Moreover, TCM not only inhibits COVID-19, but it also reduces infection rate or block infection, inhibits inflammatory action, improves immune response, and promote body repairing. Furthermore, the control measures and prevention of COVID-19 show entirely the idea of "preventive treatment of disease" [77, 66].

TCM considers Qi as a fundamental constituent of the human body that maintains normal functioning. There are two types of Qi such as pathogenic Qi and healthy Qi. Pathogenic Qi is a substance that can harm body health, while healthy Qi can regulate the body's normal functioning [78].

TCM to Prevent COVID-19 Infection

The target for COVID-19 is the lungs. Therefore, TCM treatment's purpose is to protect the lungs. Yupingfeng San is a patent TCM, selected to prevent pathogenic Qi and to improve lung Qi. TCM effectively prescribes Yupingfeng San prevent pneumonia caused by the novel coronavirus, COVID-19 [79]. It is made of herbs such as 20g of Astragalus, 15g of Fangfeng, and 15g of Atractylodes. Astragalus decreases phlegm and enhances lungs Qi [78]. Fangfeng relieves pain, removes pathogenic Qi, and prevents dampness. *Atractylodes* improve absorption and digestion by enhancing spleen Qi. Yupingfeng San can enhance the immune response of the body [75]. These herbs are mixed and then boiled for about 15 minutes in 1000ml pure water to make a tincture of about 600ml. About 200ml of tincture is orally taken three times a day by dividing it into three doses [78].

TCM to Treat the Mild Infection

According to TCM theories, lung Qi is harmed by pathogenic Qi, due to which the lung is unable to work correctly. It results in moisture and heat in the lungs and some common symptoms of mild infection of COVID-19 such as cough, fever, sore throat, and fatigue [78]. The method is used to remove moisture and lung heat for treatment. Two types of TCM, such as Yinqiao san and Sangju yin, are prescribed for clinical treatment. These prescriptions function to relieve cough, expel phlegm, remove lung heat, and restore and regulate the normal function of the lungs [80]. The medicinal herbs used in making Yinqiao san include Bamboo leaves 6g, Nepeta 6g, licorice 3g, Chinese bellflower 6g, Mint

6g, Forsythia 15g, Honeysuckle 15g, light tempeh 5g, and Burdock 6g. Medicinal herbs in Sangju yin are Mint 6g, Mulberry leaves 15 g, Chinese bellflower 6g, Chrysanthemum 10g, Reed root 15g, Forsythia10g, Almond 9g, Licorice 3g. These herbs are mixed and then boiled for about 15 minutes in 1000ml pure water to make a tincture of about 600ml. About 200ml of tincture is orally taken three times a day by dividing it into three doses [78].

Yin Qiao San improves the immune response of the respiratory tract, and it may have anti-viral and anti-bacterial activity [81]. These two medicines can be prescribed to treat patients having a mild infection of SARS CoV-2 [78].

TCM to Treat Severe Infection

During severe cases of COVID-19, respiratory and multiple organ failures occur, resulting in death [6]. If the pathogenic Qi is powerful and patients of COVID-19 are not appropriately treated, then healthy Qi is severely destroyed due to which lungs are unable to work. As a result, a large amount of sputum is produced and causes difficulty in breathing [78]. Baihegujin tang and Maxingshigan tang are TCM that can remove pathogenic Qi, improve healthy Qi, expel sputum, and allow air to enter the lungs [82]. The medicinal herbs used in Baihegujin Tang are Beimu 6g, Chinese bellflower 6g, Licorice 3g, Xuanshen 10g, Angelica 15g, Lily 6g, Dihuang 15g, Ophiopogon 6g, White peony 6g, and Shudihuang 15g. The medicinal herbs used to prepare Maxinshigan Tang include Almond 10g, Ephedra 15g, Licorice 9g, and Plaster 20g. These herbs are mixed and then boiled for about 15 minutes in 1000ml pure water to make a tincture of about 600ml. About 200ml of tincture is orally taken three times a day by dividing it into three doses [78].

Baihegujin tang is mainly used to improve lung Qi. Maxinshigan tang removes phlegm and cures lung fever. The two prescriptions should be taken together in case of severe infection to remove pathogenic Qi and enhance the healthy Qi [82].

Wild Plants against COVID-19

There are about 60,000 species of plants used for medicinal applications all across the globe. The use of approximately 28,000 is well-documented [46]. Wild plants have been used for a long time in medicine to support health care. Medicines based on plants may have no or minor side effects and toxicity. Many wild plants are well-known for their anti-viral activities and are used in herbal treatment [83]. The most important medicinal plants are *Ocimum tenuiflorum, Ocimum sanctum,* Allium sativum, Allium cepa, *Glycyrrhiza glabra, Curcuma longa, Daucus maritimus, Cinnamomum verum,* and *Piper nigrum, etc.* Using these plants' aqueous extract and honey and lemon juice is effective for the treatment of common cold and cough [84 - 93].

With the current outbreak of COVID-19, the use of wild plants in the medicinal formulation of the different medical systems such as Ayurveda, Unani, and TCM has dramatically increased [94]. It is estimated that 30% of the industrial production of TCM is obtained from sources of wild plants [95]. Over 125 species of wild plants are used in the formulation of Chinese medicines. A wild plant such as *Glycyrrhiza* spp. (Liquorice) used in more than 11 Chinese medicine formulations. Some wild species are used in more than five medicine formulations: *Pogostemon cablin, Forsythia suspensa, Atractylodes macroce phala, Armeniaca* spp., *Ephedra* spp., *cutellaria baicalensis, Magnolia officinalis,* and *Cibotium barometz, etc*., [94].

The Licorice root (*Glycyrrhiza glabra*) has an efficient anti-viral activity [96]. This is a native plant of Europe and Asia and is known as weed. This plant possesses anti-viral activity against certain viruses such as HIV-1, respiratory syncytial virus, SARS coronavirus, herpes viruses, cytomegalovirus, hepatitis viruses, varicella-zoster, HIV, Influenza A virus, H5N1, H1N1, and rotavirus, *etc*., [97 - 99]. More than 20 triterpenoids and 300 flavonoids are found in this plant which possesses anti-viral activity [96]. This plant is used in Unani, Homeopathy, and Ayurveda medicines to control COVID-19 [100]. Liquorice root is also an essential ingredient in TCM. Its aqueous extract is mainly recommended to relieve symptoms of COVID-19 such as cough, reduce body temperature, improve pulmonary infiltration absorption, and reduce corticosteroids dosage and breathing difficulties [94].

The use of medicinal herbs to treat COVID-19 infection is the same for their help to treat SARS disease, the outbreak of which happened in 2002/2003 [101]. Some of the species of wild plants most commonly used for the treatment of SARS include *Panax quinquenfolius, Angelica sinensis, Schisandra chinensis, Scutellaria baicalensis, Atractylodes macrocephala,* and *Glycyrrhiza uralensis* [94].

AYUSH issues a statement, with the help of the ministry of India, "Ayurveda's immunity-boosting measures for self-care during COVID 19 crisis", which recommended daily use of the formula of Chyavanprash containing a large number of ingredients of the wild plant [94]. Anastasiya Timoshyna, co-chairperson of a specialist group of the International Union for Conservation of Nature (IUCN) Medicinal Plant said, "Dependence of Mankind's on wild species of plants for well-being and necessary health care has never been more noticeable than the current pandemic of COVID-19" [102].

Many plant species used in medicines recommended for the treatment of COVID-19 are likely to be obtained from a wild source. The uses of these plant species provide remedies for the outbreak of COVID-19 and highlight the importance of herbal medicines, especially those from wild sources, to support health [94].

Indian Subcontinents Plants against COVID-19

Plants have been used for thousands of years in traditional systems of medicines [103, 104]. India has various agro-climatic zones and is abundant with flora of medicinal plants that have been used in the Indian medicine system for centuries to treat human diseases. India is familiar with its ethnomedicine and the use of traditional medicines [105]. The information of medicinal plants has been included in various traditional systems of medicines such as Ayurveda, Siddha, Unani, and Homeopathy, *etc*. India reported that traditional healers use 2500 species, and 100 plant species serve as regular medicine sources [106].

In various parts of India, there has been an increasing interest in the study and use of medicinal plants to treat different diseases, including viral diseases, during the last few decades. The extract of Indian medicinal plants such as *Swertia chirata* has potent anti-viral activity against the *Herpes simplex* virus [107]. The leaf extract of the mangrove plant of India, such as *Avicennia marina* has anti-viral activity against hepatitis viruses and HIV [108].

India is a center of the traditional system of alternative medicines. Therefore, it is obvious to find the solution from Indian medicinal plants to fight against COVID-19, among the sources. The following are Indian medicinal plants that have the potential to be used safely as part of therapeutic formulation for the prevention and management of COVID-19 [44].

Ashwagandha (*Withania somnifera*)

Ashwagandha (*Withania somnifera*) is a traditional Indian medicinal plant that has been used for more than 3,000 years due to its medicinal values [109]. The bioactive compounds found in this plant can prevent and treat several diseases such as impotence, arthritis, cancer, anxiety, amnesia, cardiovascular and neurodegenerative diseases, and many others [110]. The natural phytochemicals found in Ashwagandha might have potent activity against COVID-19. Receptor binding domain (RBD) found in the spike protein of COVID-19 engages the Angiotensin-converting enzyme 2 (ACE2) receptor of the host cell. Withanone, a phytochemical compound in *W. somnifera,* docks very well with the RBD-ACE2 complex binding surface and interferes with the binding of viral RBD to the host cell ACE2 receptor. Withanone decreases electrostatic binding interaction between ACE2 receptor and viral RBD; as a result, entry of COVID-19 is weakened or even blocked. In this way, Ashwagandha cures the infectivity of COVID-19 [111].

Harsinghar (*Nyctanthes Arbortristis*)

Harsinghar is one of the critical traditional plants in India, which has many medicinal values. The scientific name of Harsinghar is *Nyctanthes arbor-tristis,* and it belongs to the Oleaceae family. Commonly, it is also known as Night jasmine and Parijat [112]. It is an important source of many useful medicines against different diseases. It contains various phytochemicals that have been investigated to include significant pharmacological activities [113]. Phytochemicals of Harsinghar such as glycoside, flavonoid, oleanolic acid, tannic acid, benzoic acid, glucose, friedelin, lupeol, carotene, and essential oils have been reported. They all have anti-bacterial, anti-viral, anti-fungal, anti-malarial, anti-leishmaniasis, anti-inflammatory, anti-oxidant, anti-histaminic, hepato-protective, and antipyretic activities [114]. The n-butanol fractions, ethanolic extract as well as two pure compounds such as arbortristoside A and C extracted from Harsingar have high anti-viral activity against Semliki Forest Virus (SFV) and Encephalo Myocarditis Virus (EMCV) [115]. Lupeol(C25H26O4), astragalin (C21H20O11), and nictoflorin (C27H30O15) compound extracted from the Harsingar have been reported to possess activity against the main protease of COVID-19 and inhibit its replication. The anti-viral activity of Harsingar extract was found to be greater than hydroxychloroquine and an anti-malarial compound already studied to inhibit the main protease of COVID-19 [116].

Giloy (*Tinospora Cordifolia*)

Giloy (*Tinospora cordifolia*) is an Indian plant that is well known for possessing several medicinal properties. Giloy is an excellent stimulant of the immune system and has many antimicrobial properties [117]. The bioactive components found in Giloy have excellent immunomodulatory effects. This plant contains many phytochemicals such as choline, berberine, jatrorhizine, palmatine, palmarin, tinocordifolioside, tinosporol, tinosporin, tinosporic acid, tinosporon, tinosporon, tinosporal, tinosporic acid, tembeterine, tinosporaside, diterpenoid furano lactone, heptacosanol, chasmanthin, and columbin, *etc.* which have medicinal properties [118, 119]. It is widely used to treat various diseases such as asthma, urine disorder, rheumatoid arthritis, jaundice, dyspepsia, diabetes, excess mucus, cardiac debility, gout, inflammations, pyrexia, and spleenopathy, *etc.*, [120]. Diterpenoid and tinosporin have been used against certain viruses such as the herpes simplex virus (HSV), all kinds of retroviruses, and many other viruses [121].

The natural phytochemicals found in Giloy can suppress the infectivity of COVID-19. In-silico models reported that tinocodiside, one of the Giloy phytochemicals, docks very efficiently with the RBD-ACE2 complex binding surface and interferes with the binding of viral RBD to the host cell ACE2 receptor. Giloy extract rich in tinocordiside is one of the options available to control the entry of COVID-19. The innate immunity could also be enhanced against infection of COVID-19 due to the immunomodulatory effects of Giloy [120].

Neem (*Azadirachta indica*)

Neem (*Azadirachta indica*) is a tree that belongs to the family Meliaceae and genus Azadirachta [122]. It is a native plant of the Indian Sub-continent and is also known as Indian lilac. Neem seeds, flowers, and leaves are well known for centuries in India due to their medicinal properties [123]. In Sanskrit, Neem is known as Sarva Roga Nivarini, which means Universal healer that cures all diseases [124].

More than 10 compounds are present in different parts of the Neem, such as its roots, bark, trunk, leaves, seeds, and flowers. The compounds found in Neem leaves include Nimocinol, Meliacinanhydride, Nimbin, Nimbandiol, Zafaral, Nimbolide, Nimocinol, Desacetylnimbin, Nimbinene, and Isomeldenin have been studied [125]. The extract of Neem leaves has antiseptic, anti-bacterial, anti-viral, and anti-fungal properties [126]. Neem leaves have been reported to be effective against several viral diseases such as chickenpox, smallpox, HIV, and Herpes virus, *etc.*, [127, 128].

Ingestion of Crude Neem leaves or extracted powder of Neem leaves prevent replication of COVID-19 by targeting its main protease such as Mpro, which inhibits the virus. It also acts as an inhibitor of the host ACE-2 receptor for COVID-19. Furthermore, other compounds found in Neem leaves such as zinc, quercetin, vitamin A, B1, B2, B6, C, and E can also enhance immunity [124].

Tulsi (*Ocimum sanctum*)

In the Indian medicinal system, Tulsi (*Ocimum sanctum*) is known as "The Queen of Herbs" and "Mother Medicine of Nature" due to its spiritual and medicinal properties. Tulsi is rich in phytochemicals, which have high medicinal properties [129]. Hundreds of scientific researches on the Tulsi plant have shown its medicinal properties *in-vitro* human and animal experiments. Such studies reported a unique combination of Tulsi activities including Antimicrobial (such as anti-viral, anti-bacterial, anti-fungal, anti-malarial, antiprotozoal, and antihelmintic), anti-oxidant, anti-diabetic, antipyretic, anti-diarrheal, anti-inflammatory, anti-asthmatic, anti-allergic, anti-tussive, adaptogenic, cardio-protective, neuroprotective, hepato-protective, anti-stress and immunomodulatory actions [130].

Tulsi extracts are a good source of flavonoids and flavones. Based on the 2-phenyl-1-benzopyran-4-one backbone, flavones make the main class in the family of flavonoids. Naturally occurring flavones include 6-hydroxyflavone, scutellarein, luteolin, tangeritin, chrysin, wogonin, baicalein, and apigenin. Since the 1990s, flavones are known to have anti-viral properties when apigenin was used along with acyclovir against HSV-1 and HSV-2, which resulted in increased anti-viral effects [131].

Natural flavonoids also have anti-viral properties. Scutellarein and myricetin strongly inhibit the helicase enzyme of SARS-CoV by inhibiting the function of the ATPase enzyme. *In-silico* study using phytochemicals of Tulsi, RNA replicase of SARS-CoV was targeted. It showed that only a few phytochemicals found in Tulsi affect catalytic cleft of RNA replicase. Scutellarein, one of Tulsi phytochemicals, binds to RNA replicase with docking energy of -8.3 kcal/mol and disturbs Motif B used for polymerization. It is postulated that coronavirus replication could be inhibited by the phytochemicals of Tulsi based on these observations, to further control its spread and growth [120].

AYUSH Recommended Medicinal Plants or Extracts against COVID-19

AYUSH is an Indian medicine system implemented by the government for the treatment of various diseases. This system has five different approaches for treatment, such as Ayurveda, Yoga, Unani, Sidha, and Homeopathy, which being combined in a single term of AYUSH [132]. Among these treatment approaches, Ayurveda, Homeopathy, and Yoga are accepted worldwide and are known as an ancient system of medicine. This traditional system of medicine focuses on disease prevention through prophylactic interventions, lifestyle modification, dietary management to boost the immune system, and simple remedies for treatment based on the appearance of symptoms [133]. Based on the fact that no treatment is available against the COVID-19 in any medical system, the Indian government implemented the AYUSH system to improve respiratory health by boosting the immune system of citizens [134].

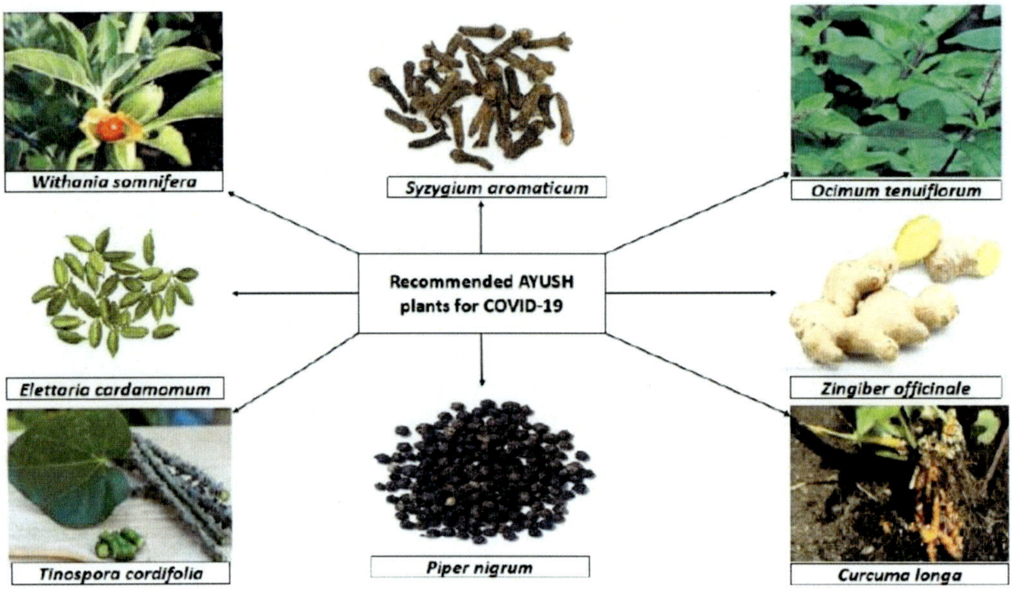

Fig. (1). AYUSH recommended plants against COVID-19.

Ayurveda Medicines

Ayurveda is a traditional medicinal system of the Indian subcontinent which is increasingly gaining importance [135]. India is a rich source of medicinal plants due to various agro-climatic zones [136]. Ayurvedic medicines have a long history since the Vedic period preceding back to over 2000 years in the Indian subcontinent [137]. Ayurvedic medicines are used for a very long time to treat several viral diseases [138]. Conventional medicines are now replacing with ayurvedic medicines for many reasons, such as low cost, easy availability, and no or fewer side effects [139].

Ayurvedic medicines work to control infection of COVID-19. The historical background suggests that if Ayurveda medicinal system is scientifically studied, it may provide an alternate solution to control and prevent COVID-19 infection [140].

Ayurveda suggested several medicines in the current pandemic of COVID-19 to boost immunity and relieve symptoms of COVID-19 [141]. These include turmeric milk, Chyavanprash, and herbal tea. Herbal tea is made from black pepper, basil, dry ginger, cinnamon, and raisin. Black peppers are traditionally used to treat the flu and cold. Holy basil benefits to treat respiratory complications including asthma, allergic bronchitis, eosinophilic lung disease, cough, and liquify phlegm [142]. Ginger target cold-causing viruses due to the presence of chemicals known as sesquiterpenes. Cinnamon contains trans-cinnamaldehyde and cinnamaldehyde, which have anti-oxidant properties. Raisins are rich in energy and a good source of minerals, vitamins, and fibers, due to which they have several medicinal values. Due to these ingredients in Herbal tea, it is recommended to enhance immunity [133].

In Ayurveda, five ways are prescribed to consume medicinal plants and herbs by Panchvidh Kashyapam in Charak Samhita [143]. These include: i) Kwath (decoction), ii) Swaras (juicing), iii) Phant (an herb-infused concoction), iv) Kalka (in paste form), v) Hima (concoction induced by herb) [144]. A valuable Ayurvedic method to enrich active agents present in pharmacological herbs includes Kadha (decoction) preparation. Kadha is made of less juice or dry ingredients such as herbs and spices. During crises of COVID 19, Kadha is recommended by AYUSH to boost immunity and reduce inflammation (Fig. **1**) [145]. Herbs commonly used in Kadha preparation include Haldi (*Curcuma longa*), Black pepper (*Piper nigrum*), Giloy (*Tinospora cordiofolia*), Ginger (*Zingiber officinale*), Ashwagandha (*Withania somnifera*), Cardamom (*Elettaria cardamomum*), Clove (*Syzygium aromaticum*), Tulsi (*Ocimum sanctum*) and lemon (*Citrus limon*) [146]. The active phytochemicals found in various herbs used in Kadha preparation were docked with various proteins of COVID-19 (include viral NSP polymerase, capsid, proteases, spike proteins), pro-inflammatory mediators (IRAK, PLA2, COX2, and NIK proteins) as well as host cell proteases and receptors (such as furin and Human receptor ACE2). The study predicted that phytochemicals possess a significant affinity for binding towards functional regions of host cell receptors, various inflammatory mediators, and viral proteins. Regular use of ayurvedic Kadha for consumption improves the host's immunity, helps prevent COVID-19 pathogenicity and infection, and reduces the severity of disease in infected individuals [144].

Ayurveda medicine system suggests a tablet known as Swasari Ras to treat respiratory tract disorders such as asthma, bronchitis, cough, excess mucous formation, and rhinitis. Swasari Ras is an herbal formulation that is used in India [147]. Swasari Ras consists of Lavanga, Akarkara, Pippali, Maricha, Ardraka, Rudanti, Karkatashringi, Dalchini, and Mulethi. Swasari Ras contains various metabolites of bioactive plants that produce anti-inflammatory actions in respiratory disorders. Swasari Ras also has mineral components of calcium such as Abhraka bhasma, Mukta shukti bhasma, Godanti bhasma, and Kapardak bhasma. These minerals are traditionally known for treating inflammation, cough, asthma, and other lung diseases. This tablet is helpful in treating respiratory symptoms caused by COVID-19 [120].

Unani Medicinal Plants for the Prevention and Management of COVID-19

The COVID-19 symptoms are almost similar to the symptoms of nazla-e-wabaiya as illustrated in Unani books as initial symptoms include cough, fever, malaise, *etc*., which may lead to diarrhea [148]. Unani medicines suggest the following management practices and preventive measures: ***Preventive measures:*** Precautionary measures of distancing, quarantine, and isolation must be followed [100]. The environment serves as a medium for spreading viruses, so special importance is given to the disinfection of the environment [149, 150]. Several disinfectants in the form of spray have been prescribed to fumigate, as sanitizers, and for applying on curtains. These mostly have aroma such as sandroos, loban, za'fran, vinegar, and rose water, *etc*., which can clear microbes [148]. Herbal disinfectants can provide a safer and cost-effective alternative to chemical drugs in the future [151]. Health care must be promoted during epidemics. Citrus fruits have immunomodulatory effects known by Unani physicians, so these fruits should be included in the diet. Take a healthy diet, avoid fish and meat, avoid starvation, and stay hydrated for promoting health [152]. Several drugs for the promotion of health may be advised, such as halela (*Terminalia chebula*), gul-e- banafsha (*Viola odorata*), and revand chini (*Rheum australe*). Gargling with a solution of arqe-gulab (*Rosa damascena*), rub-e-jauz (*Juglans regia*), rub-e-toot (*Morus nigra*), and sumaq (*Rhus coriaria*) may be advised as a prophylactic measure [148].

Suggested management: The nazla-e-wabaiya is managed with immunomodulatory, anti-inflammatory, and antipyretic drugs described in the Al Asbab wa-Alamat. These Unani medicines include unnab (Rhamnaceae; *Ziziphus jujube*), khaksi (Brassicaceae: *Sisymbrium adenophorum*), sapistan (Boraginaceae: *Cordia dichotoma G. Forst*), and behidana decoction (Rosaceae; *Cydonia oblonga*). If diarrhea is associated, tabasheer (Poaceae; *Bambusa bambos*) and habb-ul aas (Myrtaceae; *Myrtus communis*) are also prescribed. Thirst can be relieved by giving tukhm e kahu sheera (seed paste of Compositae; *Lactuca sativa L.*). If pleurisy or pneumonia develops 1g of Aloe vera sap, 1g of C. sativus abd, 10g of qairooti aarad karsana are crushed and mixed and then slightly warmed to apply on the wall of the chest. After applying, the chest is covered with a bandage of cotton [148].

Qairooti is the polyherbal ointment in Unani medicine prescribed specially for chest diseases [153]. A paste is prepared by including the following ingredients in the formulation of Qairooti aarad karsana, Aarad e Hulba (Leguminosae; *Gontsch* and *Trigonella adscendens*, flour), Aarad e Karsana (Leguminosae; *Pisum sativum L.* flour) each of 60g, Aqarqarha (Compositae; *Anacyclus pyrethrum L.*, root) of 18.g, Asl-us-Soos (Leguminosae; *Glycyrrhiza glabra* L., root), Kalonji

(Ranunculaceae, *Nigella sativa L.,* seeds) each of 24 g, an equal amount of beeswax and Roghan-e-Sosan (Iridaceae; *Iris ensata Tunb*, oil) for quantum satis. These Unani medicines are useful in relieving symptoms caused by COVID-19 [148].

Homeopathic Medicines for COVID-19: Currently, the SARS-2 patients require treatment of symptoms to cure, and hospital facilities are used to manage emergencies. The foundation of the medical system of homeopathy depends on the treatment of symptoms which plays an important role in tackling this worldwide challenge [153]. Several medicines of homeopathic are available for infection of COVID-19 patients. Pulsatilla, Calcarea carbonicum, Nitrum muriaticum, Arsenic album, Silicia, Nux vomica, Phosphorus, Lachesis, Sulphur, Hyper Sulphur, and some other homeopathic medicines are reviewed to treat COVID-19 symptoms [154]. While considering the COVID-19 symptoms of a patient, a homeopathic doctor can easily select the right choice of medicine for remedy. 'AYUSH', India's ministry recently suggested 'Arsenic albumin 30 homeopathic medicine as a prophylactic to avoid infection of COVID-19 [155] in which few have been shown in Fig. (**1**). This proposal is supported by the general secretary of LMHI (Liga Medicorum Homeopathica Internationalis) [154]. Dr. Vithoulkas pointed out that patients' access to the homeopathic physician is limited in this current outbreak [156]. Many other researchers have proved the effectiveness of homeopathic medicine for similar symptoms of respiratory tract infections and the treatment of mild pneumonia [157]. Some scholars demonstrated the prophylactic scope of homeopathic medicine and the management of flu symptoms [158]. In bronchioles of COVID-19 patients, proliferation tissues of fibero-granulation have been found by researchers; homeopathic medicines such as Arsenicum iodatum and Silicea have a role in resolving pulmonary fibrosis symptoms. In severe cases of COVID-19, many homeopathic medicines such as *Lobelia inflata*, *Zingiber officinale*, and *Cassia sophera* could be helpful along with management of the hospital. The *Cassia sophera* tincture made of leaves powder is useful in respiratory discomfort shown by aresearcher's group [154]. *Lobelia* has an antidyspnoetic effect that stimulates the respiratory system [159], and *Zingiber officinale* aqueous extract can be used as a chemotherapeutic agent for the treatment of infection of the respiratory tract. In the current outbreak of COVID-19 in Iran, a group of patients' were treated with homeopathic medicines [160]. Another study was done in Italy in which a group of patients probable and positive of COVID-19 was treated with homeopathic medicines [161]. Based on the results of these studies, homeopathic medicines are suggested for the prevention and treatment of COVID-19 infection [154].

Telemedicine and COVID-19

Since the emergence of the first case of the novel coronavirus, COVID-19, also known as SARS-CoV-2, in Wuhan city of China, new cases are rapidly emerging each day [162]. A sudden outbreak of the disease, quick spread of the virus, and the disease with unresolved nature rapidly overwhelmed the health care practice [163]. Attention was given to the new system of health care by understanding that the facilities of health care could be the cause of disease spread [164]. Therefore, telemedicine was focused on as a new health care model [165]. This method involves remote services relating to health, such as online education, advice, and monitoring, using a safe connection between patients and clinicians [166].

Types of Telemedicine

Telemedicine can be classified based on time, mode, persons engaged in communication, and communication purpose [167].

1-Communication Time

Asynchronous Telemedicine: Asynchronous telemedicine uses the technology of "store and forward" information related to health that may be medical data or questions in the form of audio, video clip or photo. They are sent to the health care provider, who responds later by giving a reasonable opinion for health [168]. Examples include email and other portals with electronic medical records [169].

Synchronous or Real-time Telemedicine: In this type of telemedicine, both health care providers and patients must be presented in real-time to communicate *via* a live video or audio telecommunication system [170]. For example, telephone or another live video or audio connection [171].

2- Communication mode

Text: Telemedicine communication based on chat, digital service for short messaging, other platforms for chat such as Google Hangout, WhatsApp, Facebook messenger, fax, and emails, *etc.*, [172].

Audio: Audio applications, phone, voice by using the protocol of the internet [173].

Video: Zoom, Skype, Facetime, and Microsoft Team, *etc.*, [174].

3-Persons engaged in teleconsultation

Doctor to doctor
Patient to doctor
Caregiver to doctor
Health care worker to doctor [167].

4-Consultation purpose

First consult: This type of telemedicine includes any patient who wants first-time consultation or any patient of follow-up who has not consulted for over six months. It may consist of follow-up patients who do not consult for the previous disease but desire to consult for another disease.

Follow-up consult: Follow-up consult includes a patient consulted to a health care provider within six months [167].

Telemedicine During the Previous Outbreak of Diseases

Telemedicine was appeared to be beneficial in the outbreaks of the diseases that occurred in the past, such as previous outbreaks of coronavirus including SARS-CoV and MERS-CoV. Other infectious diseases caused by Zika and Ebola viruses led to public health emergencies [14, 15, 175, 176]. In 2015, the first concept was published to implement telemedicine during the outbreaks of the disease [15, 177]. The framework included monitoring patients having contact cases by remote technology, tele-expertise, and teleconsultation for isolated and triage cases [162].

Telemedicine During the Pandemic of COVID-19

A new light is given to telemedicine during the pandemic of Covid-19, and the requirement for remote technologies has increased because of medical personnel's desire to stay disease-free and healthy [178]. In these situations, digital health provides an appropriate solution. Therefore, both WHO and CDC recommended monitoring patients by telemedicine to lower the risk of the virus spread that occurs by visiting patients to hospitals [179]. Telehealth is covering the gap among clinicians, people, and health care systems to enable everyone, particularly symptomatic patients to communicate with doctors and health care professionals through online digital channels while staying at home during this pandemic of COVID-19. It helps to reduce viral spread to the medical staff at the forefront and the mass population of people [180].

The American Medical Association (AMA) and the Academy of Family Physicians promote telemedicine services during the COVID-19 [181]. With the times, even companies that promote telemedicine are evolving. For example, companies such as EverlyWell and PlushCare plan to release testing kits of COVID-19 for the home that can smartly introduce their current services of remote consultation. Others such as HeyDoctor and Doctor on-demand offer free assessments of the risk of SARS-CoV-2 and then direct patients of high risk towards a phone or video consultation with a physician [182]. Telemedicine is affirmed to be at the front line in the coming times of medicine and assured to make modern health care more approachable instead of waiting in line for hours [183].

FUTURE PROSPECTIVE

Various factors influence the pandemic of COVID-19, which are needed to be evaluated in future work. There is a need to promote health literacy, a healthy lifestyle, and strong immunity through a balanced diet, physical activity, balanced micronutrients, nutraceuticals, and adequate sleep to survive COVID-19 or any other pandemic in the future [184].

Medicinal plants play an important role in the prevention and treatment of infectious diseases [185]. The use of herbal medicines must be recommended to boost immunity and fight against several problems related to health as medicines based on plants have no toxicity and side effects [186]. The proper combination of medicinal herbs in formulations of different medicinal systems and the appropriate dose for consumption is promoted and advised to prevent and treat COVID-19 and other viral diseases. The selection of a good combination of herbs against the current outbreak of COVID-19 may help health care providers to fight against any health-associated issues. During the recent outbreak of COVID-19, utilization of safer and convenient drug delivery options by using herbs such as mukhwas of herbal tonic, inhaler providing herbal immunity, proactive lozenges using herbs and patches of the herbal drug become an important area of interest. However, it requires proper care and knowledge. Patients should be properly educated about plants used in traditional medicines for their health benefits [187].

The development of vaccines is a highly effective method to reduce the burden of infectious diseases. Researchers are not trying to develop vaccines derived from plants to control the COVID-19 infection, which can be produced in high amounts with less cost. Patients readily accept carrier plants. Antigens derived from plants can be preserved for a long time and are stable [188]. At the San Diego University in California, nano-engineers are exploring a plant virus to develop a vaccine of COVID-19 that can be transported anywhere across the world without using refrigeration. This researcher group is using legume infecting virus, which is non-pathogenic to humans. They design the virus similar to the SARS-CoV-2 and then molecular signatures of COVID-19 will be placed on the virus surface to stimulate the immune system's response [189]. A green environment is needed to be conserved to store its resources keeping in view the health benefits of medicinal plants [187].

During the current outbreak of COVID-19, telemedicine using mobile apps or any other social media must be promoted to provide healthcare guidelines and prevent the spread of infectious diseases. Preventive measures, policies, and recommendations must be enforced and implemented by authorities [190].

Moreover, the new generation must be educated about science and technology to combat any such problem in the future. There must be specialized centers for research funded by all countries across the globe under the guidance of WHO. The most important centers for research are needed for insect-based diseases, viral diseases, bacterial diseases, *etc*. These research centers are necessary to combat any calamity in the world in the future [100].

CONCLUSION

The disease of COVID-19 first originated from the city of China, named Wuhan of Hubei Province, in December 2019. According to WHO, this viral disease has become pandemic by spreading to 203 counties, and the patients infected with SARS-CoV-2 present flu-like symptoms with breathing difficulties and high-grade fever. Although no treatment is still available for COVID-19, following preventive measures is the best option to prevent the spread of disease, and supportive therapy is provided. Medicinal plants used in formulations of various medicinal systems such as TCM, Ayurveda, Unani, Homeopathy may play an important role in the prevention and control of COVID-19. Telemedicine serves as a good source of providing healthcare guidelines and reduces the transmission of infectious diseases, mainly COVID-19, by close person-to-person contact. Proper management and preventive measures are important to combat this pandemic of COVID-19, and there is no need to be panic.

CONSENT FOR PUBLICATION

Not Applicable.

CONFLICT OF INTEREST

The author confirms that this chapter contents have no conflict of interest.

ACKNOWLEDGEMENT

Declared none.

REFERENCES

[1] Khan RJ, Jha RK, Amera GM, *et al.* Targeting SARS-CoV-2: a systematic drug repurposing approach to identify promising inhibitors against 3C-like proteinase and 2′-O-ribose methyltransferase. J Biomol Struct Dyn 2020; 1-4.
[PMID: 32266873]

[2] Khan SA, Zia K, Ashraf S, Uddin R, Ul-Haq Z. Identification of chymotrypsin-like protease inhibitors of SARS-CoV-2 *via* integrated computational approach. J Biomol Struct Dyn 2020; 1-0.
[PMID: 32238094]

[3] Pant S, Singh M, Ravichandiran V, Murty US, Srivastava HK. Peptide-like and small-molecule inhibitors against Covid-19. J Biomol Struct Dyn 2020; 1-0.
[PMID: 32306822]

[4] Gorbalenya AE, Baker SC, Baric RS, *et al.* The species Severe acute respiratory syndrome-related coronavirus: classifying 2019-nCoV and naming it SARS-CoV-2. Nat Microbiol 2020; 5(4): 536-44.
[PMID: 32123347]

[5] Zhong L, Mu L, Li J, Wang J, Yin Z, Liu D. Early prediction of the 2019 novel coronavirus outbreak in the mainland china based on simple mathematical model. IEEE Access 2020; 8: 51761-9.

[6] Rothan HA, Byrareddy SN. The epidemiology and pathogenesis of coronavirus disease (COVID-19) outbreak. J Autoimmun 2020; 109: 102433.
[PMID: 32113704]

[7] Wu F, Zhao S, Yu B, *et al.* A new coronavirus associated with human respiratory disease in China. Nature. 2020 Mar;579(7798):265-9.8. Velavan TP, Meyer CG. The COVID□19 epidemic. Trop Med Int Health 2020; 25(3): 278.
[PMID: 32052514]

[8] Zhou P, Yang XL, Wang XG, *et al.* A pneumonia outbreak associated with a new coronavirus of probable bat origin. Nature 2020; 579(7798): 270-3.
[PMID: 32015507]

[9] Chen N, Zhou M, Dong X, *et al.* Epidemiological and clinical characteristics of 99 cases of 2019 novel coronavirus pneumonia in Wuhan, China: a descriptive study. Lancet 2020; 395(10223): 507-13.
[PMID: 32007143]

[10] Rodríguez-Morales AJ, MacGregor K, Kanagarajah S, Patel D, Schlagenhauf P. Going global - Travel and the 2019 novel coronavirus. Travel Med Infect Dis 2020; 33: 101578.
[PMID: 32044389]

[11] Lu H. Drug treatment options for the 2019-new coronavirus (2019-nCoV). Biosci Trends 2020; 14(1): 69-71.
[PMID: 31996494]

[12] Holshue ML, DeBolt C, Lindquist S, *et al.* First case of 2019 novel coronavirus in the United States. N Engl J Med 2020; 382(10): 929-36.
[PMID: 32004427]

[13] Khaerunnisa S, Kurniawan H, Awaluddin R, Suhartati S, Soetjipto S. Potential inhibitor of COVID-19 main protease (Mpro) from several medicinal plant compounds by molecular docking study. Prepr 2020; 20944: 1-4.
[http://dx.doi.org/10]

[14] Su S, Wong G, Shi W, *et al.* Epidemiology, genetic recombination, and pathogenesis of coronaviruses. Trends Microbiol 2016; 24(6): 490-502.
[PMID: 27012512]

[15] Chen Y, Liu Q, Guo D. Emerging coronaviruses: Genome structure, replication, and pathogenesis. J Med Virol 2020; 92(4): 418-23.
[PMID: 31967327]

[16] Wu F, Zhao S, Yu B, *et al.* A new coronavirus associated with human respiratory disease in China. Nature 2020; 579(7798): 265-9.
[PMID: 32015508]

[17] Chan JF-W, Kok K-H, Zhu Z, *et al.* Genomic characterization of the 2019 novel human-pathogenic coronavirus isolated from a patient with atypical pneumonia after visiting Wuhan. Emerg Microbes Infect 2020; 9(1): 221-36.
[PMID: 31987001]

[18] Dong N, Yang X, Ye L, Chen K, Chan EW-C, Yang M, *et al.* Genomic and protein structure modelling analysis depicts the origin and infectivity of 2019-nCoV, a new coronavirus which caused a pneumonia outbreak in Wuhan, China BioRxiv 2020.

[19] Lu R, Zhao X, Li J, *et al.* Genomic characterisation and epidemiology of 2019 novel coronavirus: implications for virus origins and receptor binding. Lancet 2020; 395(10224): 565-74.
[PMID: 32007145]

[20] Xu X, Yu C, Qu J, *et al.* Imaging and clinical features of patients with 2019 novel coronavirus SARS-CoV-2. Eur J Nucl Med Mol Imaging 2020; 47(5): 1275-80.
[PMID: 32107577]

[21] Xu J, Zhao S, Teng T, *et al.* Systematic comparison of two animal-to-human transmitted human coronaviruses: SARS-CoV-2 and SARS-CoV. Viruses 2020; 12(2): 244.
[PMID: 32098422]

[22] Wu C, Liu Y, Yang Y, *et al.* Analysis of therapeutic targets for SARS-CoV-2 and discovery of potential drugs by computational methods. Acta Pharm Sin B 2020; 10(5): 766-88.
[PMID: 32292689]

[23] Wu A, Peng Y, Huang B, *et al.* Genome composition and divergence of the novel coronavirus (2019-nCoV) originating in China. Cell Host Microbe 2020; 27(3): 325-8.
[PMID: 32035028]

[24] Angeletti S, Benvenuto D, Bianchi M, Giovanetti M, Pascarella S, Ciccozzi M. COVID-2019: The role of the nsp2 and nsp3 in its pathogenesis. J Med Virol 2020; 92(6): 584-8.
[PMID: 32083328]

[25] Tsui PT, Kwok ML, Yuen H, Lai ST. Severe acute respiratory syndrome: clinical outcome and prognostic correlates. Emerg Infect Dis 2003; 9(9): 1064-9.
[PMID: 14519241]

[26] Fowler RA, Lapinsky SE, Hallett D, *et al.* Critically ill patients with severe acute respiratory syndrome. JAMA 2003; 290(3): 367-73.
[PMID: 12865378]

[27] Lew TW, Kwek T-K, Tai D, *et al.* Acute respiratory distress syndrome in critically ill patients with severe acute respiratory syndrome. JAMA 2003; 290(3): 374-80.
[PMID: 12865379]

[28] Christian MD, Poutanen SM, Loutfy MR, Muller MP, Low DE. Severe acute respiratory syndrome. Clin Infect Dis 2004; 38(10): 1420-7.
[PMID: 15156481]

[29] Zaki AM, van Boheemen S, Bestebroer TM, Osterhaus AD, Fouchier RA. Isolation of a novel coronavirus from a man with pneumonia in Saudi Arabia. N Engl J Med 2012; 367(19): 1814-20.
[PMID: 23075143]

[30] Assiri A, Al-Tawfiq JA, Al-Rabeeah AA, *et al.* Epidemiological, demographic, and clinical characteristics of 47 cases of Middle East respiratory syndrome coronavirus disease from Saudi Arabia: a descriptive study. Lancet Infect Dis 2013; 13(9): 752-61.
[PMID: 23891402]

[31] Middle East respiratory syndrome coronavirus (MERS-CoV). 2020; Available from: https://www.who.int/emergencies/mers-cov/en/

[32] Summary of probable SARS cases with onset of illness from 1 November 2002 to 31 July 2003. 2020; Available from: https://www.who.int/csr/sars/country/table2004_04_21/en/

[33] Petrosillo N, Viceconte G, Ergonul O, Ippolito G, Petersen E. COVID-19, SARS and MERS: are they closely related? Clin Microbiol Infect 2020; 26(6): 729-34.
[PMID: 32234451]

[34] Chan JF-W, Yuan S, Kok K-H, *et al.* A familial cluster of pneumonia associated with the 2019 novel coronavirus indicating person-to-person transmission: a study of a family cluster. Lancet 2020; 395(10223): 514-23.
[PMID: 31986261]

[35] Killerby ME, Biggs HM, Haynes A, *et al.* Human coronavirus circulation in the United States 2014-2017. J Clin Virol 2018; 101: 52-6.
[PMID: 29427907]

[36] Fan C, Li K, Ding Y, Lu WL, Wang J. ACE2 expression in kidney and testis may cause kidney and testis damage after 2019-nCoV infection. MedRxiv 2020.

[37] Chai X, Hu L, Zhang Y, Han W, Lu Z, Ke A, *et al.* Specific ACE2 expression in cholangiocytes may cause liver damage after 2019-nCoV infection. BioRxiv 2020.

[38] Wang Y, Wang Y, Chen Y, Qin Q. Unique epidemiological and clinical features of the emerging 2019 novel coronavirus pneumonia (COVID-19) implicate special control measures. J Med Virol 2020; 92(6): 568-76.
[PMID: 32134116]

[39] Hani C, Trieu NH, Saab I, *et al.* COVID-19 pneumonia: A review of typical CT findings and differential diagnosis. Diagn Interv Imaging 2020; 101(5): 263-8.
[PMID: 32291197]

[40] Holshue ML, DeBolt C, Lindquist S, *et al.* First case of 2019 novel coronavirus in the United States. N Engl J Med 2020; 382(10): 929-36.
[PMID: 32004427]

[41] Sohrabi C, Alsafi Z, O'Neill N, *et al.* World Health Organization declares global emergency: A review of the 2019 novel coronavirus (COVID-19). Int J Surg 2020; 77: 217.
[PMID: 32305321]

[42] Chan KH, Poon LL, Cheng VC, *et al.* Detection of SARS coronavirus in patients with suspected SARS. Emerg Infect Dis 2004; 10(2): 294-9.
[PMID: 15030700]

[43] Zhang Y, Li J, Zhan Y, *et al.* Analysis of serum cytokines in patients with severe acute respiratory syndrome. Infect Immun 2004; 72(8): 4410-5.
[PMID: 15271897]

[44] Parasuraman S, Thing GS, Dhanaraj SA. Polyherbal formulation: Concept of ayurveda. Pharmacogn Rev 2014; 8(16): 73-80.
[PMID: 25125878]

[45] Mohammad Ejaz SJ. Muhammad Hamza, Sadia Tabassum, Muhammad Abubakar, Irfan, Ullah. Fungal Endophytes are Effective Alternatives and Novel Sources of Anticancer Drugs. Punjab Univ J Zool 2020; 35(1): 13-24.

[46] Jenkins M, Timoshyna A, Cornthwaite M. Wild at Home: Exploring the global harvest, trade and use of wild plant ingredients. Retrieved 2018: 26.

[47] Gomathi M, Padmapriya S, Balachandar V. Drug studies on Rett syndrome: from bench to bedside. J Autism Dev Disord 2020; 50(8): 2740-64.

[PMID: 32016693]

[48] Ni L, Zhou L, Zhou M, Zhao J, Wang DW. Combination of western medicine and Chinese traditional patent medicine in treating a family case of COVID-19. Front Med 2020; 14(2): 210-4. [PMID: 32170559]

[49] Yarnell E. Herbs for Viral Respiratory Infections. J Altern Complement Med 2018; 24(1): 35-43.

[50] Liu Z, Xiao X, Wei X, *et al.* Composition and divergence of coronavirus spike proteins and host ACE2 receptors predict potential intermediate hosts of SARS-CoV-2. J Med Virol 2020; 92(6): 595-601. [PMID: 32100877]

[51] Keyaerts E, Li S, Vijgen L, *et al.* Antiviral activity of chloroquine against human coronavirus OC43 infection in newborn mice. Antimicrob Agents Chemother 2009; 53(8): 3416-21. [PMID: 19506054]

[52] Nourazarian SM, Nourazarian A, Majidinia M, Roshaniasl E. Effect of root extracts of medicinal herb *Glycyrrhiza glabra* on HSP90 gene expression and apoptosis in the HT-29 colon cancer cell line. Asian Pac J Cancer Prev 2015; 16(18): 8563-6. [PMID: 26745117]

[53] Olivieri F, Prasad V, Valbonesi P, *et al.* A systemic antiviral resistance-inducing protein isolated from Clerodendrum inerme Gaertn. is a polynucleotide:adenosine glycosidase (ribosome-inactivating protein). FEBS Lett 1996; 396(2-3): 132-4. [PMID: 8914973]

[54] Galani VJ, Patel BG, Rana DG. Sphaeranthus indicus Linn.: A phytopharmacological review. Int J Ayurveda Res 2010; 1(4): 247-53. [PMID: 21455454]

[55] Ganjhu RK, Mudgal PP, Maity H, *et al.* Herbal plants and plant preparations as remedial approach for viral diseases. Virusdisease 2015; 26(4): 225-36. [PMID: 26645032]

[56] Dabeek WM, Marra MV. Dietary Quercetin and Kaempferol: bioavailability and potential cardiovascular-related bioactivity in humans. Nutrients 2019; 11(10): 2288. [PMID: 31557798]

[57] Andarwulan N, Batari R, Sandrasari DA, Bolling B, Wijaya H. Flavonoid content and antioxidant activity of vegetables from Indonesia. Food Chem 2010; 121(4): 1231-5. [PMID: 28814820]

[58] Lau TF, Leung PC, Wong EL, *et al.* Using herbal medicine as a means of prevention experience during the SARS crisis. Am J Chin Med 2005; 33(3): 345-56. [PMID: 16047553]

[59] Poon PM, Wong CK, Fung KP, *et al.* Immunomodulatory effects of a traditional Chinese medicine with potential antiviral activity: a self-control study. Am J Chin Med 2006; 34(1): 13-21. [PMID: 16437735]

[60] Cinatl J, Morgenstern B, Bauer G, Chandra P, Rabenau H, Doerr HW. Glycyrrhizin, an active component of liquorice roots, and replication of SARS-associated coronavirus. Lancet 2003; 361(9374): 2045-6. [PMID: 12814717]

[61] Lau K-M, Lee K-M, Koon C-M, *et al.* Immunomodulatory and anti-SARS activities of Houttuynia cordata. J Ethnopharmacol 2008; 118(1): 79-85. [PMID: 18479853]

[62] Gong S, Su X, Wu H, Li J, Qin Y, Xu Q, *et al.* A study on anti-SARS-CoV 3CL protein of flavonoids from Litchi chinensis sonn core. J Chin Pharm Sci 2008; 24(5): 699-700.

[63] Lin C-W, Tsai F-J, Tsai C-H, *et al.* Anti-SARS coronavirus 3C-like protease effects of Isatis indigotica root and plant-derived phenolic compounds. Antiviral Res 2005; 68(1): 36-42. [PMID: 16115693]

[64] Luo W, Su X, Gong S, *et al.* Anti-SARS coronavirus 3C-like protease effects of *Rheum palmatum* L. extracts. Biosci Trends 2009; 3(4): 124-6. [PMID: 20103835]

[65] Li GQ, Duke CC, Roufogalis BD. Aust Prescr 2003; 26(6): 128-302003.

[66] Ren JL, Zhang AH, Wang XJ. Traditional Chinese medicine for COVID-19 treatment. Pharmacol Res 2020; 155: 104743. [PMID: 32145402]

[67] Luo Y, Wang CZ, Hesse-Fong J, Lin JG, Yuan CS. Application of Chinese medicine in acute and critical medical conditions. Am J Chin Med 2019; 47(6): 1223-35. [PMID: 31505937]

[68] Chen Z, Nakamura T. Statistical evidence for the usefulness of Chinese medicine in the treatment of SARS. Phytother Res 2004; 18(7): 592-4. [PMID: 15305324]

[69] Wan S, Xiang Y, Fang W, *et al.* Clinical features and treatment of COVID-19 patients in northeast Chongqing. J Med Virol 2020; 92(7): 797-806. [PMID: 32198776]

[70] Ho LTF, Chan KKH, Chung VCH, Leung TH. Highlights of traditional Chinese medicine frontline expert advice in the China national guideline for COVID-19. Eur J Integr Med 2020; 36: 101116. [PMID: 32292529]

[71] Wang Z, Chen X, Lu Y, Chen F, Zhang W. Clinical characteristics and therapeutic procedure for four cases with 2019 novel coronavirus pneumonia receiving combined Chinese and Western medicine treatment. Biosci Trends 2020; 14(1): 64-8. [PMID: 32037389]

[72] Li W. The curative effect observation of shuanghuanglian and penicillin on acute tonsillitis. J Clin Otolaryngol 2002; 16(9): 475-6. [PMID: 15515537]

[73] Chen X, Howard OM, Yang X, Wang L, Oppenheim JJ, Krakauer T. Effects of Shuanghuanglian and Qingkailing, two multi-components of traditional Chinese medicinal preparations, on human leukocyte function. Life Sci 2002; 70(24): 2897-913. [PMID: 12269401]

[74] Wang L, Wang Y, Ye D, Liu Q. A review of the 2019 Novel Coronavirus (COVID-19) based on current evidence. Int J Antimicrob Agents 2020; 56(3): 106137. [PMID: 32826129]

[75] Shahrajabian MH, Sun W, Shen H, Cheng Q. Chinese herbal medicine for SARS and SARS-CoV-2 treatment and prevention, encouraging using herbal medicine for COVID-19 outbreak. Acta Agr Scand B-S P. 2020: 1-7.

[76] Gao K, Song YP, Chen H, Zhao LT, Ma L. Therapeutic efficacy of Qingfei Paidu decoction combined with antiviral drugs in the treatment of corona virus disease 2019: A protocol for systematic review and meta analysis. Medicine (Baltimore) 2020; 99(22): e20489. [PMID: 32481460]

[77] Luo E, Zhang D, Luo H, *et al.* Treatment efficacy analysis of traditional Chinese medicine for novel coronavirus pneumonia (COVID-19): an empirical study from Wuhan, Hubei Province, China. Chin Med 2020; 15: 34. [PMID: 32308732]

[78] Xu J, Zhang Y. Traditional Chinese Medicine treatment of COVID-19. Complement Ther Clin Pract 2020; 39: 101165.
[PMID: 32379692]

[79] Huang R, Zhang Y, Zhang Y, *et al.* Evaluation of the synergetic effect of Yupingfeng san and Flos Sophorae Immaturus based on free radical scavenging capacity. Biomed Pharmacother 2020; 128: 110265.
[PMID: 32425327]

[80] Luo H, Tang QL, Shang YX, *et al.* Can Chinese medicine be used for prevention of corona virus disease 2019 (COVID-19)? A review of historical classics, research evidence and current prevention programs. Chin J Integr Med 2020; 26(4): 243-50.
[PMID: 32065348]

[81] Liu LS, Lei N, Lin Q, Wang WL, Yan HW, Duan XH. The effects and mechanism of Yinqiao Powder on upper respiratory tract infection. Int J Biotechnol Wellness Ind 2015; 4(2): 57-60.

[82] Das A, Ahmed R, Akhtar S, Begum K, Banu S. An overview of basic molecular biology of SARS-CoV-2 and current COVID-19 prevention strategies Preprints 2020.

[83] Lin LT, Hsu WC, Lin CC. Antiviral natural products and herbal medicines. J Tradit Complement Med 2014; 4(1): 24-35.
[PMID: 24872930]

[84] Bano N, Ahmed A, Tanveer M, Khan GM, Ansari MT. Pharmacological evaluation of *Ocimum sanctum*. J Bioequivalence Bioavailab 2017; 9(3): 387-492.

[85] Chang JS, Wang KC, Yeh CF, Shieh DE, Chiang LC. Fresh ginger (*Zingiber officinale*) has anti-viral activity against human respiratory syncytial virus in human respiratory tract cell lines. J Ethnopharmacol 2013; 145(1): 146-51.
[PMID: 23123794]

[86] Bayan L, Koulivand PH, Gorji A. Garlic: a review of potential therapeutic effects. Avicenna J Phytomed 2014; 4(1): 1-14.
[PMID: 25050296]

[87] Fatima M, Zaidi NU, Amraiz D, Afzal F. *In-vitro* anti-viral activity of *Cinnamomum cassia* and its nanoparticles against H7N3 influenza a virus. Microb Biotechnol 2016; 26(1): 151-9.
[PMID: 27860310]

[88] Ghoke SS, Sood R, Kumar N, *et al.* Evaluation of antiviral activity of *Ocimum sanctum* and Acacia arabica leaves extracts against H9N2 virus using embryonated chicken egg model. BMC Complement Altern Med 2018; 18(1): 174.
[PMID: 29866088]

[89] Hashemipour MA, Tavakolineghad Z, Arabzadeh SA, Iranmanesh Z, Nassab SA. Antiviral Activities of Honey, Royal Jelly, and Acyclovir Against HSV-1. Wounds 2014; 26(2): 47-54.
[PMID: 25860226]

[90] Jiang ZY, Liu WF, Zhang XM, Luo J, Ma YB, Chen JJ. Anti-HBV active constituents from Piper longum. Bioorg Med Chem Lett 2013; 23(7): 2123-7.
[PMID: 23434420]

[91] Lee JB, Miyake S, Umetsu R, Hayashi K, Chijimatsu T, Hayashi T. Anti-influenza A virus effects of fructan from Welsh onion (*Allium fistulosum* L.). Food Chem 2012; 134(4): 2164-8.
[PMID: 23442670]

[92] Omer MO, Almalki WH, Shahid I, Khuram S, Altaf I, Imran S. Comparative study to evaluate the anti-viral efficacy of *Glycyrrhiza glabra* extract and ribavirin against the Newcastle disease virus. Pharmacognosy Res 2014; 6(1): 6-11.
[PMID: 24497736]

[93] Praditya D, Kirchhoff L, Brüning J, Rachmawati H, Steinmann J, Steinmann E. Anti-infective properties of the golden spice curcumin. Front Microbiol 2019; 10: 912. [PMID: 31130924]

[94] COVID-19-the role of wild plants in health treatment and why sustainability of their trade matters. 2020; Available from: https://www.traffic.org/news/covid-19-the-role- of-wild-plants-in-he-lth-treatment/

[95] Brinckmann JA. Sustainable Sourcing: Markets for certified Chinese medicinal and aromatic Plants. Geneva: International Trade Centre 2016; p. 22.

[96] Wang L, Yang R, Yuan B, Liu Y, Liu C. The antiviral and antimicrobial activities of licorice, a widely-used Chinese herb. Acta Pharm Sin B 2015; 5(4): 310-5. [PMID: 26579460]

[97] Fiore C, Eisenhut M, Krausse R, *et al.* Antiviral effects of Glycyrrhiza species. Phytother Res 2008; 22(2): 141-8. [PMID: 17886224]

[98] Asl NN, Hosseinzadeh H. Review of anti-viral effects of *Glycyrrhiza glabra* L. and its active component, glycyrrhizin. Faslnamah-i Giyahan-i Daruyi 2007; 6(22).

[99] Anagha K, Manasi D, Priya L, Meera M. Scope of *Glycyrrhiza glabra* (Yashtimadhu) as an Anti-viral agent: A Review. Int J Curr Microbiol Appl Sci 2014; 3(12): 657-65.

[100] Ali I, Alharbi OML. COVID-19: Disease, management, treatment, and social impact. Sci Total Environ 2020; 728: 138861. [PMID: 32344226]

[101] Chinese herbs combined with Western medicine for severe acute respiratory syndrome (SARS). Cochrane Database Syst Rev 2012; (10).

[102] NGO sounds alarm on use of wild plants to cure COVID-19 2020. https://www.aa.com.tr/en/environment/ngo-sounds-alarm-on-use-of-wild-plants-to-cure-covid-19/1881782

[103] Hosseinzadeh S, Jafarikukhdan A, Hosseini A, Armand R. The application of medicinal plants in traditional and modern medicine: a review of *Thymus vulgaris*. Int J Clin Med 2015; 6(09): 635.

[104] Azaizeh H, Fulder S, Khalil K, Said O. Ethnobotanical knowledge of local Arab practitioners in the Middle Eastern region. Fitoterapia 2003; 74(1-2): 98-108. [PMID: 12628401]

[105] Srinivasan D, Nathan S, Suresh T, Lakshmana Perumalsamy P. Antimicrobial activity of certain Indian medicinal plants used in folkloric medicine. J Ethnopharmacol 2001; 74(3): 217-20. [PMID: 11274820]

[106] Muthu C, Ayyanar M, Raja N, Ignacimuthu S. Medicinal plants used by traditional healers in Kancheepuram district of Tamil Nadu, India. J Ethnobiol Ethnomed 2006; 2(1): 43. [PMID: 17026769]

[107] Verma H, Patil PR, Kolhapure RM, Gopalkrishna V. Antiviral activity of the Indian medicinal plant extract Swertia chirata against herpes simplex viruses: a study by *in-vitro* and molecular approach. Indian J Med Microbiol 2008; 26(4): 322-6. [PMID: 18974483]

[108] Beula JM, Gnanadesigan M, Rajkumar PB, Ravikumar S, Anand M. Antiviral, anti-oxidant and toxicological evaluation of mangrove plant from South East coast of India. Asian Pac J Trop Biomed 2012; 2(1): 352-7.

[109] Verma SK, Kumar A. Therapeutic uses of *Withania somnifera* (ashwagandha) with a note on withanolides and its pharmacological actions. Asian J Pharm Clin Res 2011; 4(1): 1-4.

[110] Mir BA, Khazir J, Mir NA, Hasan TU, Koul S. Botanical, chemical and pharmacological review of *Withania somnifera* (Indian ginseng): an ayurvedic medicinal plant. Indian J Drugs Dis 2012; 1: 147-60.

[111] Balkrishna A. Withanone from *Withania somnifera* may inhibit novel Coronavirus (COVID-19) entry by disrupting interactions between viral S-protein receptor binding domain and host ACE2 receptor. Drug Des Devel Ther 2021; 11;15: 1111-33.

[112] Bansal S, Bharati AJ, Bansal YK. *In-vitro* callogenesis and phytochemical screening of harsingar (Nyctanthes arbor-tristis) a multipotent medicinal tree. Int J Pharm Tech Res 2015; 5(4): 1786-93.

[113] Jain PK, Pandey A. The wonder of Ayurvedic medicine-*Nyctanthes Arbortristis*. Int J Herb Med 2016; 4(4): 9-17.

[114] Chamoli RT, Minj S, Singh V. Phytochemical chemical characters of Nyctanthes arbor-tristis Linn.: A promising medicinal plant. J Med Plants Res 2019; 7(6): 141-3.

[115] Bhosale AV, Abhyankar MM, Pawar SJ, Khan S, Patil N. *Nyctanthes Arbortristis*: A pharmacognostic review. J Pharmacogn Phytochem 2009; 1(2): 91-7.

[116] Srivastava AK, Kumar A, Misra N. On the inhibition of covid-19 protease by indian herbal plants: an *in silico* investigation. 2020.

[117] Dhama K, Sachan S, Khandia R, *et al.* Medicinal and beneficial health applications of Tinospora cordifolia (Guduchi): a miraculous herb countering various diseases/disorders and its Immunomodulatory effects. Recent Pat Endocr Metab Immune Drug Discov 2017; 10(2): 96-111. [PMID: 28260522]

[118] Mishra A, Gond SK, Kumar A, *et al.* Season and tissue type affect fungal endophyte communities of the Indian medicinal plant Tinospora cordifolia more strongly than geographic location. Microb Ecol 2012; 64(2): 388-98. [PMID: 22430503]

[119] Sharma P, Dwivedee BP, Bisht D, Dash AK, Kumar D. The chemical constituents and diverse pharmacological importance of *Tinospora cordifolia.* Heliyon 2019; 5(9): e02437. [PMID: 31701036]

[120] Balkrishna A. Indian traditional ayurvedic treatment regime for novel coronavirus, COVID-19. 2020.

[121] Gyawali R, Paudel PN, Basyal D, *et al.* A review on ayurvedic medicinal herbs as remedial perspective for COVID-19. 2020; 3.

[122] Jafari S, Saeidnia S, Ardekani MR, Hadjiakhoondi A, Khanavi M. Micromorphological and preliminary phytochemical studies of *Azadirachta indica* and Melia azedarach. Turk J Bot 2013; 37(4): 690-7.

[123] Uchegbu M, Okoli I, Esonu B, Iloeje M. The grovving importance of neem (*Azadirachta indica* A. Juss) in agriculture, industry, medicine and Eenvironment: A review. Res J Med Plant 2011; 5(3): 230-45.

[124] Gurung AB, Ali MA, Lee J, Farah MA, Al-Anazi KM. Unravelling lead antiviral phytochemicals for the inhibition of SARS-CoV-2 M^{pro} enzyme through in silico approach. Life Sci 2020; 255: 117831. [PMID: 32450166]

[125] Alzohairy MA. Therapeutics role of *Azadirachta indica* (Neem) and their active constituents in diseases prevention and treatment. Evid Based Complement Alternat Med 2016; 2016: 7382506. [PMID: 27034694]

[126] Ahmad S, Maqbool A, Srivastava A, Gogoi S. Biological detail and therapeutic effect of *Azadirachta indica* (neem tree) products-a review. J Evid Based Med Healthc 2019; 6(22): 1607-12.

[127] Younus I, Siddiq A, Ishaq H, Anwer L, Badar S, Ashraf M. Evaluation of antiviral activity of plant extracts against foot and mouth disease virus *in vitro*. Pak J Pharm Sci 2016; 29(4): 1263-8.

[PMID: 27393440]

[128] Schang LM. Cyclin-dependent kinases as cellular targets for antiviral drugs. J Antimicrob Chemother 2002; 50(6): 779-92.
[PMID: 12460995]

[129] Cohen MM. Tulsi - *Ocimum sanctum*: A herb for all reasons. J Ayurveda Integr Med 2014; 5(4): 251-9.
[PMID: 25624701]

[130] Mahajan N, Rawal S, Verma M, Poddar M, Alok S. A phytopharmacological overview on Ocimum species with special emphasis on *Ocimum sanctum*. Biomed Prev Nutr 2013; 3(2): 185-92.

[131] Mucsi I, Gyulai Z, Béládi I. Combined effects of flavonoids and acyclovir against herpesviruses in cell cultures. Acta Microbiol Hung 1992; 39(2): 137-47.
[PMID: 1339152]

[132] Tiwari Rakesh R, Chaudhari K. Role of AYUSH Workers in Active G COVID19. Indian J Basic Appl Med Res 2020; 2(9): 277-9.

[133] Prajapati S, Kumar NG. SARS-CoV-2 pandemic: an opportunity for Indian traditional medicines (AYUSH). Int J Complement Altern Med 2020; 13(3): 103-5.

[134] Priya R, Sujatha V. AYUSH for COVID-19: Science or Superstition? Indian J Public Health 2020; 64(6) (Suppl.): S105-7.
[PMID: 32496237]

[135] Golechha M. Time to realise the true potential of Ayurveda against COVID-19. Brain Behav Immun 2020; 87: 130-1.
[PMID: 32389701]

[136] Jatawa S, Paul R, Tiwari A. Indian medicinal plants: a rich source of natural immuno-modulator. Int J Pharmacol 2011; 7(2): 198-205.

[137] Saini A. Physicians of ancient India. J Family Med Prim Care 2016; 5(2): 254-8.
[PMID: 27843823]

[138] Arora R, Chawla R, Marwah R, *et al.* Potential of complementary and alternative medicine in preventive management of novel H1N1 flu (Swine flu) pandemic: thwarting potential disasters in the bud. Evid Based Complement Alternat Med 2010; 2011.

[139] Pandey MM, Rastogi S, Rawat AK. Indian traditional ayurvedic system of medicine and nutritional supplementation. Evid Based Complement Alternat Med 2013; 2013.

[140] Rastogi S, Pandey DN, Singh RH. COVID-19 pandemic: A pragmatic plan for ayurveda intervention. J Ayurveda Integr Med 2020; S0975-9476(20): 30019-X.
[PMID: 32382220]

[141] Acharyya A. Prospect of ayurveda system of medicine in recent COVID-19 pandemic in India. Int J Ayurveda Res 2020; 2(2): 26-9.

[142] Roka DB, Ayu BD. Ayurveda guidelines of preventive measures and curative management protocol for COVID 19 in Nepal. 2020.

[143] Shingadiya RK, Agrawal SB, Bedarkar PB, Patgiri BJ, Prajapati PK. Unique methods of swarasa (Juice) extraction in ayurveda. JISM 2016; 4(4): 230.

[144] Maurya DK, Sharma D. Evaluation of traditional ayurvedic preparation for prevention and management of the novel Coronavirus (SARS-CoV-2) using molecular docking approach. 2020.

[145] Khanal P, Duyu T, Dey YN, Patil BM, Pasha I, Wanjari M. Network pharmacology of AYUSH recommended immune-boosting medicinal plants against COVID-19. J Ayurveda Integr Med 2020.

[146] Singh R. Diet and COVID-19. Int J Food Sci Nutr 2020; 9(1): 20.

[147] Balkrishna A, Solleti SK, Singh H, Tomer M, Sharma N, Varshney A. Calcio-herbal formulation, Divya-Swasari-Ras, alleviates chronic inflammation and suppresses airway remodelling in mouse model of allergic asthma by modulating pro-inflammatory cytokine response. Biomed Pharmacother 2020; 126: 110063.
[PMID: 32145582]

[148] Nikhat S, Fazil M. Overview of Covid-19; its prevention and management in the light of Unani medicine. Sci Total Environ 2020; 728: 138859.
[PMID: 32334163]

[149] Kumar V, Singh SB, Singh S. COVID-19: Environment concern and impact of Indian medicinal system. J Environ Chem Eng 2020; 8(5): 104144.
[PMID: 33520648]

[150] Parvez A, Ahmed Z, Anwar N, Ahmed K. 'Razi's unique approach to Amraz-e-Wabaiya (Infectious Diseases): An overview. Int J Herb Med 2016; 4(6): 176-8.

[151] Bhatwalkar SB, Shukla P, Srivastava RK, Mondal R, Anupam R. Validation of environmental disinfection efficiency of traditional Ayurvedic fumigation practices. J Ayurveda Integr Med 2019; 10(3): 203-6.
[PMID: 31427141]

[152] Rhazi Z, Tibb AH. Central council for research in unani medicine New Delhi. Ministry of health & family welfare. Govt of India 1997; 1: 11-48.

[153] Baranifard M, Khazaei MM, Jamshidi S, Zarshenas MM, Zargaran A. A critical comparison between dosage forms in traditional Persian pharmacy and those reported in current pharmaceutical sciences. Int J Pharmacogn Phytochem 2017; 4(3): 67-74.

[154] Hasan N, Nayem MU, Mohshinuzzaman M, *et al.* Homeopathic Approach to COVID-19: A Review. Malays J Med Biol Res 2020; 7(1): 39-44.

[155] Indra S, Vijayasankari A, Kalpana S. Current scenerio of management on COVID-19–a global review. IJMBS 2020; 4(6).

[156] Chaudhary A, Khurana A. A review on the role of homoeopathy in epidemics with some reflections on COVID-19 (SARS-CoV-2). Indian J Res Homoeopathy 2020; 14(2): 100.

[157] Beghi GM, Morselli-Labate AM. Does homeopathic medicine have a preventive effect on respiratory tract infections? A real life observational study. Multidiscip Respir Med 2016; 11(1): 12.
[PMID: 27004125]

[158] Siqueira CM, Homsani F, da Veiga VF, *et al.* Homeopathic medicines for prevention of influenza and acute respiratory tract infections in children: blind, randomized, placebo-controlled clinical trial. Homeopathy 2016; 105(1): 71-7.
[PMID: 26828000]

[159] Pizzorno JE, Murray MT, Joiner-Bey H. The Clinician's Handbook of Natural Medicine E-Book. Elsevier Health Sciences 2016.

[160] Okiki Pius A, Oluwadunsin O, Benjamin O. Antibacterial activity of ginger (*Zingiber officinale*) against isolated bacteria from the respiratory tract infections. J Biol Agric Healthcare Res 2015; 19(5): 2224-3208.

[161] Valeri A. Symptomatic COVID-19 Positive and Likely Patients Treated by Homeopathic Physicians-An Italian Descriptive Study. Researchgate 2020.

[162] Moazzami B, Razavi-Khorasani N, Dooghaie Moghadam A, Farokhi E, Rezaei N. COVID-19 and telemedicine: Immediate action required for maintaining healthcare providers well-being. J Clin Virol 2020; 126: 104345.
[PMID: 32278298]

[163] Sanei Taheri M, Falahati F, Radpour A, Karimi V, Sedaghat A, Karimi MA. Role of social media and

telemedicine in diagnosis & management of COVID-19; an experience of the Iranian Society of Radiology. Arch Iran Med 2020; 23(4): 285-6.
[PMID: 32271607]

[164] Ohannessian R, Duong TA, Odone A. Global telemedicine implementation and integration within health systems to fight the COVID-19 pandemic: a call to action. JMIR Public Health Surveill 2020; 6(2): e18810.
[PMID: 32238336]

[165] Portnoy J, Waller M, Elliott T. Telemedicine in the Era of COVID-19. J Allergy Clin Immunol Pract 2020; 8(5): 1489-91.
[PMID: 32220575]

[166] Rockwell KL, Gilroy AS. Incorporating telemedicine as part of COVID-19 outbreak response systems. Am J Manag Care 2020; 26(4): 147-8.
[PMID: 32270980]

[167] Ghosh A, Gupta R, Misra A. Telemedicine for diabetes care in India during COVID19 pandemic and national lockdown period: guidelines for physicians. 2020.

[168] von Wangenheim A, de Souza Nobre LF, Tognoli H, Nassar SM, Ho K. User satisfaction with asynchronous telemedicine: a study of users of Santa Catarina's system of telemedicine and telehealth. Telemed J E Health 2012; 18(5): 339-46.
[PMID: 22703378]

[169] Lee I, Kovarik C, Tejasvi T, Pizarro M, Lipoff JB. Telehealth: Helping your patients and practice survive and thrive during the COVID-19 crisis with rapid quality implementation. J Am Acad Dermatol 2020; 82(5): 1213-4.
[PMID: 32229278]

[170] Pollock K, Setzen M, Svider PF. Embracing telemedicine into your otolaryngology practice amid the COVID-19 crisis: An invited commentary. Am J Otolaryngol 2020; 41(3): 102490.
[PMID: 32307192]

[171] Loeb AE, Rao SS, Ficke JR, Morris CD, Riley LH III, Levin AS. Departmental experience and lessons learned with accelerated introduction of telemedicine during the COVID-19 crisis. J Am Acad Orthop Surg 2020; 28(11): e469-76.
[PMID: 32301818]

[172] Hollander JE, Carr BG. Virtually perfect? Telemedicine for COVID-19. N Engl J Med 2020; 382(18): 1679-81.
[PMID: 32160451]

[173] Nord G, Rising KL, Band RA, Carr BG, Hollander JE. On-demand synchronous audio video telemedicine visits are cost effective. Am J Emerg Med 2019; 37(5): 890-4.
[PMID: 30100333]

[174] Barton C, Morris R, Rothlind J, Yaffe K. Video-telemedicine in a memory disorders clinic: evaluation and management of rural elders with cognitive impairment. Telemed J E Health 2011; 17(10): 789-93.
[PMID: 22023458]

[175] Welsh TS. Organizational structure of telehealth care: An examination of four types of telemedicine systems. The University of Tennessee 2002.

[176] Ohannessian R, Mattos S, Paranhos-Baccalà G, Vanhems P. The role of telemedicine in response to the Zika virus outbreak in Brazil. Zika Summit 2016.

[177] Ohannessian R. Telemedicine: potential applications in epidemic situations. European Research in Telemedicine/La Recherche Européenne en Télémédecine 2015; 4(3): 8-95.

[178] Bashshur R, Doarn CR, Frenk JM, Kvedar JC, Woolliscroft JO. Telemedicine and the COVID-19 Pandemic, Lessons for the Future. Telemed J E Health 2020; 26(5): 571-3.
[PMID: 32275485]

[179] Chauhan V, Galwankar S, Arquilla B, *et al.* Novel coronavirus (COVID-19): Leveraging telemedicine to optimize care while minimizing exposures and viral transmission. J Emerg Trauma Shock 2020; 13(1): 20-4.
[PMID: 32308272]

[180] Webster P. Virtual health care in the era of COVID-19. Lancet 2020; 395(10231): 1180-1.
[PMID: 32278374]

[181] 2020.https://www.pulmonologyadvisor.com/home/topics/lung-infection/seven-things-to-consider-when-transitioning-to-telemedicine-during-covid-19/4/

[182] 2020.https://medicalfuturist.com/covid-19-was-needed-for-telemedicine-to-finally-go-mainstream/

[183] Mann DM, Chen J, Chunara R, Testa PA, Nov O. COVID-19 transforms health care through telemedicine: evidence from the field. J Am Med Inform Assoc. J Am Med Inform 2020; 27: pp. (7)1132-5.

[184] Bloukh SH, Shaikh AA, Pathan HM, Edis Z. Prevalence of COVID-19: A Look behind the Scenes Preprints 2020.

[185] Udayakumar R, Begum VH. Elemental analysis of Medicinal Plants used in controlling infectious diseases. Hamdard Med 2004; 67: 35-6.

[186] Hadady L, Ac D. Asian health secrets: the complete guide to Asian herbal medicine. Crown Archetype 2020.

[187] Desai A, Desai C, Desai DH, Mansuri A, Desai J. Possible role of medicinal plants in COVID-19: a brief review. IJERD 2020; 5(4): 2455-631.

[188] Pocket K. COVID-19 treatment efforts using plant technologies. 2020; Available from: http://www.isaaa.org/resources/publications/pocketk/58/ default.asp

[189] Nanoengineers combine molecular farming and advanced manufacturing to develop COVID-19 vaccine. crop biotech update. 2020; Available from: http://www.isaaa.org/kc/cropbiotechupdate /article/default.asp?ID=18090

[190] Setzen M, Svider PF, Pollock K. COVID-19 and rhinology: A look at the future. Am J Otolaryngol 2020; 41(3): 102491.
[PMID: 32327218]

CHAPTER 10

Role of Blood Plasma Transfusion Against COVID-19

Muhammad Ibrar[1], Abdullah[2], Iyad Ibrahim Shaqura[3,4], Ahmed Abdelmajed Alkhodary[4,5] and **Fazlullah Khan[6,*]**

[1] *Department of Allied Health Sciences, Iqra National University Peshawar, Swat Campus, KP, Pakistan*

[2] *Department of Pharmacy, University of Malakand, Chakdara Dir Lower, KP, Pakistan*

[3] *Department of Health Management and Economics, School of Public Health, Tehran University of Medical Sciences, Tehran, Iran*

[4] *Ministry of Health, Gaza Governorates, Palestine*

[5] *International Centre for Casemix and Clinical Coding, Faculty of Medicine, National University of Malaysia, Kuala Lumpur, Malaysia*

[6] *Department of Allied Health Sciences, Bashir Institute of Health Sciences, Bharakahu, Islamabad, Pakistan*

Abstract: Historically, convalescent plasma (CP) has been successfully used in pandemics caused by the influenza A (H1N1) virus, severe acute respiratory syndrome (SARS), Middle East respiratory syndrome (MERS), and Ebola. As the current pandemic by SARS-CoV-2 poses an unprecedented threat to humanity. The number of infections is increasing exponentially day by day. Identifying, qualifying, collecting, and preparing plasma from convalescents with sufficient SARS-CoV-2 neutralizing antibody titers in this pandemic may be challenging but within the approach of most blood establishments. Careful clinical evaluation may rapidly establish whether CP therapy at the early onset of disease in patients of high risk may improve symptoms, reduce hospital stay and decrease mortality due to COVID-19. Moreover, CP is an excellent therapeutic option due to the lack of specific treatment for COVID-19, as the availability of anti-viral drugs/vaccines may take more time.

Keywords: Adverse effects, Antibody titer, Convalescent plasma, Safety and efficacy, Transfusion.

* **Corresponding author Fazlullah Khan:** Department of Allied Health Sciences, Bashir Institute of Health Sciences, Bharakahu, Islamabad, Pakistan; Tel: +92 3469 433 155; E-mail: fazlullahdr@gmail.com

Kamal Niaz & Muhammad Farrukh Nisar (Eds.)

INTRODUCTION

Many patients were suffering from chest infections of unknown cause in December 2019 in Wuhan, China. The causative agent was found to be a new coronavirus (CoV), named nCoV2019 (2019 novel coronavirus) by the World Health Organization (WHO) on January 7, 2020 [1]. Subsequently, the virus was retitled severe acute respiratory syndrome coronavirus-2 (SARS-CoV-2), and the resulting infection was named coronavirus disease-2019 (COVID-19). This disease spread in many countries within three months, and the WHO declared it a global pandemic on March 11, 2020 [1].

Convalescent plasma (CP) therapy, prime adoptive immunotherapy that has been used in the treatment and prevention of various diseases for more than one century [2]. In the last two decades, CP therapy has been successfully applied with satisfactory efficacy and safety in the treatment and prevention of the Middle East respiratory syndrome (MERS), severe acute respiratory syndrome (SARS), and H1N1 pandemic [3]. In passive immunization therapy, the antibodies are administered to the susceptible person to treat or prevent the infectious disease caused by the same agent

On the contrary, active immunization requires the inductance of an immune response which takes time to develop and varies depending on the recipient. Therefore, for providing prompt immunity to a susceptible person, passive immunization is considered the only way [4]. For therapeutic purposes, passive immunization is the most effective way to administer in a short time after the appearance of symptoms. Passive administration of antibodies works by neutralization of the initial inoculation in which the amount is much smaller than that of established disease [5]. A sufficient amount of antibodies must be administered for passive immunization therapy to be effective. When given to a susceptible individual, the antibodies circulate in the bloodstream for some time. After it reaches the tissues, and provides proper protection against an infectious agent.

According to WHO, the current management and treatment of COVID-19 have been mainly centered on case detection, treatment, monitoring, prevention of infection, and supportive care [6]. Currently, due to the lack of evidence, no specific treatment against nCOV-19 has been recommended [7]. So CP therapy is the only choice for the treatment of severe patients infected with nCOV-19. In the current pandemic of SARS-CoV-2, CP therapy was tested to treat COVID-19 patients in China, as claimed in several studies [8, 9], as shown in Fig. (**1**) . A research study on 10 COVID-19 patients with severe symptoms, CP with neutralizing antibody titers equal to or greater than a 1:640 dilution, was collected and transfused to all severe COVID-19 patients [10]. No serious side effects were reported in the recipients of CP transfusion. Moreover, the improvement in radiological pulmonary lesions and other symptoms was observed in all 10 patients within 1-3 days of CP transfusion. Studies revealed that CP obtained from COVID-19 recovered patients could be used for the treatment without producing severe adverse effects. Recently, Food and Drug Administration (FDA) has recommended the administration of investigational CP may result in clinical benefits for the management of COVID-19 patients during public health emergencies [11]. The current chapter aimed to summarize all the possible CP transfusion studies that might be beneficial for the treatment and management of individuals infected with SARS-CoV-2.

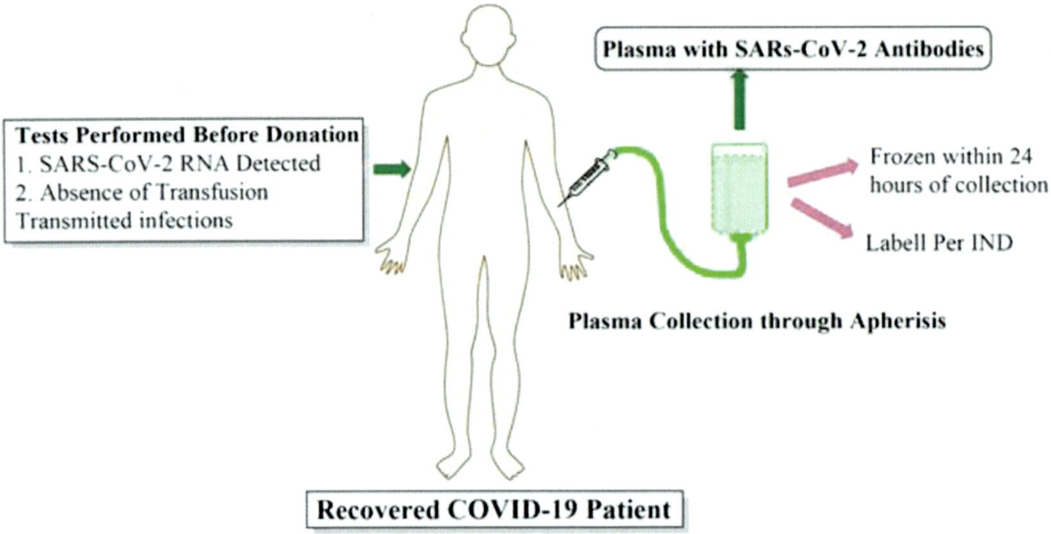

Fig. (1). Flow diagram of blood plasma preparation from infected individuals.

Therapeutic Agents (Convalescent Plasma and Immune Globulin)

Convalescent plasma, convalescent serum, and hyperimmune immunoglobulin prepared from convalescent plasma are interventions that have been used in the past to treat conditions when no vaccine or pharmacological interventions were available. Diphtheria, pneumococcal pneumonia, mumps, measles, hepatitis A and B, rabies, and polio are conditions where convalescent plasma is effective [12].

CP contains pathogen-specific neutralizing antibodies, which can neutralize viral particles, and treatment with CP or hyperimmune immunoglobulin confers passive immunity to recipients. The duration of granted protection can differ depending on the timing of administration, ranging from weeks to months after treatment [13]. Apheresis is the approved technique to obtain plasma. Blood from the donor is continuously centrifuged to allow the selective collection of plasma for COVID-19 patients. From a single apheresis donation, the efficiency of this method is about 400–800 mL. The amount of plasma received from the blood through apheresis is frozen and stored in units ranging from 200 to 250 ml which can be used for transfusion to severe patients [14]. Natural defense (antibodies) to the disease is developed in the blood of the patients recovered from COVID-19 present in the plasma portion of the blood.

Plasma from the blood of recovered patients, which contains antibodies against SARS-CoV-2, can be utilized to make two preparations that include CP and hyperimmune immunoglobulin. Later on, it is more concentrated and therefore has more antibodies. The main objective of CP therapy is to neutralize the infectious agent to combat the disease [15]. The composition of CP obtained is variable and may consist of a wide variety of components present in the blood.

It consists of a mixture of organic and inorganic salts, water, and above one thousand proteins, including immunoglobulins, albumin, coagulation, and antithrombotic factors and complement [16]. These components are responsible for the immunomodulatory potential of CP in COVID-19 patients with severe symptoms. It is suggested that plasma obtained from healthy volunteers exerts immunomodulatory actions *via* the infusion of antibodies and anti-inflammatory cytokines that blocks autoantibodies, cytokines, and complement proteins [17].

After the onset of infection, the first antibody produced is IgM by day-7 and is detectable in serum till day-21. IgG antibody production starts at around day-14 and continues for a longer time [18]. Plasma rich in IgG antibodies is usually collected after 14 days from the date of recovery for convalescent plasma therapy. The first high antibody titers can be observed in recovered patients' serum on the 21st day because the immune system starts developing antibodies from day 0 of exposure to the antigen (SARS-CoV-2). A rise in antibody production can be observed 14th day. A significant increase in these specific antibodies (raised against COVID-19) in the serum of the recovered patients can be determined upon further antibody development in the host immune system by the 21st day. Hence, it can be recommended to use the plasma collected during this peak of antibody increase period for therapeutic purposes effectively [19]. Hyperimmune immunoglobulin has the advantage of preventing harmful coagulation factors from transferring present in plasma products compared to convalescent plasma. The amount and antibody concentration can be more accurately dosed compared to convalescent plasma. Hyperimmune immunoglobulin can be prepared in a consistent manner [20]. The primary accepted mechanism of action for convalescent plasma therapy is the clearance of viremia, which typically happens 10–14 days after infection [21]. For the first time, Shen *et al.* [9] reported the experience of critically ill patients who received a single dose of 400 mL CP with neutralizing antibody titer in the range of 1:80- 1:480. This increased anti-SAR--CoV-2 IgG and IgM titers in recipients in a time-dependent manner. All the patients were recovered in a short time with improvement in fever and other biochemical parameters. CP therapy in COVID-19 patients is considered an effective and safe technique for the prophylaxis and treatment of COVID-19; however, it needs further investigation in randomized clinical studies.

Safety and Efficacy of CP for COVID-19 patients

Till the discovery of proper drugs for treating COVID-19 or the development of vaccines, the therapeutic strategy is primarily supportive. Several medications, including anti-HIV and anti-viral agents, are clinically effective, but their efficacy was not found satisfactory [22, 23]. The alternate strategy to overcome this viral infection is the use of convalescent plasma. Studies revealed that the patients treated with CP had a short stay in the hospital and lower mortality than those treated with other drugs [24].

The safety and efficacy of CP for COVID 19 were reviewed from 12 different studies [25]. Out of these, 9 studies have shown improvement in clinical symptoms due to CP therapy, while research carried out by Joyner *et al* [26] did not notice much improvement. About 75 patients in 9 studies required different forms of respiratory support at baseline. The efficacy and safety of CP were significant after therapy initiation in the early stages of viremia as shown by the results. In another study, the patient was clinically stable before and after CP therapy [3].

Pathways Use for Investigational COVID-19 CP

As the Federal Drug Administration (FDA) has not yet approved the CP treatment of COVID-19 patients, so it is regulated under the status of "investigational product". FDA released the guidelines for investigational COVID-19 CP in March 2020 [27]. These guidelines plan three different pathways for access to CP. The first pathway includes the application of an investigational new drug (IND) in an emergency. It grants permission to the providers to apply for compassionate use of this treatment in a patient having life-threatening COVID-19 with severe symptoms [28]. It should be noted that this pathway does not allow the use of this treatment in individuals for prophylactic purposes. Minimum requirements for requesting permission for the first pathway include a brief history and a description of indications. The first pathway has been allowed in the current situation to cope with the given public health emergency that the COVID-19 pandemic presents [29].

The second pathway relates to the clinical trial research for the management of COVID-19 with CP. Under this pathway, providers are required to request an IND for clinical trials in a traditional pathway as it is for other clinical trials [29]. The third pathway is that of expanded access under the government-led initiative. According to this pathway, expanded access of CP to collaborative research institutes following a master protocol can be provided through a government-led initiative. This pathway would enable the institutions to collect extensive data through a non-randomized study pattern [30].

Collection of COVID-19 Plasma and Eligibility to Donate Blood Plasma (Precautionary Measures)

Convalescent plasma needs immobilization using the blood collection and transfusion infrastructure. The collection and administration of convalescent plasma require standard practices of collection and transfusion [31]. The following points should be noted while collecting CP for administration into COVID-19 patients.

Eligibility of Donors

The first important thing for treating the COVID-19 patients with CP is the determination of the right donor. The eligibility criteria for CP include a person with a history previously confirmed case of COVID-19 with approved laboratory test from nasopharyngeal swab sample, have passed not less than two weeks after the resolution of symptoms such as cough, fever, and SOB. Finally, have a negative COVID-19 history confirmed by standard molecular test in nasopharyngeal swab sample [32]. The donors should be confirmed to be virus-free; negligence in this regard can cause potential problems for the target patients or receivers and the health staff dealing with the donors for the collection of plasma. Approaches for the recruitment of donors include community outreach in places with robust epidemics, communication, and advertising directly *via* providers, professional organizations, or media. Patients can also be contacted directly; however, this approach poses the issue of patient confidentiality. Blood centers having well-developed and well-equipped infrastructure can be the best option for recruiting donors [33].

Pre-screening of Donors

Pre-screening of donors before donating plasma is the prerequisite for successful therapy of COVID-19 patients with CP. Clinical providers are responsible for the pre-screening of donors. They collect a nasopharyngeal swab sample from the donor and test it for the virus's nucleic acid to ensure the donors are free from the virus. If the donors are free from the virus, they further collect the blood samples from donors for testing antibodies before referring to a collection facility [33].

Antibody Screening

When reflecting on FDA guidance, the tests for antibodies have their challenges. Generally, an individual cannot qualify to be an appropriate donor while using tests that have not been carefully and appropriately examined. It is still not known that which types of antibodies are maximally effective COVID-19 contexts [14]. Antibody neutralization assay is required to be correlated better with its function. However, these assays are not widely available in clinical laboratories. Though quantitative assays such as enzyme-linked immunosorbent assay (ELISA), however, commercially available assays cannot be trusted as they are not appropriately validated [34].

There is limited data available on ELISA. Similarly, the correlation between neutralizing anti-SARS-CoV-2 antibodies and total anti-SARS-CoV-2 antibodies is still not clear. Furthermore, more spike proteins have been tested and used to see if subclasses such as IgG, IgM, or IgA and total antibodies are optimal measures [35]. Thus, an urgent need for an assay is highly validated and a refined treatment modality.

Blood Collection and Testing

Upon qualification of the donors, they are referred to the blood centers that are specialized and well-equipped. A specialized form designed for ensuring the meeting of pre-screening criteria is sent to the blood center. This also ensures that the donors have been appropriately examined. At this stage, the FDA specifies that the donors should go through a complete questionnaire about donor history and standard physical screening. This process helps in preventing the spread of other communicable diseases [36]. For optimizing the yield of CP, apheresis is recommended rather than whole blood donation. This helps in the targeted collection of the required blood volume fraction, and the other components to the donor are returned during the process [36].

Dosing and Transfusion

CP dosing has been considerably variable due to severity and different indications (*i.e.,* treatment *vs* . prevention). Recently, during the COVID-19 pandemic in china, an investigative study used a single dose (200 mL) of CP [10]. The dose that has been suggested for treatment is 1-2 units, while for post-exposure prophylaxis, the suggested dose 1 unit in the planned clinical trials. The duration of the efficacy of antibodies is not known but has been suggested to last for few weeks [37]. The dosing regimen selected was based on a previous study with the use of CP therapy in SARS, wherein plasma (5 mL/kg) was used at a titer of >1:160 [21]. Previously it has been reported that the prophylactic doses successfully used were only in a short time than the proposed treatment dose. This experience was utilized even in the designing of clinical investigations. The amount of plasma 3.125 mL/kg with a titer of >1:64 would provide an equivalent immunoglobulin level to one-quarter of 5ml/kg plasma with a titer of > 1:160 following first-order linear proportionality. For a typical patient (~80 Kg), this would result in 250 mL of plasma (3.125 ml/kg x 80 kg = 250 mL > 1:64), approximately the same as the amount of a standard unit of plasma in the United States. This stratagem provides logistical ease in the preparation of the product for adult transfusions [31]. Clinical investigations are being programmed for pediatrics where transfusions will be needed to aliquot large volume units and CP dose per body weight. Based on the latest degree of situations, accurate models to determine the bioavailability of CP dose in tissues where virus and host interactions are not yet possible [38].

Patient Eligibility

Patient eligibility criteria are essential to meet FDA requirements for successful treatment of COVID-19 with CP. FDA has suggested the following criteria for patient eligibility for treating COVID-19 with CP.

1. COVID-19confirmed in laboratory.
2. Severe, life-threatening COVID-19: Patients having blood oxygen saturation less than 93%, shortness of breath, respiratory frequency less than 30 per minute, lung infiltrates greater than 50% within 24 to 48 hours, septic shock, and multiple organs failures.
3. Informed consent is provided by the patient or healthcare proxy [28].

Labeling and Recordkeeping

The CP labeled container of COVID-19 units shall have the following statement, “Caution: New Drug--Limited by Federal (or the United States) law to investigational use with reference to the circular of information”. FDA considers that label for COVID-19 CP container does not provide specific information about CP concerning dosage information, indications, cautions, or contraindications. A uniform container label for COVID-19 CP is recommended, especially using the format recommended by the International Society of Blood Transfusion (ISBT) for the Uniform labeling using ISBT 128.

COVID-19 CP should be stored below or at -18°C, frozen within 8 hours, and have an expiry date one year from the collection date. Expiry date and the manufacturing process applied on the label must be the same and for other plasma products of the same type. Health professionals participating in an IND or an expanded access IND (eIND), must keep a record of the units of COVID-19 CP given to the patient suffering from COVID-19. A unique identification number(s) must be a part of such records.

Adverse Effects of CP Therapy

The most common side effects observed with CP therapy include transfusion-related events, such as fever, chills, acute lung injury relating to transfusion, anaphylactic reactions, hemolysis, and cardiovascular problems, *etc* [39, 40]. Moreover, the risk of infections transmitted by transfusions, such as the hepatitis C virus, human immunodeficiency virus, syphilis, and hepatitis B virus, should not be neglected. Therefore, we need to pay attention to the proper use of CP therapy [41]. The following adverse effects have been noted in several studies. Many of the CP transfusion studies did not report the grade of adverse reactions. Reportedly the participants involved in two studies have experienced adverse reactions data, presumably grades 3 or 4 [42]. A case of severe anaphylactic shock was recorded in another study (3 participants). In contrast, 4 studies (19 participants) have recorded no moderate or severe adverse reaction [43]. A participant in one case study reported mild fever (38.9 °C). One serious adverse event (anaphylactic reaction) was reported in one study (3 participants) after receiving CP. Additionally, 6 case studies described the occurrence of no serious adverse reactions. We are unsure whether or not CP therapy increases the risk of severe adverse reactions (very low-certainty evidence) [42].

Optimal Dose and Clinical Benefits of CP Therapy

CP should be administered to high-risk patients in the early course of the disease. The high-risk patients have an oxygen saturation level below 94% or have an age of more than 70 years [44]. The most appropriate time for CP transfusion is within 5 days after the onset of the disease. The main objective of the treatment of such patients is survival, while secondary outcomes are avoiding the need for ICU and shortening the length of hospital stay [45]. Transfusion (200-250 ml CP/patient/50-80 kg) earlier in the course of the disease or even up to days of the onset of the disease is required. The volume of CP may be adjusted for patients weighing the range of 50-80 kg. The infusion should be slow and closely monitored to avoid circulatory overload and other immediate side effects related to transfusion. After confirmation of sufficient tolerance, 2 units after 24-48 h may be administered [27]. Almost all COVID-19 patients exhibited improvement of symptoms after the transfusion of CP. The acute respiratory distress syndrome was resolved; body temperature became normal, varying degrees of absorption of lung lesion, weaning from ventilator within 1 to a maximum of 5 weeks after transfusion of CP [11].

FUTURE PERSPECTIVE

The convalescent plasma of COVID-19 can be used to treat people having early symptoms and prevent disease in exposed individuals. Healthcare professionals, including physicians and nurses, are exposed to COVID-19 and are being quarantined, collapsing [46]. It is hoped that CP will prevent SARS-CoV-2 infection and if it gets established. It may prevent the health care providers from getting quarantined, and therefore, they will play their critical role. CP may be used prophylactically to prevent COVID-19 among individuals caring for patients of the disease [31].

CONCLUSION

There is a dire need to control the unprecedented global calamity of public health due to the pandemic of COVID-19. At present, no reliable therapeutic option is available for COVID-19 patients having severe symptoms. Based on the aforementioned facts and figures, it may be concluded that CP may be an effective therapeutic option in addition to anti-viral drugs, with some evidence of a reduction in mortality, safety, and improvement of clinical symptoms. However, conclusive evidence on the optimum dose and time-point of treatment for CP to COVID-19 are not available, for which large multicenter clinical trials are urgently required to combat this pandemic.

CONSENT FOR PUBLICATION

Not Applicable.

CONFLICT OF INTEREST

The authors confirm that this chapter contents have no conflict of interest.

ACKNOWLEDGEMENT

Declared none.

REFERENCES

[1] 2020. Organization, W.H., Naming the coronavirus disease (COVID-19) and the virus that causes it. 2020. URL https://www. who. int/emergencies/diseases/novel-coronavirus-2019/technical-guidance/naming-the-coronavirus-disease-(covid-2019)-and-the- virus-that-causes-it

[2] Marano G, Vaglio S, Pupella S, *et al.* Convalescent plasma: new evidence for an old therapeutic tool? Blood Transfus 2016; 14(2): 152-7.
[PMID: 26674811]

[3] Duan K, Liu B, Li C, *et al.* Effectiveness of convalescent plasma therapy in severe COVID-19 patients. Proc Natl Acad Sci USA 2020; 117(17): 9490-6.
[http://dx.doi.org/10.1073/pnas.2004168117] [PMID: 32253318]

[4] Casadevall A, Scharff MD. Return to the past: the case for antibody-based therapies in infectious diseases. Clin Infect Dis 1995; 21(1): 150-61.
[http://dx.doi.org/10.1093/clinids/21.1.150] [PMID: 7578724]

[5] Robbins JB, Schneerson R, Szu SC. Perspective: hypothesis: serum IgG antibody is sufficient to confer protection against infectious diseases by inactivating the inoculum. J Infect Dis 1995; 171(6): 1387-98.
[http://dx.doi.org/10.1093/infdis/171.6.1387] [PMID: 7769272]

[6] Chen H, Guo J, Wang C, *et al.* Clinical characteristics and intrauterine vertical transmission potential of COVID-19 infection in nine pregnant women: a retrospective review of medical records. Lancet 2020; 395(10226): 809-15.
[http://dx.doi.org/10.1016/S0140-6736(20)30360-3] [PMID: 32151335]

[7] Russell CD, Millar JE, Baillie JK. Clinical evidence does not support corticosteroid treatment for 2019-nCoV lung injury. Lancet 2020; 395(10223): 473-5.
[http://dx.doi.org/10.1016/S0140-6736(20)30317-2] [PMID: 32043983]

[8] Casadevall A, Pirofski LA. The convalescent sera option for containing COVID-19. J Clin Invest 2020; 130(4): 1545-8.
[http://dx.doi.org/10.1172/JCI138003] [PMID: 32167489]

[9] Shen C, Wang Z, Zhao F, *et al.* Treatment of 5 critically ill patients with COVID-19 with convalescent plasma. JAMA 2020; 323(16): 1582-9.
[http://dx.doi.org/10.1001/jama.2020.4783] [PMID: 32219428]

[10] Duan K, Liu B, Li C, *et al.* The feasibility of convalescent plasma therapy in severe COVID-19 patients: a pilot study medRxiv 2020.
[http://dx.doi.org/10.1101/2020.03.16.20036145]

[11] Rajendran K, Krishnasamy N, Rangarajan J, Rathinam J, Natarajan M, Ramachandran A. Convalescent plasma transfusion for the treatment of COVID-19: Systematic review. J Med Virol 2020; 92(9): 1475-83.
[http://dx.doi.org/10.1002/jmv.25961] [PMID: 32356910]

[12] Eibl MM. History of immunoglobulin replacement. Immunol Allergy Clin North Am 2008; 28(4): 737-764, viii.
[http://dx.doi.org/10.1016/j.iac.2008.06.004] [PMID: 18940572]

[13] Keller MA, Stiehm ER. Passive immunity in prevention and treatment of infectious diseases. Clin Microbiol Rev 2000; 13(4): 602-14.
[http://dx.doi.org/10.1128/CMR.13.4.602] [PMID: 11023960]

[14] Bloch EM, Shoham S, Casadevall A, *et al.* Deployment of convalescent plasma for the prevention and treatment of COVID-19. J Clin Invest 2020; 130(6): 2757-65.
[http://dx.doi.org/10.1172/JCI138745] [PMID: 32254064]

[15] Burnouf T, Seghatchian J. Ebola virus convalescent blood products: where we are now and where we may need to go. Transfus Apheresis Sci 2014; 51(2): 120-5.
[http://dx.doi.org/10.1016/j.transci.2014.10.003] [PMID: 25457751]

[16] Benjamin RJ, McLaughlin LS. Plasma components: properties, differences, and uses. Transfusion .2012; 52 (Suppl. 1): 9S-19S.
[http://dx.doi.org/10.1111/j.1537-2995.2012.03622.x] [PMID: 22578375]

[17] Lünemann JD, Nimmerjahn F, Dalakas MC. Intravenous immunoglobulin in neurology--mode of action and clinical efficacy. Nat Rev Neurol 2015; 11(2): 80-9. [http://dx.doi.org/10.1038/nrneurol.2014.253] [PMID: 25561275]

[18] Wölfel R, Corman VM, Guggemos W, *et al.* Virological assessment of hospitalized patients with COVID-2019. Nature 2020; 581(7809): 465-9. [http://dx.doi.org/10.1038/s41586-020-2196-x] [PMID: 32235945]

[19] Anudeep T, Jeyaraman M, Shetty DU, *et al.* Convalescent Plasma as a plausible therapeutic option in nCOVID-19–A Review 2020.

[20] Gan CT-J, Lankhaar J-W, Westerhof N, *et al.* Noninvasively assessed pulmonary artery stiffness predicts mortality in pulmonary arterial hypertension. Chest 2007; 132(6): 1906-12. [http://dx.doi.org/10.1378/chest.07-1246] [PMID: 17989161]

[21] Cheng Y, Wong R, Soo YO, *et al.* Use of convalescent plasma therapy in SARS patients in Hong Kong. Eur J Clin Microbiol Infect Dis 2005; 24(1): 44-6. [http://dx.doi.org/10.1007/s10096-004-1271-9] [PMID: 15616839]

[22] Matthay MA, Aldrich JM, Gotts JE. Treatment for severe acute respiratory distress syndrome from COVID-19. Lancet Respir Med 2020; 8(5): 433-4. [http://dx.doi.org/10.1016/S2213-2600(20)30127-2] [PMID: 32203709]

[23] Kalil AC. Treating COVID-19—off-label drug use, compassionate use, and randomized clinical trials during pandemics. JAMA 2020; 323(19): 1897-8. [http://dx.doi.org/10.1001/jama.2020.4742] [PMID: 32208486]

[24] Chen L, Xiong J, Bao L, Shi Y. Convalescent plasma as a potential therapy for COVID-19. Lancet Infect Dis 2020; 20(4): 398-400. [http://dx.doi.org/10.1016/S1473-3099(20)30141-9] [PMID: 32113510]

[25] Devasenapathy N, Ye Z, Loeb M, *et al.* Efficacy and safety of convalescent plasma for severe COVID-19 based on evidence in other severe respiratory viral infections: a systematic review and meta-analysis. CMAJ 2020; 192(27): E745-55. [http://dx.doi.org/10.1503/cmaj.200642] [PMID: 32444482]

[26] Joyner MJ, Senefeld JW, Klassen SA, *et al.* Effect of Convalescent Plasma on Mortality among Hospitalized Patients with COVID-19: Initial Three-Month Experience medRxiv 2020. [http://dx.doi.org/10.1101/2020.08.12.20169359]

[27] FDA. 2020. Investigational-covid-19-convalescent-plasma-emergency-inds. US Food and Drug Administration. 2020; https://www.fda.gov/vaccines-blood

[28] Tanne JH. Covid-19: FDA approves use of convalescent plasma to treat critically ill patients. BMJ 2020; 368: m1256. [http://dx.doi.org/10.1136/bmj.m1256] [PMID: 32217555]

[29] Sahu KK, Jindal V, Siddiqui AD, Cerny J, Gerber JM. Convalescent plasma therapy: A passive therapy for an aggressive COVID-19. J Med Virol 2020; 92(11): 2251-3. [http://dx.doi.org/10.1002/jmv.26047] [PMID: 32437024]

[30] Barone P, DeSimone RA. Convalescent plasma to treat coronavirus disease 2019 (COVID-19): considerations for clinical trial design. Transfusion 2020; 60(6): 1123-7. [http://dx.doi.org/10.1111/trf.15843] [PMID: 32374891]

[31] Bloch EM, Shoham S, Casadevall A, *et al.* Deployment of convalescent plasma for the prevention and treatment of COVID-19. J Clin Invest 2020; 130(6): 2757-65. [http://dx.doi.org/10.1172/JCI138745] [PMID: 32254064]

[32] Long Q-X, Tang X-J, Shi Q-L, *et al.* Clinical and immunological assessment of asymptomatic SARS-CoV-2 infections. Nat Med 2020; 26(8): 1200-4. [http://dx.doi.org/10.1038/s41591-020-0965-6] [PMID: 32555424]

[33] Zaheer HA, Waheed U. Blood transfusion service in disasters. Transfus Apheresis Sci 2016; 55(2): 186-90.
[http://dx.doi.org/10.1016/j.transci.2016.09.007] [PMID: 27665156]

[34] Peeling RW, Artsob H, Pelegrino JL, *et al.* Evaluation of diagnostic tests: dengue. Nat Rev Microbiol 2010; 8(12) (Suppl.): S30-8.
[http://dx.doi.org/10.1038/nrmicro2459] [PMID: 21548185]

[35] Okba NM, Muller MA, Li W, Wang C. GeurtsvanKessel, C.H.; Corman, V.M.; Lamers, M.M.; Sikkema, R.S.; de Bruin, E.; Chandler, F.D., SARS-CoV-2 specific antibody responses in COVID-19 patients medRxiv 2020.

[36] Kamel HT, Bassett MB, Custer B, *et al.* Safety and donor acceptance of an abbreviated donor history questionnaire. Transfusion 2006; 46(10): 1745-53.
[http://dx.doi.org/10.1111/j.1537-2995.2006.00967.x] [PMID: 17002631]

[37] Casadevall A. Passive antibody administration (immediate immunity) as a specific defense against biological weapons. Emerg Infect Dis 2002; 8(8): 833-41.
[http://dx.doi.org/10.3201/eid0808.010516] [PMID: 12141970]

[38] Tatara AM. Role of Tissue Engineering in COVID-19 and Future Viral Outbreaks. Tissue Eng Part A 2020; 26(9-10): 468-74.
[http://dx.doi.org/10.1089/ten.tea.2020.0094] [PMID: 32272857]

[39] Luke TC, Kilbane EM, Jackson JL, Hoffman SL. Meta-analysis: convalescent blood products for Spanish influenza pneumonia: a future H5N1 treatment? Ann Intern Med 2006; 145(8): 599-609.
[http://dx.doi.org/10.7326/0003-4819-145-8-200610170-00139] [PMID: 16940336]

[40] MacLennan S, Barbara JA. Risks and side effects of therapy with plasma and plasma fractions. Best Pract Res Clin Haematol 2006; 19(1): 169-89.
[http://dx.doi.org/10.1016/j.beha.2005.01.033] [PMID: 16377549]

[41] Organization WH. Use of convalescent whole blood or plasma collected from patients recovered from Ebola virus disease for transfusion, as an empirical treatment during outbreaks: interim guidance for national health authorities and blood transfusion services. World Health Organization 2014.

[42] Valk SJ, Piechotta V, Chai KL, *et al.* Convalescent plasma or hyperimmune immunoglobulin for people with COVID-19: a rapid review. Cochrane Database Syst Rev 2020; 5(5): CD013600.

[43] Casadevall A, Joyner MJ, Pirofski L-A. A randomized trial of convalescent plasma for COVID-1--potentially hopeful signals. JAMA 2020; 324(5): 455-7.
[http://dx.doi.org/10.1001/jama.2020.10218] [PMID: 32492105]

[44] Zhou F, Yu T, Du R, *et al.* Clinical course and risk factors for mortality of adult inpatients with COVID-19 in Wuhan, China: a retrospective cohort study. Lancet 2020; 395(10229): 1054-62.
[http://dx.doi.org/10.1016/S0140-6736(20)30566-3] [PMID: 32171076]

[45] Salazar E, Perez KK, Ashraf M, *et al.* Treatment of COVID-19 Patients with Convalescent Plasma. Am J Pathol 2020; 190(8): 1680-90.
[PMID: 32473109]

[46] Moazzami B, Razavi-Khorasani N, Dooghaie Moghadam A, Farokhi E, Rezaei N. COVID-19 and telemedicine: Immediate action required for maintaining healthcare providers well-being. J Clin Virol 2020; 126: 104345.
[http://dx.doi.org/10.1016/j.jcv.2020.104345] [PMID: 32278298]

CHAPTER 11

Stem Cell Therapy for COVID-19

Ovais Sideeq[1,2,*], Kamal Niaz[3], Kashif Rahim[4] and **Aadil Javed[5]**

[1] *School of Medicine, Tehran University of Medical Sciences (TUMS), Tehran, Iran*

[2] *Universal Scientific Education and Research Network (USERN), Tehran, Iran*

[3] *Department of Pharmacology & Toxicology, Faculty of Bio-Sciences, Cholistan University of Veterinary and Animal Sciences, Bahawalpur-63100, Pakistan*

[4] *Department of Microbiology, Cholistan University of Veterinary and Animal Sciences (CUVAS), Punjab, Bahawalpur-63100, Pakistan*

[5] *Department of Biotechnology, Graduate School of Natural and Applied Sciences, Ege University, Bornova, Izmir, Turkey*

Abstract: Stem cells have long been a topic of interest around the globe. Now and then, stem cells are being studied for revealing their beneficial effects. Countries around the world are in a race in stem cell research. Stem cells possess some unique and considerable qualities that hardly any other cell to date has. The outbreak of novel coronavirus or coronavirus disease-19 (COVID-19) was located in Wuhan, China. After a few months, the episode was declared Pandemic by the World Health Organization (WHO) as it engulfed many countries worldwide. Since then, stem cells have gained more push in clinical as well as pre-clinical stage research studies. COVID-19 shares some molecular properties with other coronaviruses like severe acute respiratory syndrome (SARS) and the Middle East respiratory syndrome (MERS). Stem cells surprisingly showed some good outcomes in many patients infected with COVID-19. A lot of laboratory evaluation is being carried out to check the feasibility of different stem cells to be used in COVID-19 infected patients. This chapter discusses and highlights the possible interventions in COVID-19 using different lineages and bio-cultured stem cells.

Keywords: Bone marrow, Coronavirus, Cytokines, Hematopoietic, Mesenchymal, Patients, SARS-CoV-2, Stem cells.

INTRODUCTION

Since decades of extensive research, hematopoietic stem cells (HSCs) have been shown to exhibit tissue-specific stem cell characteristics and have been continuously used in many clinical procedures. Upon clinical application, they

* **Corresponding author Ovais Sideeq:** School of Medicine, Tehran University of Medical Sciences (TUMS), Tehran, Iran, E-mail: owasesiddique@gmail.com

provide a deep understanding of the fundamentals of stem cell sciences. The different fields of HSCs being studied and their clinical applications are believed to benefit significantly. The properties of self-renewal and differentiation have put stem cells at the center of regenerative medicine. The combination of these features is leading to improve ways to treat many medical conditions [1]. The undifferentiated stem cells have their origin in the different stages of life. They can be found in the embryonic, fetal, and adult stages of life. They give rise to different lineages of cells that are necessary for building up various organs and tissues. Many studies have shown the use of stem cells in cellular therapy. In the regeneration of organs and the replacement of damaged cells, these cells are highly valued. Some recent research has shown that stem cell-associated specific cells in some diseases can be transformed to develop drugs [2]. In the jewels of medicine, cellular therapy is considered a favorable and encouraging approach that, instead of generating a new organ, focuses on the regeneration and restoration of various injured tissues [3]. Genetically modified stem cells and the production of engrafts with bio cultures scaffolds have enhanced therapeutic outcomes in animal models.

However, several vigorous pre-clinical studies are required to move forward in the field of stem cell therapy [4]. There are a lot of researches that have shown assuring effects of stem cell therapy. The scope of stem cell therapy can be seen during the developing phase of the embryo in various cardiovascular diseases, including cardiomyopathies, degenerative nervous disorders, metabolic diseases like diabetes, and osteoarthritis [5]. MSCs induce immunomodulatory and anti-inflammatory effects and have ascertained a dynamic role in the cure of COVID-19. The MSCs therapy has been a cost-effective treatment in COVID-19 [6]. This chapter will discuss the fundamentals of stem cells, their origin, and their types. Also, we will discuss the use of stem cells in novel coronavirus (COVID-19), the immune reactions, and the future perspective of HSCs for COVID-19.

Overview of Stem Cells

The term stem cell denotes a type of cell that holds the property to differentiate into several other types of cells while maintaining the self-renewal feature. Stem cells have the following main characteristics: a). The capability of expansive proliferation, *i.e.,* the process of renewing itself b). Potentiality to form different types of cells and c). The ability to grow from a single cell [2]. Going afar and crossing the limitations of cell lineages, hematopoietic stem cells possess a versatile nature to proliferate and give rise to abundant cell types. This process is also called transdifferentiation [7]. Different components in the blood are a reason for the differentiation of the multipotency feature of hematopoietic stem cells. HSCs are solely in charge of forming blood and its elements in all the spans of life. They develop, maintain, and regenerate a major portion of blood which itself is connective tissue. Multipotent stem cells act as the origin to give rise to the lineage of myeloid and lymphoid cells. Myeloid lineage then differentiates to common myeloid progenitors or CMP, while lymphoid lineage gives rise to common lymphoid progenitors or CLP. CMP and CLL themselves are left with no or negligible transdifferentiating characteristics reaching the stage of these progenitors. They also lose self-renewal ability and show very little division. From the CLP arise the cells that are essential components of cellular immunity. The cells that arise from CLP include T cells, B cells, natural killer cells (NK), lymphocyte subset forming lineages, and antigen-presenting cells like dendritic cells.

CMP differentiates into granulocyte monocyte progenitors (GMP), which can differentiate into granulocytes and monocytes. CMP also gives rise to megakaryocyte erythrocyte progenitors (MEP), which further develops a change to megakaryocytes and erythrocytes [8]. Outbreaking research has been conducted on HSC circulation under different conditions. HSCs don't follow a haphazard path circulating in the blood, but they distribute under proper physiologic rhythmic regulatory signals. The central nervous system has a major part in regulating the circadian clock, which draws the HSCs to the bone marrow [9]. High resistance to viral infections has been found in different stem cells. It has been noticed that stem cells can protect themselves from viruses by inducing interferon stimulating genes (ISGs). Interferon reaction is the first main mechanism of many cells against viral invasion. It has been reported that when stem cells differentiate into other types of cells, as they cannot differentiate any further, the ISGs become lower. Different types of stem cells have a particular way of expressing the ISGs [10]. The stem cells are generated when the embryo cells migrate and specify in multiple sites during its developmental phase. In upper-class vertebrates, various locations can be seen to undergo hematopoiesis, the process of blood formation. Hematopoiesis can be consecutively seen in the yolk sac, aorta gonad mesonephros region that encircles the dorsal aorta, the fetus's liver, and lastly, the bone marrow. Placental tissue has been recently recognized as another spot for the development of HSCs [11]. HSCs can be transplanted in two different ways, *i.e.,* autologous and allogenic. Therapeutically autologous transplantation of stem cells is related to radiotherapy and chemotherapy. This has been regulated to kill the tumor cells and recover the patient later on by Stem cell therapy. Allogenic stem cell transplantation is different from autologous. It uses stem cells of hematopoietic origin from a matched donor to revive the patient without using chemotherapy. The allogeneic transfer can lead to a graft-versus-tumor effect [12]. The hematopoietic stem cell lineages have been illustrated in Fig. (**1**) .

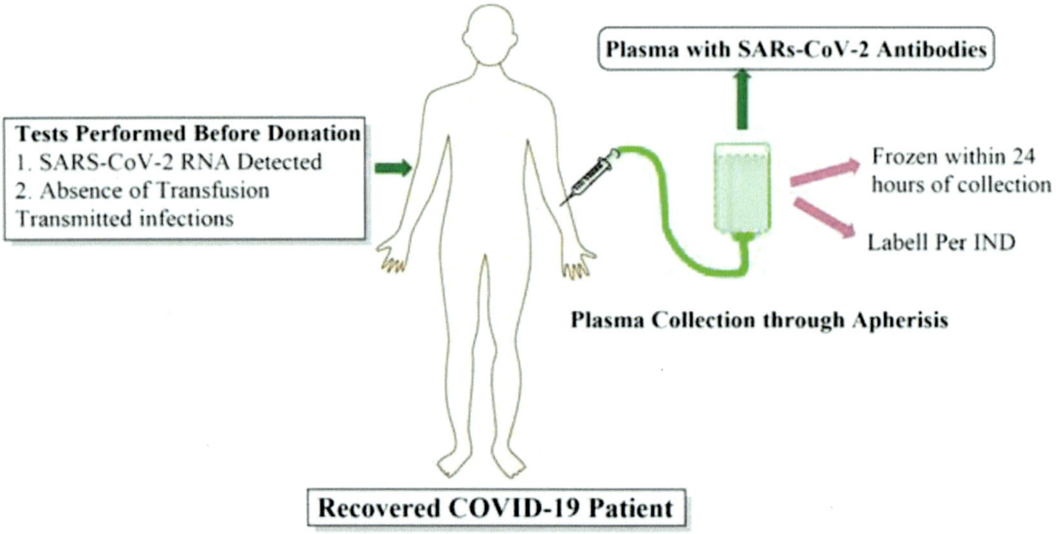

Fig. (1). LT-HSC: Long Term Hematopoietic Stem Cells, ST-HSC: Short Term Hematopoietic Stem Cells, CMP: Common Myeloid Progenitor, CLP: Common Lymphoid Progenitor, GMP: Granulocyte-Monocyte Progenitor, MEP: Megakaryocyte-Erythroid Progenitor, RBC: Red Blood Cells, NK: Natural Killer Cell, PDCs: Plasmacytoid Dendritic Cells, MDC: Monocyte Dendritic Cell.

Different Stem Cells

Although Stem cells can be divided into different types, two main types have been broadly categorized, namely the Pluripotent cells and Multipotent cells. The cells that have the property to differentiate into cells forming the endoderm, ectoderm, and mesoderm are known as pluripotent cells. These cells include embryonic stem cells, embryonic germ cells and also share some properties with induced pluripotent stem cells (iPSCs). The other types of stem cells based on potency are multipotent stem cells. These cells are different from embryonic or pluripotent cells in the way that they can be isolated from many fetal and animal tissues. HSCs, hepatic stem cells, neuronal stem cells are all lineages of multipotent cells [12]. HSCs have the characteristic to proliferate into both myeloid and lymphoid cell types. Multipotent stem cells can differentiate into a single layer of germ cells. Mesenchymal stem cells (MSCs) also belong to the cell types of multipotent stem cells. Several tissues are a source of multipotent stem cells, including peripheral blood, adipose tissue, bone marrow, bone, Wharton's jelly, and umbilical cord blood [2]. A cluster of stem cells has been recorded and hierarchized into different types based on potency and origin.

The different types of stem cells based on the potency to differentiate are as follows:

a. Totipotent or omnipotent cells are differentiable into embryonic as well as extra-embryonic tissues. Examples include an oocyte that has undergone fertilization. Embryonic and extra-embryonic tissues with development form into the embryo and the placenta.
b. Pluripotent stem cells including embryonic stem cells.
c. Multipotent stem cells include Mesenchymal stem cells.
d. Oligopotent stem cells can form two or more cell lineages belonging to a particular tissue. Hematopoietic stem cells can be included in this group.
e. Unipotent stem cells for example muscle stem cells which differentiate into only one type of cell.

Based on the origin of stem cells, they can be classified as:

a. ***Embryonic stem cells:*** The source of these cells is a 5-6-day stage of embryo known as the blastocyst. The blastocyst is formed of two cell types, i.e.., the inner cell mass developing inti embryo and the outer cell mass, also known as trophoblasts, give rise to the placenta.
b. ***Fetal stem cells:*** Whose source is terminated pregnancy fetus. Fetal stem cells lack many features ascribed to embryonic stem cells. They cannot differentiate indeterminately unless forced to do so under certain conditions in biological cultures. Neural stem cells can identify lineages that can be increased using fetal stem cells.
c. ***Perinatal stem cells*:** The origin of these cells may be the umbilical cord, placenta, and amniotic fluid. The blood of the placenta is a rich source of stem cells. Fetal epithelial cells are commonly found in amniotic fluid.
d. ***Adult stem cells:*** They are also known as resident stem cells or tissue-restricted stem cells. They can be found in the tissues and organs of an adult. Adult stem cells can be sourced to originate from bone marrow, menstrual blood, and adipose tissue, as shown in Table **1**.
e. ***Induced Pluripotent stem cells (iPS):*** Which shares the features of embryonic stem cells and adheres to their *in vitro* indefinite division [13]. In Table **1** below most important types of stem cells with their sources and/or examples are shown.

Table 1. Various stem cells originated from cell types.

Type of Stem Cell	Examples
1. Totipotent	Zygote
2. Pluripotent	Embryonic Stem Cells (ESCs) and induced Pluripotent Stem Cells (iPSCs)
3. Multipotent	Mesenchymal Stem Cells (MSCs)
4. Oligopotent	Lymphoid or Myeloid Stem Cells
5. Nullipotent	Osteoblasts
	Osteocytes

Stem Cells and Immune System Responses During COVID-19

Among the different stem cells, mainly mesenchymal stem cells have shown beneficial effects in COVID-19. MSCs inhibit many lymphocytes like T lymphocytes, monocytes, and macrophages. MSCs stimulate the differentiation of these cells into regulatory T cells (Treg). They also induce anti-inflammatory effects on macrophages. Mesenchymal stem cell therapy impedes the secretion of different cytokines, *e.g.,* IL-1, TNF-a, IL-6, IL-12, and IFN-g. Inhibition of such cytokines decreases the occurrence of cytokine storms in COVID-19 patients. MSCs protect the damaged respiratory tissue and pulmonary fibrosis; also relieve the COVID-19 patient from acute respiratory distress syndrome (ARDS). This effect has been reported based on the secretion of some factors by MSCs such as IL-10, vascular endothelial growth factor (VEGF), hepatocyte growth factor, and keratinocyte growth factor [14]. MSCs act through paracrine secretions, interacting with different cells of the immune system and regulating immunomodulatory effects. In various disease settings, the condition was improved after MSC transplantation. In such clinical settings, immune cells that secrete multiple cytokines have shown a decline in the blood. These cells include CXCR3+ NK cells, CXCR3+ CD4+ T cells, and CXCR3+ CD8+ T cells. MSCs also help in the proliferation of peripheral lymphocytes. In addition to the mentioned immune responses, CD14+ CD11c+ CD11bmid dendritic cells (DCs) have surged after the infusion of MSC therapy. Other immune responses found in many trials showed a reduction in TNF-a and an increment in IL-1 [15]. It should be noted that whenever the virus gets entry into the cells, it first presents its antigen to antigen-presenting cells (APCs). The peptides of antigen are presented by human leukocyte antigen (HLA) or major histocompatibility complex (MHC) in humans. Cytotoxic T lymphocytes (CTLs) then recognize these antigens. CD8+ and CD4+ T cells are reduced in COVID-19 [16]. It has been noted that there is a strong affinity of HLA molecules to bind to COVID-19 viral peptides [17]. Embryonic stem (ES) cells can be used in transplantation against MHC barriers without provoking an immune response [18]. Some studies reveal that mesenchymal stem cells inhibit the proliferation and differentiation of dendritic cells from CD34+ cells in humans while stimulating the regulatory dendritic cell differentiation [19]. It is known that lymphocytes and their subsets have a major role in regulating cellular immunity, and these cells work by restricting and regulating their common cascade. In novel coronavirus pneumonia, CD4+ T cells show a serene decrement in mild symptomatic COVID-19 patients, whereas in severely ill patients, this number is further decreased. Similarly, the CD8+ T cells are shown a gentle reduction in mild patients while a high drop is found in severe reported cases. This shows that immune system suppression was more noted in severe patients [20]. In the earlier course of the disease, activated partial thromboplastin time (aPTT) was considerable of shorter duration in more severe forms of COVID-19 affected patients. The quantity of D-dimer has also been reported to be elevated in novel coronavirus. Some other monitored findings are reduced number of B cells and higher than normal levels of NK cells, respectively more in severe cases than milder ones. Reduction in the levels of Treg subsets such as CD4+, CD25+, and CD127+ has also been reported in mild and severe forms of the disease. CD45RA+ Treg is decreased rapidly in severe cases as compared to mild reported cases [21]. Naïve Th cell count is increased, and memory Th cell count is reduced in COVID-19 patients who are severely infected. Cytotoxic suppressor T cells, which are CD28+, are also decreased below the normal levels. There is no big difference in the count of activated T cells, which are CD3+, HLA-DR+, and activated suppressor T cells which are CD8+, HLA-DR+, and CD3+. It was observed in seriously ill patients that regulatory T cells are decreased. No major change was seen in Treg cells and naïve T cells [22]. Much clinical analysis reported in certain cases of COVID 19 was explored for immune responses. These reports revealed high levels of immune factors in the serum of COVID-19 infected patients. One sample has shown high M-CSF, IL-10, IL-2, IL-4, IL-7, IL-12, IL-13, IL-14, IL-1a, IL-1ra, IL-1B, IP-10, IFN-a2, IFN-g, G-CSF, and HGF. Further immune-stimulating factors including cytokines and chemokines such as TRAIL, IL-16, IL-18, TNF-B, IL-2Ra, CTACK, LIF, GRO-a, MIF, MCP-3, b-NGF, SCF, SDF-1a, and SCGF-B have also been noticed. One study reveals the excess number of CD14+ and CD16+ monocytes responsible for the secretion of IL-6, which has also been accounted for in COVID-19 [23]. SARS-CoV2/COVID-19 suppresses and inhibits the TNF receptor-associated factors (TRAF), such as TRAF3 and TRAF6. Both of them have a crucial role in inducing TLR3/7 with the help of stimulating IRF-3/7. TRAF indirectly activates the RIG-I, MDA-5, and NFKB pathways. COVID-19 hinders the signaling pathway of T1IFN and activates phosphorylation reactions to inhibit the STAT family factors [24]. An early phase of the disease in hospitalized patients revealed low levels of IgM and IgG. Later on, with the course of the disease, IgM, and IgG, both immunoglobulin levels were reported to be positive, *i.e.,* there was an increment in the levels of IgG and IgM [25].

Mesenchymal Stem Cells in COVID-19

In various clinical studies, it has been put forth that MSCs can be used therapeutically as these cells treat *via* immunomodulation. Several clinical trials have shown an increasing amount of interest in MSCs. A study reveals that post mesenchymal stem cell transplantation, the lungs' alveolar lining is protected. It has also shown that pulmonary fibrosis can also be prevented, and the dysfunction of lungs can also be treated. As the immune system releases a storm of cytokines in COVID-19, mesenchymal stem cell therapy can prevent this phenomenon by promoting endogenous repair, which is a characteristic of stem cells. MSCs are a group of multipotent stem cells. They can be stored and then used repetitively for therapeutic purposes. MSCs are safe and effective with no nasty effects [26].

MSCs have been known to drift towards injured and inflammatory tissues and upregulate receptors like CCR2, CCR3, CCR4, and CXCR4 for RANTES and MDC. They also express PDGF and IGF receptor tyrosine kinase [27]. Bone marrow mesenchymal stem cells secrete FAS-regulated monocyte chemotactic protein 1 (MCP-1) and cause FASL-mediated T cell apoptosis. These T cells that undergo apoptosis recruit macrophages. Macrophages, in turn, secrete TGFB, which expresses CD4+ CD25+ and FOXP3 Treg cells. Treg cells mediate immune tolerance paving a way to affect the functioning of the immune system [28]. Mesenchymal Stem cells, which have been recently known as mesenchymal stromal cells, have been found to adhere to their immunomodulatory properties. They affect the T cells and show an interaction with B cells. This mechanism of mesenchymal stem cells shows that they can reduce inflammation in COVID-19 patients [29]. MSCs increase the activity of phagocytosis and secrete antimicrobial peptides and proteins (AMPs). In this way, they employ antimicrobial activity by coordinating pro and anti-inflammatory components of the immune system. While circulating in the bloodstream, mesenchymal stem cells invade the parenchyma of the lung and start refining the alveolar structure of the lungs. They also improve lung compliance and avoid further fibrosis of the respiratory tissue. They have inhibitory properties against the overstated reaction of the immune system, which helps to promote, revitalize, and regenerate the microenvironment. The mesenchymal stem cells derived from the umbilical cord are allogenic and are available in sparse quantity.

In contrast, the mesenchymal stem cells from bone marrow and adipose tissue can be accessed easily with ample quantity possessing autologous nature. The cells can regenerate epithelium and meshwork of alveoli in the lungs, thus bringing down mortality and morbidity and helping to boost the quality of life in patients with COVID-19 [30]. Among many sources of MSCs, umbilical cord blood and placenta are two excellent references from where MSCs can be derived. MSCs have been studied in a range of studies and clinical applications and have shown positive outcomes in treating the ARDS, acute lung injury and enhancing the repair of tissues [31]. Intravenous administration of human umbilical cord mesenchymal stem cells (hUCMSCs) helps to return the levels of CD3+ T cell, CD4+ T cell, and CD8+ T cell to normal. Thymosin a1, in combination with hUCMSCs, can significantly induce anti-inflammatory effects and regenerate the damaged organs and help in regaining the activity of antiviral cells of the immune system. These cells also have the potency to inhibit the inflammatory cytokines as G-CSF and IL-6 by activating homing receptors to heal the tissues injured due to abnormal immune responses in COVID-19 [32].

Recently, the infusion of mesenchymal stem cells of haploid nature represses graft *versus* host disease (GVHD). Hematopoietic mesenchymal stem cells interact with the APCs. They change the APCs to deletional APCs, which display immunomodulatory features. Stem cells of mesenchymal origin with the expression of HLA-DR17 and CD80-10 stimulate T cells [33]. MSCs express integrin-A and B-subunits, which interact with extracellular matrix receptors of collagen, laminin, fibronectin, and vitronectin. In this way, they can manage the extracellular matrix. MSCs can upregulate the ligands for interaction with hematopoietic stem cells. They upregulate cell-binding factors such as ICAM-1, ICAM-2, vascular cell adhesion molecule 1, lymphocyte-associated antigen-3, CD72, and leukocyte adhesion molecule. All these features help to generate a scaffold for hematopoietic stem cells. MSCs can evade the immune system as the major histocompatibility complex is expressed at low levels or is not expressed. The communication *via* the FAS ligand cannot be seen in MSCs. Costimulatory elements like B7-1, B7-1, CD40, or CD40L are not expressed as well. Thus mesenchymal stem cells can form a backbone to develop a stem cell niche *ex vivo* and can be infused in COVID-19 patients to lessen their complications [34].

Synthetic Stem Cells for COVID-19

Stem cells are available throughout life. Their function is to sustain and form functional tissues with their self-renewal mechanism. Stem cells are used to get a particular and vastly applicable synthetic tissue. Bioengineered stem cells are cultivated in humanized materials mimicking the bodily compartments of the extracellular matrix in which stem cells proliferate quickly. By providing such an environment, stem cells can be easily allowed to proliferate and differentiate. Some of the materials that are known to be compatible to synthesize stem cells such as peptide hydrogels, polylactic acids (LGA and PLA), and hydroxyapatite (HA) like bioceramics [35]. 3D hydrogel scaffold has been utilized to preserve the characteristics of different stem cells. This 3D culture system mimics the microenvironment and extracellular matrix of stem cells *in vivo*. This scaffold can be used to generate stem cells that proliferate and differentiate easily in this 3D architecture hydrogel [36]. Silk-derived fibroin proteins can be used *in vitro* in biomaterials for synthesizing stem cells. Silk fibroin provides adhesive support to stem cells; regulates the molecular mechanism and structure of these cells. Silk-based microenvironments drive the proliferation, differentiation of stem cells which can then be infused into damaged tissues to repair them [37].

Nanotechnology's use of bioengineered stem cells known as "LIFNano" has been made available. With mesenchymal stem cell therapy, advantages of LIFNano have been registered in COVID-19 subjects suffering from pneumonia. LIFNano has shown useful properties in revitalizing the damaged tissues and reducing the cytokine release in pneumonia [38]. Secretome is a Mesenchymal Stem Cell derivative consisting of biological products that primarily include lipid derivatives, nucleic acids, soluble proteins, and extracellular vesicles. Secretome-based MSC therapy has been noted as a novel way to treat degenerative and inflammatory diseases. Several research groups have registered the major effects of MSC-derived secretome in suppressing the myofibroblastic differentiation, reducing the production of cytokines, and initiating immunosuppression. In the COVID-19 patients, secretome-based MSC therapy can be of great use. MSC sourced secretome reduces the influx of monocyte, neutrophil, and eosinophil infiltration. They also decrease and overturn the activation of T cells and Dendritic cells, thus helping to rejuvenate the microenvironment in the lungs [39]. MSC-derived secretome is becoming a new research tool for cell-free treatment therapy in acute and chronic pulmonary disorders. Anti-protease, promoting angiogenesis, modulating immune responses, and stopping inflammation are some features of mesenchymal stem cells that can be seen in the secretome as well. Many cytokines can be acted upon at the same time by the secretome. It also possesses some synergistic activity. Many have reported secretomes to be safer than cells. Another feature that can be related to secretome is that they lack the power of self-replication, thus cannot generate tumors. Secretomes yield low immune responses and, on intravenous infusion, has a low possibility of embolism [40].

Synthetic stem cells can be used in multiple therapeutic possibilities for treating a disease. A biosynthesized stem cell niche can be used to generate a unique type of cell population from pluripotent stem cells (PSCs) *in vitro* [41]. Thus, making a stable stem cell niche for the therapeutic purpose in COVID-19 adhering to the complex nature and interactions between HSCs can provide a vital foundation of microenvironment *ex vivo*.

Stem Cells in Clinical and Preclinical Research Stage

Stem cells are known for their peculiar biological characteristics. They are the only cells needed for engrafting while considering tissue transplantations. Pre-clinical and clinical studies have to lead to detrimental observations with experimental employing of hematopoietic stem cells. Hematopoietic stem cell transplantation (HSCT) has been beneficial therapeutically in graft *versus* tumor (GVT) in common hematology-related malignancies. HSC infusion restores graft *versus* tumor without GVHD. Some of the pre-clinical and clinical case studies indicate if HSCs can improve autoimmune diseases keeping in view the donors are regular. In the case of solid organ transplantation, grafts of HDCs permit a long duration for survival. This has been presented in heart grafts of neonates who are matched with the donor [8]. Hematopoietic and mesenchymal stem cells have also been reported to be the progenitor for many cells, which can give rise and differentiate to form cardiac muscle cells. Injured myocardium can be refurbished with bone marrow cells. These bone marrow cells are attributed to plasticity and differentiate into endothelial cells, smooth muscle cells, and myocytes [42]. Many pre-clinical studies have been carried out on the use of umbilical stem cells for multiple sclerosis, ataxia, motor nervous system disorders, atrophy, and paraplegia without eliciting an acute immune response. Stem cells originating from the placenta are in Phase 3 of clinical-stage research to treat ischemia of limbs. In multiple sclerosis, CD34+ HSCs have shown immunosuppression and are considered to inhibit the immune responses of autoreactive T lymphocytes. Umbilical cord cells are indicated to generate *in vitro* neurons according to some pre-clinical data. Clinical research on HSC therapy is going on for genetic disorders blood like b-thalassemia and sickle cell disease. Adipose derives stromal stem cells are found in abundant quantities and can be accessed with ease. They have the property of soft tissue reconstruction and regeneration. The fetus, neonate, or brain of the adult can be a source of neural stem cells (NSCs). These cells have been reported in pre-clinical studies to divide into cells like astrocytes, oligodendrocytes, and neurons. They undergo clinical trials for lysosomal storage disease, Parkinson's disease, glioma, and other disorders. Pluripotent human embryonic stem cells (ESCs) are also undergoing clinical research and are considered safe in thoracic spinal cord injury diseases [43]. Testicular or spermatogonial stem cells possess a significant part in constituting germ cell lineage. These cells are diploid and are thought to have eternal nature. Testicular stem cell grafting has proven beneficial in the generation of sperm. This innovative approach can help retain fertility in young patients who are at potential risk of developing fertility disorders due to undergoing treatment for cancers or being exposed to many toxins that affect gonads [44]. A combination of cell-based therapy using different sourced stem cells is a new clinical and pre-clinical trial experimented with by different researchers. Animal-based studies using such therapies with a combination of multipotent MSCs, adipose-derived stem cells, bone marrow mononuclear stem cells, and induced pluripotent stem cells have been used together with angiogenic and/or growth factors. This approach in animals has resulted in intensified vasculogenesis, decreased automatic cell death, and improved heart function [45]. Pre-clinical results and clinical study of stem cell-based therapy infused in Myocardial infarction and ischemic cardiac diseases have proven beneficial with improved left ventricular ejection fraction and has been marked safe [46]. Stem cells in combination with biomaterials can provide relief in terms of available bone engrafts. Bone marrow has been found to inherit an abundant amount of osteoprogenitors and growth factors in addition to stromal stem cells. MSCs can be sourced in the bone marrow and have been recognized as the most persuading cells with osteogenic activity. Stem cells of mesenchymal or adipose origin have the vital capacity to regenerate the bone. Pre-clinical trials have shown that these cells play a vital role in bone regeneration *via* secreting factors needed for angiogenesis while maintaining the environment of hypoxia and inflammation. Stem cells can be stimulated by inducing bioceramic materials and osteoinduction to develop bone [47].

Serum Cytokine/Chemokine/Growth factors Up- and Down-Regulation During Stem Cell Therapy

As with the previous strains of coronavirus like SARS and MERS, we have seen dysregulation of immune responses. The same is true for the novel COVID-19 or SARS-CoV-2. Various studies across the globe have noted the irregularities of different immune responses in novel coronavirus patients. There has been upregulation of many cytokines and chemokines in COVID-19. It includes IL6, CXCL1, CXCL5, CXCL10, and CCl2. IL-10 and TNFa were higher in Intensive Care Unit patients than those who had moderate clinical progress. The term "Cytokine storm" has been commonly associated with recent studies regarding novel coronavirus [48]. These immune responses stimulated by COVID-19 occur in two phases, first during the incubation period second during the non-severe phase of the disease when the patient has been discharged from the hospital. Higher levels of pro-inflammatory cytokines TNF and IL-1 lead to the induction of EpCAM+ in the alveolar tissue of the lungs. Also are potent inducers of fibroblasts and hyaluronan (HA-synthase-2) in CD31+ endothelial cells [17]. Acute phase reactants like fibrinogen, serum amyloid A, CRP (C-reactive protein), hepcidin, and inhibiting the synthesis of albumin have been associated with the elevations of IL-6. Thus IL-6 serves as an essential biomarker for inflammation and can conduct us to early severity of COVID-19 [49]. Laboratory data reveals an abnormally high level of CRP and hyperferritinemia in many COVID-19 reported cases. Elevated CRP can lead to macrophage activation syndrome (MAS) or haemophagocytic lymphohistiocytosis (HLH) [50]. High plasma levels TNFa, IL2, IL6, IL7, IL10, IP10, GCSF, MAP1a, and MCP1, have been reported in COVID-19 patients. The different growth factors are also highlighted to be involved in novel coronavirus infection having viral protein interactions between cytokines and cytokine receptor pathways. According to one study 15 chemokines include CCL2, CCL4L1, CCL4L2, CCL5, CCL10, CCL12, CCL16, CCL17, CCL27, CCL28, CCL32, CXC3CL1, and BAFF. They are involved with 12 cytokines, including IL3, IL6, IL12, IL13, IL17A, IL17B, IL17E, IL19, IL20, IL21, IL32, and IFNG. Growth factors involved in COVID-19 infection have been found as TGFB1 and NGF. In the onset of the acute phase of COVID-19 immunoregulatory pathways like MAPK, ERK1/ERK2, JAK-STAT, and PI3K are also activated. These studies reveal a more precise understanding of inflammation and immune signaling pathways in COVID-19 [51]. Dysfunctional T cells express PD-1, which inherits inhibitory functions. This leads to the immune dysregulation commonly seen in COVID-19. The responses of the immune system are directed from immunoregulatory T cells towards immunosuppressive T cells. It has been clear from many types of research immune dysfunction is the main target in COVID-19 and still needs to be observed precisely to understand the mechanism behind the cytokine storm [52].

Role of ACE2-Mesenchymal Stem Cells for COVID-19

Angiotensin-converting enzyme (ACE2) is a host protein in which COVID-19 uses a co-receptor to enter the human body tissues. Its path is intracellular and usually targets the respiratory system and brain. The expression of ACE2 can be found in almost all body tissues. High expression of ACE2 can be seen in the kidney and ileum. In comparison, the moderate expression has been reported in nasal and oral mucosa, liver, stomach, vasculature, adipose tissue, brain stem, heart, and lungs. SPIKE or S protein is expressed on the coating of COVID-19, which has a high affinity to the ACE2. ACE2 also binds to peptides in maternal and fetal circulation [53]. Many researchers have received the interaction of COVID-19 and ACE2.

ACE2 helps COVID-19 to enter the cells. ACE2 also interacts with the kallikrein-kinin system. It has been proposed that the downregulation of ACE2 by COVID-19 leads to the failure of inactivating the B1 bradykinin receptor, a receptor attributed to endothelial cells. The loss to downregulate the B1 receptor is mutually related to the downregulation of ACE2. This mechanism of COVID 19, *via* downregulation of ACE2 and failure in the inactivation of B1 ligand, has been related to a severe form of infections [54]. A study conducted on the genetic profiling of mesenchymal stem cells indicated that MSCs are ACE-, proving the virus-free nature of mesenchymal stem cells. Henceforth mesenchymal stem cells are efficient in treating COVID-19 induced pneumonia [26]. Mesenchymal stem cells have the trait of not showing the ACE2 [30]. Many benefits have been registered for ACE2- the nature of mesenchymal stem cells. Some of which we will discuss in this section. After the infusion of MSCs, COVID 19 patients with acute onset have shown improvement in pulmonary function, protection of respiratory epithelium, and healing of fibrosis. MSCs refurbish the immune cell compartments and their functions. ACE2(-) mesenchymal stem cells prevent the cytokine storm by inhibiting T and B lymphocyte proliferation and secreting anti-inflammatory factors. They also normalize the immunomodulatory functions of different cytokines [55]. Some research on mice reveals that the ACE2 gene is overexpressed with bone marrow mesenchymal stem cells offering protection of endothelium and anti-inflammatory effects in response to lung injury caused by endotoxins [56]. ACE2 binds to the Fc domain of IgG in COVID-19 patients. MSCs with neutralizing antibodies can target ACE2-Fc and prove to help treat the COVID-19 by inhibiting the mentioned binding domains [57]. Responding to the beneficial effects of immune cells and their immunoregulatory and immunomodulatory effects in antiviral activities, ACE2- MSCs may provide a breakthrough to combat the COVID-19 [58].

Clinical Outcomes of Stem Cells for COVID-19

Many cases can be illustrated based on the overall outcome of stem cell transplantation for COVID-19 in different hospitals worldwide. A 65-year-old female COVID-19 patient with a critical condition was hospitalized in China. hUCMSCs were infused intravenously in three phases for the mentioned case. At the end of the 2nd phase, autoimmune responses were greatly changed. SGOT/SGPT, CRP, and bilirubin levels in serum were notably decreased. T lymphocyte subsets like CD3+, CD4+, and CD*+ T cells were also noted to return to normal levels. After the treatment, pneumonia in the patient was relieved. WBC count was normal. But the neutrophil count was increased. There was a decrease in lymphocyte numbers.

The patient was taken out of ICU with normal vital signs, and the swab sample taken from the throat was also reported negative. hUCMSCs have displayed potent capabilities to regulate immune system responses and heal tissue damage without any side effects [32]. Several clinical trials have been carried out in China on the safety of stem cells in COVID-19 pneumonia patients. A trial conducted on 7 patients who were infected with novel coronavirus revealed some beneficial effects in treating COVID-19 complications. All 7 patients have infused stem cells and are observed for 14 days. These patients recovered after receiving stem cell therapy without any notable complications. Another pre-clinical trial was conducted in Wuhan on MSCs in mice, which revealed a significant reduction of viral load, reduced pulmonary injury, anti-inflammatory characteristics, and decreased the mortality rate [59]. RNA sequencing performed on MSCs therapy of COVID-19 patients showed the safe and infectious-free nature of MSCs. In many patients after MSCs therapy, the levels of pro-inflammatory cytokines like TNF-a were decreased, and anti-inflammatory cytokines like IL-10 were increased. Biomarkers of dendritic cells, *i.e.,* CD14+CD11bmid, were also alleviated after the infusion of MSCs [60]. Investigations of 7 COVID-19 patients after MSC therapy showed improvement in pulmonary functions. All the pulmonary complications have been reported to have diminished in 2-4 days after MSC introduction [61]. In a clinical trial of 48 COVID-19 patients with severe pneumonia in Wuhan Union Hospital, 24 patients received conventional treatment while 24 others were infused with MSCs. The investigation was based on the fact that MSCs induce anti-inflammatory and immunoregulatory effects. MSCs helped to promote tissue repair and protect from apoptosis and fibrosis of lung tissue. The patients who received MSC therapy showed better outcomes than those getting conventional treatment. Another trial has been carried out in Puren Hospital to demonstrate the safety of MSCs in COVID-19 [30].

FDA/WHO Approved Stem Cells Therapy for COVID-19

Owing to the growing clinical research and safety of stem cells, Food and Drugs Association (FDA) has given a green signal to many projects to be carried out on stem cell therapy for their use in COVID-19. 4 projects have been approved in China, and another one has also registered their project of interest to FDA [62]. Many changes have been made in FDA regulations in response to stem cell providers. Under the current FDA guidelines, autologous bone marrow transplantation of stem cells has taken over stem therapy in the US [59]. Hope Biosciences' has been given a green signal by the US Food and Drug Administration (FDA) to evaluate the mesenchymal stem cells as a treatment type in COVID-19 patients. Based on the trial, patients with severe signs and symptoms of COVID-19 will be infused with adipose-originated mesenchymal stem cells [63]. The FDA has also approved the Global Institute of Stem Cell Therapy and Research (GIOSTAR) to carry on the clinical trials of mesenchymal mesenchymal-based stem cell therapy for their utilization in critical cases COVID-19 the new guidelines keeping in view some important outcomes of mesenchymal stem cells and "expanded access for compassionate use" project [64]. Authority to test the protective characteristics and effectiveness of umbilical cord mesenchymal stem cells has been granted to a team of scientists by the US FDA. They will explore the benefits of these cells by intravenous administration in COVID-19 patients suffering from inflammatory responses in the lungs [65]. RESTEM company has received authentication from the FDA to conduct a trial of umbilical cord stem cells on 60 patient studies in response to the treatment of COVID-19. This study will assess the success of systemized umbilical cord mesenchymal stem cells in COVID-19 patients with acute respiratory distress syndrome (ARDS) [66]. A biotech-linked company, mesoblast, has received acceptance from the FDA for the clinical application of their stem cell remestemcel-L. Remestemcel-L has its origin from allogeneic mesenchymal stem cells.

Several hospitals and COVID-19 patients with ARDS are going to be part of this study [67]. FDA has also approved Caladrius Biosciences, which proposed CLBS119 CD34+ cell therapy for lung injury in COVID-19. Organicell™ Flow, a stem cell product of Organicell Regenerative Medicine, has been agreed upon by the FDA to undergo clinical trials in moderate and severely suffering COVID-19 patients. The aforementioned trial will be one of its kind to involve randomized, placebo-controlled, and multicenter investigations to prove the usefulness of amniotic fluid sourced stem cells for novel coronavirus [68]. After the outbreak of novel coronavirus worldwide, the US FDA changed their policies and guidelines and came up with proper issuances to help many benefactors carry on clinical and pre-clinical trials on participants while maintaining passivity during the pandemic trials. FDA formed a unique platform and database for potential cell therapies named the Coronavirus Treatment Acceleration Program (CTAP) [69]. World Health Organization (WHO) has mentioned the use of umbilical cord mesenchymal stem cells, human dental pulp stem cells, and bone marrow-derived mesenchymal stem cells as experimental non-drug treatment under advanced therapy medicinal products (ATMPs) [70].

FUTURE PERSPECTIVE OF HSC FOR COVID-19

Hematopoietic stem cell therapy is a novel approach to treat many diseases. The research on stem cells to be used in COVID-19 has been geared up and is still undergoing many clinical and pre-clinical trials. UCMSCs have been successful in repairing lung tissue and renovating the airway permeability in endothelial cells. MSC therapy has also successfully treated the alveolar damage in various strains of influenza-induced viral pneumonia such as ARDS induced by H7N9. This can serve as a platform to induce MSCs *in vitro* for clinical trials in COVID-19 infected patients [56]. Stem cells from a patient may prove to be a conceivable cornerstone in cellular therapies and a novel approach of treatment in molecular science [71]. Different sourced stem cells can suppress the immune system, regulate the levels of serum cytokines and chemokines. Stem cells have also been shown to reduce the number of macrophages in the damaged pulmonary tissue. They increase the number of regulatory dendritic cells in the tissue undergoing inflammation. MSCs can help enhance the recovery in COVID-19 patients in obligation to regenerative, renewal, and rejuvenate features of these cells [55]. Stem cells can have promising effects to treat acute lung injury in COVID-19.

MSCs reduce the pro-inflammatory cytokines. This can serve as an integral approach to treat the cytokine storm in novel coronavirus [31]. ACE2 is expressed in multiple tissues of the body like the heart, lungs, and gastrointestinal tract *et al.* In COVID-19, ACE2 has been observed to express itself on lymphocytes. Thrombocytopenia and venous thromboembolism have been reported in COVID-19 patients with the expression of ACE2. MSCs can suppress the expression of ACE2 and thus prevent many complications in COVID-19 patients. There is the necessity of stem cell donors, which over time, will increase the need for blood donors to prevent severe complications and disorders in seriously infected patients with COVID-19 [72].

MSCs act *via* paracrine routes and can disperse in the lungs. These factors help to reduce and save the mugs from further fibrosis. The respiratory tract microenvironment in COVID-19, especially in elderly patients, is well preserved with the intravenous infusion of stem cells. The elderly population is at high risk of respiratory suppression, and morbidity is also high in these individuals. A thorough understanding of stem cells will prove essential to save the COVID-19 induced respiratory disorders [15]. Clinical use of recombinant stem cells that can be viewed in future use for COVID-19 is adipose tissue-derived stromal stem cells, embryonic stem cells derived from amnion, and umbilical cord stem cells. Umbilical cord mesenchymal stem cells have been studied thoroughly and have yielded positive outcomes in various patients.

Further studies to use cell therapy in combination with other drugs to alleviate the condition of the COVID-19 infected patients will bring a new perspective and challenging techniques ahead [59]. Although different stem cells have shown combating promises to regulate and rejuvenate the immune system in COVID-19, these cell therapies also have some side effects noted by many researchers. To have a clear understanding of the mechanism of hematopoietic stem cell therapy in COVID-19 patients, a vigorous qualitative and quantitative analysis is the requirement of the time. Extra evaluation of stem cells on the clinical applications will uncover many mysteries that cover up the treatment plans of COVID-19 [73].

CONCLUSION

Stem cell therapy is valid cell therapy in many diseases. Stem cell therapy has yielded surprising outcomes in some clinical trials conducted on COVID-19 patients. It has been noted that COVID-19 is more of a respiratory viral infection causing damage to the lungs. COVID-19 causes inflammation, fibrosis, and pneumonia. Stem cell infusion suppresses the cytokine storm, a process that causes leakage of cytokines and chemokines responsible for the severity of disease in the pulmonary system. This can help to reduce the complications of

COVID-19. Different stem cells exert a particular mechanism to deal with COVID-19. A more prosperous outlook of stem cells in clinical trials can be of great benefit in decreasing mortality and morbidity in COVID-19. Mesenchymal stem cells derived from the umbilical cord can be a breakthrough to modulate the immune responses in COVID-19. WHO and FDA should allow researchers and clinicians to evaluate clinical trials and the potent effects of stem cells in COVID-19. Timely interventions of stem cell therapies can prevent rising cases of COVID-19, thus provide a sigh of relief to the millions of people worldwide.

CONSENT FOR PUBLICATION

Not Applicable.

CONFLICT OF INTEREST

The author confirms that this chapter contents have no conflict of interest.

ACKNOWLEDGEMENT

Declared none.

REFERENCES

[1] Bryder D, Rossi DJ, Weissman IL. Hematopoietic stem cells: the paradigmatic tissue-specific stem cell. Am J Pathol 2006; 169(2): 338-46. [http://dx.doi.org/10.2353/ajpath.2006.060312] [PMID: 16877336]

[2] Kolios G, Moodley Y. Introduction to stem cells and regenerative medicine. Respiration 2013; 85(1): 3-10. [http://dx.doi.org/10.1159/000345615] [PMID: 23257690]

[3] Sánchez A, Schimmang T, García-Sancho J. In Stem Cell Transplantation. Springer 2012; pp. 89-102. [http://dx.doi.org/10.1007/978-1-4614-2098-9_7]

[4] O'Brien T. Barry, F.P. Mayo Clinic Proceedings. Elsevier 2009; Vol. 84: pp. 859-61.

[5] Andrades JA, Becerra J, Muñoz-Chápuli R, *et al.* Stem cells therapy for regenerative medicine: Principles of present and future practice. J Biomed Sci Eng 2014; 07(02): 49-57.

[6] Kumar P. COVID-19 Cure through Stem Cells. J Regen Biol Med 2020; 2(3): 1-15.

[7] Alison MR, Poulsom R, Forbes S, Wright NA. An introduction to stem cells. J Pathol 2002; 197(4): 419-23. [http://dx.doi.org/10.1002/path.1187]

[8] Shizuru JA, Negrin RS, Weissman IL. Hematopoietic stem and progenitor cells: clinical and preclinical regeneration of the hematolymphoid system. Annu Rev Med 2005; 56: 509-38. [http://dx.doi.org/10.1146/annurev.med.54.101601.152334] [PMID: 15660525]

[9] Méndez-Ferrer S, Lucas D, Battista M, Frenette PS. Haematopoietic stem cell release is regulated by circadian oscillations. Nature 2008; 452(7186): 442-7. [http://dx.doi.org/10.1038/nature06685] [PMID: 18256599]

[10] Wu X, Thi VLD, Huang Y, *et al.* Intrinsic immunity shapes viral resistance of stem cells. 2018. [http://dx.doi.org/10.1016/j.cell.2017.11.018]

[11] Orkin SH, Zon LI. Hematopoiesis: an evolving paradigm for stem cell biology. Cell 2008; 132(4): 631-44.
[http://dx.doi.org/10.1016/j.cell.2008.01.025] [PMID: 18295580]

[12] Kondo M, Wagers AJ, Manz MG, *et al.* Biology of hematopoietic stem cells and progenitors: implications for clinical application. Annu Rev Immunol 2003; 21(1): 759-806.
[http://dx.doi.org/10.1146/annurev.immunol.21.120601.141007] [PMID: 12615892]

[13] Ilic D, Polak JM. Stem cells in regenerative medicine: introduction. Br Med Bull 2011; 98(1): 117-26.
[http://dx.doi.org/10.1093/bmb/ldr012] [PMID: 21565803]

[14] Ye Q, Wang B, Mao J. The pathogenesis and treatment of the 'Cytokine Storm'in COVID-19. J Infect 2020; 80(6): 607-613.

[15] Shetty AK. Mesenchymal stem cell infusion shows promise for combating coronavirus (COVID-19--induced pneumonia. Aging Dis 2020; 11(2): 462-4.
[http://dx.doi.org/10.14336/AD.2020.0301] [PMID: 32257554]

[16] Li X, Geng M, Peng Y, Meng L, Lu S. Molecular immune pathogenesis and diagnosis of COVID-19. J Pharm Anal 2020; 10(2): 102-8.
[http://dx.doi.org/10.1016/j.jpha.2020.03.001] [PMID: 32282863]

[17] Mondal M, Sarkar K, Nath PP, Paul G. Monosodium glutamate suppresses the female reproductive function by impairing the functions of ovary and uterus in rat. Environ Toxicol 2017; 33(2): 198-208.
[PMID: 29119727]

[18] Heng TS, Dudakov JA, Khong DM, Chidgey AP, Boyd RL. Stem cells--meet immunity. J Mol Med (Berl) 2009; 87(11): 1061-9.
[http://dx.doi.org/10.1007/s00109-009-0539-z] [PMID: 19841876]

[19] Zhao RC. Stem cell-based therapy for coronavirus disease 2019.. Stem Cells Dev 29(11): 679-81.

[20] Wan S, Yi Q, Fan S, *et al.* Characteristics of lymphocyte subsets and cytokines in peripheral blood of 123 hospitalized patients with 2019 novel coronavirus pneumonia (NCP) MedRxiv 2020.
[http://dx.doi.org/10.1101/2020.02.10.20021832]

[21] Chen G, Wu D, Guo W, *et al.* Clinical and immunological features of severe and moderate coronavirus disease 2019. J Clin Invest 2020; 130(5): 2620-9.
[http://dx.doi.org/10.1172/JCI137244] [PMID: 32217835]

[22] Qin C, Zhou L, Hu Z, *et al.* Dysregulation of immune response in patients with COVID-19 in Wuhan, China. Clin Infect Dis 2020; ciaa248.

[23] Liu Y, Zhang C, Huang F, *et al.* Elevated plasma level of selective cytokines in COVID-19 patients reflect viral load and lung injury. Natl Sci Rev 2020; 7(6): 1003-11.

[24] Felsenstein S, Herbert JA, McNamara PS, Hedrich CM. COVID-19: Immunology and treatment options. Clin Immunol 2020; 215: 108448.
[http://dx.doi.org/10.1016/j.clim.2020.108448] [PMID: 32353634]

[25] Zhang W, Du R-H, Li B, *et al.* Molecular and serological investigation of 2019-nCoV infected patients: implication of multiple shedding routes. Emerg Microbes Infect 2020; 9(1): 386-9.
[http://dx.doi.org/10.1080/22221751.2020.1729071] [PMID: 32065057]

[26] Golchin A, Seyedjafari E, Ardeshirylajimi A. Mesenchymal Stem Cell Therapy for COVID-19: Present or Future. Stem Cell Reviews and Reports, 1-7. Stem Cell Rev Rep 2020; 1-7.

[27] Eggenhofer E, Luk F, Dahlke MH, Hoogduijn MJ. The life and fate of mesenchymal stem cells. Front Immunol 2014; 5: 148.
[http://dx.doi.org/10.3389/fimmu.2014.00148]

[28] Akiyama K, Chen C, Wang D, *et al.* Mesenchymal-stem-cell-induced immunoregulation involves FAS-ligand-/FAS-mediated T cell apoptosis. Cell Stem Cell 2012; 10(5): 544-55.

[http://dx.doi.org/10.1016/j.stem.2012.03.007] [PMID: 22542159]

[29] Rada G, Corbalan J, Rojas P. Mesenchymal stromal cells for COVID-19: A living systematic review protocol medRxiv 2020.
[http://dx.doi.org/10.1101/2020.04.13.20064162]

[30] Jeyaraman M, Somasundaram R, Anudeep TC, *et al.* Mesenchymal stem cells (MSCs) as a novel therapeutic option for nCOVID-19-A Review. Open Journal of Regenerative Medicine 2020; 09(02): 20-35.
[http://dx.doi.org/10.4236/ojrm.2020.92004]

[31] Li H, Liu S-M, Yu X-H, Tang S-L, Tang C-K. Coronavirus disease 2019 (COVID-19): current status and future perspectives.

[32] Liang B, Chen J, Li T, *et al.* Clinical remission of a critically ill COVID-19 patient treated by human umbilical cord mesenchymal stem cells. ChinaXiv 2020.

[33] Beyth S, Borovsky Z, Mevorach D, *et al.* Human mesenchymal stem cells alter antigen-presenting cell maturation and induce T-cell unresponsiveness. Blood 2005; 105(5): 2214-9.
[http://dx.doi.org/10.1182/blood-2004-07-2921] [PMID: 15514012]

[34] Le Blanc K, Ringdén O. Immunobiology of human mesenchymal stem cells and future use in hematopoietic stem cell transplantation. Biol Blood Marrow Transplant 2005; 11(5): 321-34.
[http://dx.doi.org/10.1016/j.bbmt.2005.01.005] [PMID: 15846285]

[35] Semino CE. Can we build artificial stem cell compartments? J Biomed Biotechnol 2003; 2003(3): 164-9.
[http://dx.doi.org/10.1155/S1110724303208019] [PMID: 12975532]

[36] Raic A, Rödling L, Kalbacher H, Lee-Thedieck C. Biomimetic macroporous PEG hydrogels as 3D scaffolds for the multiplication of human hematopoietic stem and progenitor cells. Biomaterials 2014; 35(3): 929-40.
[http://dx.doi.org/10.1016/j.biomaterials.2013.10.038] [PMID: 24176196]

[37] Wang Y, Kim H-J, Vunjak-Novakovic G, Kaplan DL. Stem cell-based tissue engineering with silk biomaterials. Biomaterials 2006; 27(36): 6064-82.
[http://dx.doi.org/10.1016/j.biomaterials.2006.07.008] [PMID: 16890988]

[38] Metcalfe Su M. Mesenchymal stem cells and management of COVID-19 pneumonia. Med Drug Discov 2020; 5: 100019.

[39] Harrell CR, Fellabaum C, Jovicic N, Djonov V, Arsenijevic N, Volarevic V. Molecular mechanisms responsible for therapeutic potential of mesenchymal stem cell-derived secretome. Cells 2019; 8(5): 467.
[http://dx.doi.org/10.3390/cells8050467] [PMID: 31100966]

[40] Bari E, Ferrarotti I, Saracino L, Perteghella S, Torre ML, Corsico AG. Mesenchymal stromal cell secretome for severe COVID-19 infections: premises for the therapeutic use. Cells 2020; 9(4): 924.
[http://dx.doi.org/10.3390/cells9040924] [PMID: 32283815]

[41] Peerani R, Zandstra PW. Enabling stem cell therapies through synthetic stem cell–niche engineering. J Clin Invest 120(1): 60-70.
[http://dx.doi.org/10.1172/JCI41158]

[42] Strauer BE, Kornowski R. Stem cell therapy in perspective. Circulation 2003; 107(7): 929-34.
[http://dx.doi.org/10.1161/01.CIR.0000057525.13182.24] [PMID: 12600901]

[43] Trounson A, Thakar RG, Lomax G, Gibbons D. Clinical trials for stem cell therapies. BMC Med 2011; 9(1): 52.
[http://dx.doi.org/10.1186/1741-7015-9-52] [PMID: 21569277]

[44] Schlatt S, Ehmcke J, Jahnukainen K. Testicular stem cells for fertility preservation: preclinical studies on male germ cell transplantation and testicular grafting. Pediatr Blood Cancer 2009; 53(2): 274-80.

[http://dx.doi.org/10.1002/pbc.22002] [PMID: 19415740]

[45] Tompkins BA, Balkan W, Winkler J, *et al.* Pre-clinical studies of stem cell therapy for heart disease. Circ Res 2018; 122(7): 1006-20. [http://dx.doi.org/10.1161/CIRCRESAHA.117.312486] [PMID: 29599277]

[46] van der Spoel TI, Jansen of Lorkeers SJ, Agostoni P, *et al.* Human relevance of pre-clinical studies in stem cell therapy: systematic review and meta-analysis of large animal models of ischaemic heart disease. Cardiovasc Res 2011; 91(4): 649-58. [http://dx.doi.org/10.1093/cvr/cvr113] [PMID: 21498423]

[47] Gómez-Barrena E, Rosset P, Müller I, *et al.* Bone regeneration: stem cell therapies and clinical studies in orthopaedics and traumatology. J Cell Mol Med 2011; 15(6): 1266-86. [http://dx.doi.org/10.1111/j.1582-4934.2011.01265.x] [PMID: 21251219]

[48] Coperchini F, Chiovato L, Croce L, Magri F, Rotondi M. The cytokine storm in COVID-19: An overview of the involvement of the chemokine/chemokine-receptor system. Cytokine Growth Factor Rev 2020; 53: 25-32. [http://dx.doi.org/10.1016/j.cytogfr.2020.05.003] [PMID: 32446778]

[49] Aziz M, Fatima R, Assaly R. Elevated interleukin-6 and severe COVID-19: A meta-analysis. J Med Virol 2020; 92(11): 2283-5. [http://dx.doi.org/10.1002/jmv.25948] [PMID: 32343429]

[50] McGonagle D, O'Donnell JS, Sharif K, Emery P, Bridgewood C. Immune mechanisms of pulmonary intravascular coagulopathy in COVID-19 pneumonia. Lancet Rheumatol 2020; 2(7): e437-45. [http://dx.doi.org/10.1016/S2665-9913(20)30121-1] [PMID: 32835247]

[51] Hou X, Zhang X, Wu X, *et al.* Serum protein profiling reveals a landscape of inflammation and immune signaling in early-stage COVID-19 infection. MedRxiv 2020.

[52] Sarzi-Puttini P, Giorgi V, Sirotti S, *et al.* COVID-19, cytokines and immunosuppression: what can we learn from severe acute respiratory syndrome? Clin Exp Rheumatol 2020; 38(2): 337-42. [PMID: 32202240]

[53] South AM, Diz DI, Chappell MC. COVID-19, ACE2, and the cardiovascular consequences. Am J Physiol Heart Circ Physiol 2020; 318(5): H1084-90. [http://dx.doi.org/10.1152/ajpheart.00217.2020] [PMID: 32228252]

[54] van de Veerdonk F, Netea MG, van Deuren M, *et al.* Kinins and cytokines in COVID-19: a comprehensive pathophysiological approach. eLife 2020; 9: e57555.

[55] Leng Z, Zhu R, Hou W, *et al.* Transplantation of ACE2-mesenchymal stem cells improves the outcome of patients with COVID-19 pneumonia. Aging Dis 2020; 11(2): 216-28. [http://dx.doi.org/10.14336/AD.2020.0228] [PMID: 32257537]

[56] Khoury M, Cuenca J, Cruz FF, Figueroa FE, Rocco PRM, Weiss DJ. Current status of cell-based therapies for respiratory virus infections: applicability to COVID-19. Eur Respir J 2020; 55(6): 2000858. [http://dx.doi.org/10.1183/13993003.00858-2020] [PMID: 32265310]

[57] Vellingiri B, Jayaramayya K, Iyer M, *et al.* COVID-19: A promising cure for the global panic. Sci Total Environ 2020; 725: 138277. [http://dx.doi.org/10.1016/j.scitotenv.2020.138277] [PMID: 32278175]

[58] Dong X, Wang M, Liu S, *et al.* Immune Characteristics of Patients with Coronavirus Disease. (COVID-19). Aging Dis 2019; 2020: 465-71. [PMID: 32489708]

[59] Atluri S, Manchikanti L, Hirsch JA. Is Vice, H.; Manchikanti, L., Expanded umbilical cord mesenchymal stem cells (UC-MSCs) as a therapeutic strategy in managing critically ill COVID-19 patients: the case for compassionate use. Pain Physician 2020; 23(2): E71-83. [PMID: 32214286]

[60] Ray S, Rajarshi K, Chatterjee A. Combating COVID-19 with mesenchymal stem cell therapy. Biotechnol Rep (Amst) 2020; 26: e00467.
[http://dx.doi.org/10.31219/osf.io/3ecda]

[61] Gentile P, Sterodimas A. Adipose-Derived Stromal Stem Cells (ASCs) as a new regenerative immediate therapy combating Coronavirus (COVID-19)-Induced Pneumonia. Expert Opinion on Biological Therapy, 2020, (just-accepted) Expert Opin Biol Ther 20(7): 711-6.

[62] Zhu S, Guo X, Geary K, Zhang D. Emerging therapeutic strategies for COVID-19 patients. Discoveries 2020; 8(1): e105.
[http://dx.doi.org/10.15190/d.2020.2.]

[63] Arbillaga L, Azqueta A, van Delft JH, López de Cerain A. *In vitro* gene expression data supporting a DNA non-reactive genotoxic mechanism for ochratoxin A. Toxicol Appl Pharmacol 2007; 220(2): 216-24.
[http://dx.doi.org/10.1016/j.taap.2007.01.008] [PMID: 17316727]

[64] Sutken E, Aral E, Ozdemir F, Uslu S, Alatas O, Colak O. Protective role of melatonin and coenzyme Q10 in ochratoxin A toxicity in rat liver and kidney. Int J Toxicol 2007; 26(1): 81-7.
[http://dx.doi.org/10.1080/10915810601122893] [PMID: 17365150]

[65] Sava V, Velasquez A, Song S, Sanchez-Ramos J. Adult hippocampal neural stem/progenitor cells *in vitro* are vulnerable to the mycotoxin ochratoxin-A. Toxicol Sci 2007; 98(1): 187-97.
[http://dx.doi.org/10.1093/toxsci/kfm093] [PMID: 17449898]

[66] Lambert D, Padfield PJ, McLaughlin J, Cannell S, O'Neill CA. Ochratoxin A displaces claudins from detergent resistant membrane microdomains. Biochem Biophys Res Commun 2007; 358(2): 632-6.
[http://dx.doi.org/10.1016/j.bbrc.2007.04.180] [PMID: 17499213]

[67] Costa S, Utan A, Cervellati R, Speroni E, Guerra MC. Catechins: natural free-radical scavengers against ochratoxin A-induced cell damage in a pig kidney cell line (LLC-PK1). Food Chem Toxicol 2007; 45(10): 1910-7.
[http://dx.doi.org/10.1016/j.fct.2007.04.008] [PMID: 17548142]

[68] Di Giacomo C, Acquaviva R, Piva A, *et al.* Protective effect of cyanidin 3-O-β-D-glucoside on ochratoxin A-mediated damage in the rat. Br J Nutr 2007; 98(5): 937-43.
[http://dx.doi.org/10.1017/S0007114507756908] [PMID: 17562227]

[69] Khoury M, Rocco PR, Phinney DG, *et al.* Cell-based therapies for COVID-19: proper clinical investigations are essential. Cytotherapy 2020; 22(11): 602-5.

[70] Domijan AM, Peraica M, Vrdoljak AL, Radić B, Žlender V, Fuchs R. The involvement of oxidative stress in ochratoxin A and fumonisin B1 toxicity in rats. Mol Nutr Food Res 2007; 51(9): 1147-51.
[http://dx.doi.org/10.1002/mnfr.200700079] [PMID: 17688296]

[71] Caplan AI. Mesenchymal stem cells. J Orthop Res 1991; 9(5): 641-50.
[http://dx.doi.org/10.1002/jor.1100090504] [PMID: 1870029]

[72] Terpos E, Ntanasis-Stathopoulos I, Elalamy I, *et al.* Hematological findings and complications of COVID-19. American J Hematology. Am J Hematol 2020; 10.1002-ajh.25829.

[73] Chena J, Hua C, Chena L, *et al.* Clinical study of mesenchymal stem cell treating acute respiratory distress syndrome induced by epidemic Influenza A (H7N9) infection, a hint for COVID-19 treatment. Engineering (Beijing) 6(10): 1153-61.

CHAPTER 12

Computational Methods for COVID-19 Treatment

Zahid Manzoor[1,*], **Shaukat Hussain Munawar**[1], **Muhammad Farrukh Nisar**[2], **Muhammad Yasir Waqas**[2] and **Muhammad Mazhar Munir**[1]

[1] *Department of Pharmacology & Toxicology, Faculty of Bio-Sciences, Cholistan University of Veterinary & Animal Sciences, Bahawalpur, Pakistan*

[2] *Department of Physiology & Biochemistry, Faculty of Bio-Sciences, Cholistan University of Veterinary & Animal Sciences, Bahawalpur, Pakistan*

Abstract: Computational approaches efficiently design the drugs to prevent diseases for which no drug is available. These techniques are also used for the development of new drugs. It involves using a variety of computer software for drug modeling and simulation, hence usually known as computer-aided drug designing (CADD). The computational tools provide crucial drug designing in a short period. These techniques are time and cost-effective as compared to conventional drug development methods. Computational methods can effectively model the suitable drug candidate by optimizing ligand-target interactions and observing the deep insight of cellular processes by its powerful tools. Several studies have applied these modern computational techniques to find out the possible therapy against the pandemic disease of COVID-19. The critical proteins of COVID-19, including 3C-like protease, papain-like protease, and RNA polymerase, are targeted to model the effective drug. CADD approaches suggest anti-viral drugs, anti-coagulant, anti-HIV drugs, and anti-fungal drugs to have little effect against COVID-19. This chapter aims to overview the different CADD approaches to design the possible drug for the treatment of COVID-19.

Keywords: CADD, Computational methods, COVID-19, Treatment.

INTRODUCTION

The development of a novel drug usually takes a long time and is often associated with a high risk of failure and high cost. Typically, the complete drug development procedure, from the drug concept to the market, may take about 14 years [1]. The drug development procedure is not an easy task, and the whole process may involve a very high cost ranges from 0.8 to 1.0 billion USD [2]. However, advanced scientific approaches expedite this time-consuming procedure

* **Corresponding author Zahid Manzoor:** Department of Pharmacology & Toxicology, Faculty of Bio-sciences, Cholistan University of Veterinary & Animal Sciences, Bahawalpur, Pakistan; E-mail: zahidmanzoor@cuvas.edu.pk

Kamal Niaz & Muhammad Farrukh Nisar (Eds.)

in a short time [3, 4]. In the last few years, heavy investment has been made in the drug discovery procedure, but the output was not up to the expectations because of the low efficiency and high failure rate in the process [3].

Consequently, scientists and researchers searched for alternate tools to increase the success rate with high accuracy in a short research period. Various scientific approaches have been developed for this purpose. Among these techniques, computer-aided drug design (CADD) is one of the most effective methods for drug discovery. CADD is a widely used term that refers to the different computational tools for designing the compounds. It usually includes the analysis, storage, management, and modeling of compounds. CADD covers almost all of the essential aspects of the drug discovery and development process. Different computer-integrated programs are used to design compounds, assess the most appropriate candidate, and develop digital repositories for studying chemical interactions [4]. The application of CADD has altered the pipeline for drug discovery and development. CADD tools potentially identify the drug targets, validate and optimize the procedures, and may be applied in preclinical studies [5, 6].

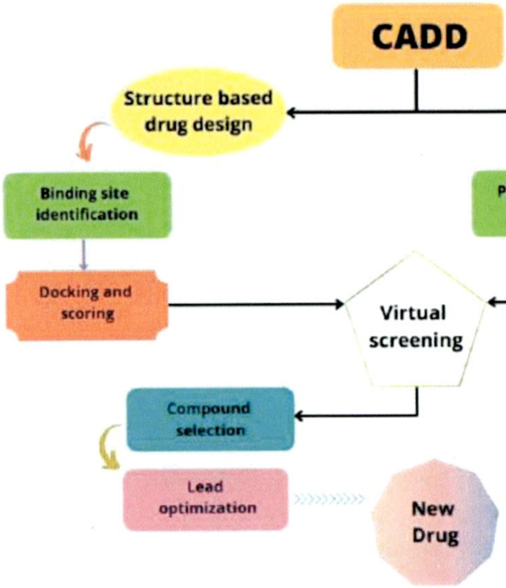

Fig. (1). The major steps involved in the CADD.

CADD approach is cost-effective and could reduce costs by half than conventional drug discovery and development [7]. The standard approaches of CADD can be divided into structure-based drug design and ligand-based drug design techniques.

The important steps involved in the CADD approach are shown in Fig. (**1**) . The CADD technique is generally divided into two important categories. The first category is the structure-based drug design, while the other refers to the ligand-based drug design. Structure-based design is usually applied to the availability of the 3D structure of a molecule. In this technique, the *de novo* approach provides valuable information. If the 3D structure of the target is unknown, then a ligand-based drug design can be applied. In this approach, pharmacophore modeling and quantitative structure-activity relationship (QSAR) can provide a deep insight into ligand-target interactions, which may be further processed by Virtual screening, selection of suitable compound, lead discovery, and ultimately the modeling of the new drug [8]. The purpose of this chapter is to highlight the importance of CADD approaches and the possible use of these tools in exploring the novel treatment for COVID-19.

Integrated Pipelines of COVID-19

Computational methods are more convenient in terms of less time-consuming and more cost-effective. These modern techniques have advantages over the historical practices of drug development in the pharmaceutical industry. In conventional methods, a series of experiments must be performed to find the suitable compound with desired properties. These experiments are usually time-consuming. With the advancement of technology, CADD tools efficiently analyze several compounds and quickly sort out the compound of interest to be evaluated for further biochemical reactions. Modern technology enables us to search for the drug target by the visual image of the 3D structure of the compounds.

In the current scenario of COVID-19, it is crucial to find an effective and safe drug very quickly; however, the potential drug candidate for the treatment of COVID-19 could be identified by using the modern computational screening of drug libraries. Virtual screening (VS) of ligand databases plays a vital role in exploring suitable molecules and has accelerated the initial stages of drug discovery [9, 10]. The purpose of *vs* is to rapidly recognize the potential hit molecules and can be tested experimentally and clinically. The crystal structure of molecules provides essential information in the identification process of potential drug molecules. *vs* is used by docking drug fragment libraries where the crystal structure of molecules is available. If the crystal structure is not available, then homology models are used. *vs* is used to identify the inhibitors in this scenario [11].

Virtual Screening of COVID-19

Two important proteases are coded by SARS-CoV-2 polyprotein. These proteases play an essential role in the process of non-structural protein (NSPs) and their release. The main protease is 3C like protease, also known as M_{pro}, whereas the other is a papain-like protease called Pl_{pro} [12]. Both proteases are considered to play a vital role in SARS-CoV-2 pathogenesis and hence an important target for drugs against SARS-CoV-2 and other coronaviruses [13, 14]. The crystal structure of only M_{pro} of SARS-CoV-2 is available and published in Feb 2020 (PDB ID 6lu7). The leading virtual screening against COVID-19 was performed in this study. The findings of this study will provide useful information to apply further CADD approaches to design possible effective drugs against COVID-19.

Another study employing virtual screening and targeting the crystal structure of M_{pro} of SARS-CoV-2 was conducted. Many drugs that the FDA approved were screened in this study. The study also provides important information about SARS-CoV-2 by conducting sequence statistics and phylogenetics. The results showed that SARS-CoV-2 M_{pro} formed a distinct phylogenetic group with SARS COV. It was different from MERS-COV. Sequence comparison analysis revealed that SARS-CoV-2 resembles about 96.06% with SARS and about 51% with MERS-COV. Some important drugs that were virtually screened against COVID-19 include telbivudine (used against the hepatitis-B virus), ribavirin (anti-viral drug), nicotinamide (vitamin), and vitamin B_{12}, *etc* . Data from the study revealed that one of these combinations of these essential drugs could provide better protection against COVID-19 [15].

Drug Libraries for COVID-19

To combat the SARS-CoV-2 infection, some drugs that inhibit the HIV protease such as Lopinavir, are suggested. Though their therapeutic potential against coronaviruses has not been determined up till now. In SARS-CoV-2, the protease protein is an important target to inhibit the pathogenesis of this pandemic disease. In the current study, CADD techniques are used to model an appropriate drug by screening the Marine Natural Product (MNP) library. Two important CADD techniques, molecular docking and the hyphenated pharmacophore model, were used to screen the MNP library. Molecular dynamics and re-docking techniques further confirmed the results of the study. The study proposed the 17 important protease inhibitors originated from natural marine origin. The crucial CADD technique identified these substances. Hence, it is suggested that one of these substances could provide better protection against COVID-19 [16].

Drug Repurposing Approach for COVID-19

Drug repurposing or repositioning is a promising approach to find out the possible ways to improve the therapeutic potential of the existing drugs. It may involve the failed developing compounds for further clinical trials. This approach is expanding rapidly for the treatment of rare and neglected diseases. Drug repurposing mainly focuses on drug-drug interaction (DDI) and drug-drug target interaction (DTI). One of the surveys on DTIs collected by the Drug Bank databases showed that a drug has many drug targets. A drug can bind to three different sites present on the other drug molecule [17]. The study concludes that polypharmacology is a common phenomenon of most drugs. Hence, it is crucial to find out the potential DTIs for both drug candidates and approved drugs. The basis of drug repurposing is to identify the DTIs. If a drug is selected without knowing the DTIs, it may cause specific side effects. Polypharmacology provides a new approach to drug designing with the least side effects and is more useful therapeutically. CADD has been playing a vital role in modern drug designing. A hieratical strategy consisting of various types of scoring functions has been implemented during drug lead identification and optimization phases to enhance the computational efficiency and accuracy of CADD. In addition, certain docking scoring functions, such as one employed by the Glide docking program, are very efficient for screening an extensive drug library [18]. However, it is not so much accurate in functioning. Another scoring function is the molecular mechanical force field (MMFF)-based scoring functions. It is more accurate, but the efficiency of MMFF is poor.

A hierarchical virtual screening (HVS) has recently been developed to improve the efficiency, accuracy, and success rate of rational drug designing [19, 20]. The crystal structure of SARS-CoV-2 revealed the target protein where different drugs might interact to decrease the pathogenicity of SARS-CoV-2 infection. Multiscale modeling techniques such as Flexible docking and MM-PBSA-WSAS were applied as filters to identify the potential drugs as inhibitors of COVID-19. CADD-based approaches are more efficient than experimental techniques in exploring the possible treatment for epidemic disease outbreaks like COVID-19.

Drug repurposing is an effective tool of CADD that can shorten the time and cost for the discovery of the new drug. This technique modifies the existing drug to model the structure of the new drug. An experimental study was performed on the available anti-viral drugs by applying the drug repurposing approach. The drug target, protein-protein interaction (PPI), and structural sequence were also evaluated. The results of the phylogenetic analysis showed that the SARS-CoV-2 genome was about 79% similar to the SARS-COV. Notably, the sequence of viral envelops and nucleocapsid of SARS-CoV-2 and SARS-COV were very similar and shared about 96% and 89% similarities. In this study, 16 different drugs were repurposed, including sirolimus, mercaptopurine, and melatonin against SARS-CoV-2, further validated by different CADD techniques. Data from the study proposed three different drug combinations emodin with toremifene, melatonin plus mercaptopurine, and dactinomycin with sirolimus that can show effective protection against COVID-19 [21].

Molecular Databases of COVID-19

In a study, *in silico* approach was used to predict the potential drugs against COVID-19 using molecular databases such as the ZINC database and CHEMBL database. The co-crystallized structures of 6W63 and 6Y2F from the protein data bank (PDB) were studied. Approximately 700 various compounds from CHEMBL/ZINC databases and 1400 substances from PDB were chosen based upon their possible interactions with the documented binding site. Various computational approaches were applied to screen about 300 potential candidates from different databases. Also, approximately 66 FDA-approved drugs were screened by employing these techniques. Some of the essential drugs include darunavir, lopinavir, ritonavir, and cobicistat, *etc* . These drugs and compounds may provide adequate control against COVID-19 after further CADD analysis [22].

Genomic Information of SARS-CoV-2 (COVID-19)

The genomic studies of SARS-CoV-2 revealed that the 3-chymotrypsin-like cysteine protease ($3CL_{pro}$) enzyme is vital in controlling the viral replication, and the virus requires this enzyme to complete its life cycle. It was proposed in the recent studies that $3CL_{pro}$ could be the right target for new drug development against MERS-COV and SARS-COV infections. In recent studies, it was suggested that the genome sequence of SARS-CoV-2 is parallel to the genomic sequence of SARS-COV. Hence, the sequence of $3CL_{pro}$ was analyzed, and the 3D model was constructed using the homology model. The constructed model was screened against a huge Data Bank of the medicinal plant containing about 32,297 potential anti-viral and bio-active phytocompounds. It was proposed in the study that the top nine screened compounds may provide useful information for the drug development process against COVID-19 [23].

Homology Modeling and Molecular Docking of COVID-19

Homology modeling refers to the comparative modeling of protein. It involves identifying one or more protein structures that show a similar structure to the query sequence. The residues are aligned in the query sequence to make the template sequence-structure [16]. Proteins with similar structures are evolved to have a similar sequence as naturally occurred homologous protein and thus are more conserved to generate a structural model of the target with the help of template structure and sequence alignment techniques.

Molecular Docking

Molecular docking is a computational method that predicts the best orientation of a molecule to the other molecule during the formation of a complex. The other molecule may be a protein or a ligand. Docking refers to the ligand-binding either to its target protein or to its receptor. This technique is mainly used to predict the interaction of stable drug molecules by observing and modeling the interactions of drug molecules between drugs or their target proteins. Many possible ligand conformations and orientations are developed during the molecular docking process, and the most suitable ones are selected for further research [24].

There are numerous tools for molecular docking; some of the common tools include FRED, AutoDOCK, FTDock, and eHITS. Docking studies are helpful in a deep understanding of the type of interaction between the different drug molecules and proteins. Novel algorithms are available at present, which provide a deep insight into the microenvironment during an interaction. These tools also predict the presence or absence of water molecules during the exchange. The available computational tools have remarkably increased the flexibility of computation possibilities. Molecular docking has enabled us to study the small molecule docking such as protein-protein, protein-RAN, and protein-DNA interactions considering the associated cellular complexities [25, 26]. Studying complex interaction using a distributed computation is a common practice in computational biology. Recently, homology modeling and *in silico* docking are applied to some possible medications to determine the potential treatment of the pandemic outbreak of COVID-19.

The structure of SARS-CoV-2 closely resembles SARS-COV. The advantage of these known proteins is to build a proposed model for the treatment of COVID-19 [27] quickly. The drug development by the conventional method may take many years for COVID-19; hence the CADD approach was used to develop the model drug. The two important proteins of SARS-CoV-2 were targeted for *in silico* docking model. These include spike glycoprotein and the SARS-CoV-2 3CL main protease.

The spike protein of SARS-CoV-2 interacts with the receptor protein of the host cells and enters into the cells. The CADD tools revealed that the entrance mechanism of the SARS-CoV-2 spike protein is similar to the SARS virus. The COV spike protein interacts with the host cell receptor, which allows the spike protein to enter into the host cell. The interaction of the COV spike protein to the host receptor is also similar to that of the SARS virus. The ligand-protein has a great affinity to the angiotensin-converting enzyme2 (ACE2) [28]. The modern computational approaches revealed that the COV spike protein is structurally similar to the SARS spike protein. The receptor interaction of both proteins is also very similar. However, a 27% variation exists between the interaction mechanisms of both proteins. These variations are mostly from the host cell. There is no crystal structure COV spike protein available until now; hence, homology modeling is used to predict COV spike protein crystal structure using SARS spike protein (PDB; 2GHV) as a model template.

The second important protein of SARS-CoV-2 is the $3CL_{pro}$ main protease (PDB: 6LU7) [29] associated with many controlling mechanisms of the virus. This protein is highly conserved in SARS-CoV-2 as compared to the SARS virus [30]. An essential function of $3CL_{pro}$ protease is linked with the replication of viruses which may be an ideal target for the action of new drugs [31].

Spike proteins and protease equally contribute to viral transmission and pathogenesis. To decrease the virulence of SARS-CoV-2, both of these proteins or anyone protein can be targeted. Some efforts have been made in this regard. A large data of bioactive compounds with known structures were run to attach different binding sites of COV spike protein and catalytic sites of protease protein using computational techniques. One of the possible solutions to combat SARS-CoV-2 virulence is to conduct quick trials with approved compounds by the FDA with modern computational approaches. CADD tools revealed that saquinavir, indinavir, remdesivir, and zanamivir are potential candidates to target $3CL_{pro}$ main protease of SARS-CoV-2. It is important to note that adeflavin, flavin adenine dinucleotide (FAD), coenzyme-A, and B_2 deficiency medicine may protect against COVID-19.

Protein Modeling

Protein modeling is an important tool in CADD to predict the 3D structure of most of the proteins from their amino-acid sequence. Various techniques such as NMR spectroscopy and X-ray crystallography have been used worldwide to determine the protein structures in detail. Characterization of the amino-acid sequence in protein structure is one of the challenging tasks. This difficulty is usually addressed by the careful observation of the 3D structure of a protein. Two important principles of science: the theory of evolution and the laws of Physics have provided much guidance in studying the 3D structure of natural proteins. The application of both these principles gave rise to different prediction approaches for a protein structure [32].

Many protein conformations are made to assess the lifespan of protein. The first method mostly relies on the amino-acid sequence and is called *ab initio* or *de novo* method. This type of prediction mainly focuses on the sequence pattern and does not depend upon the similarity of folded protein between the modeled protein and any other known structures [33]. The *de novo* approach assumes that the native biomolecule structure corresponds to the free energy; hence, it is challenging to predict the life span of the protein. There are two main components of the *de novo* method. One is the efficient procedure to carry out the conformational search, and the other is the free energy function which is used for the evaluation purpose of conformational changes.

The second method is mostly associated with the detectable similarities between the model sequences with any known structure. Comparative modeling and threading are some examples of this method [34, 35]. The structure of one protein in a family is determined experimentally. It will provide a guide to model the other protein members of the family. The primary alignment structure plays a vital role in this phenomenon. In the process of protein modeling, a 3D structure of unknown protein usually target protein is built depending on one or more related known structures of protein which are referred to as templates [36, 37]. For successful modeling, the detectable similarity between the template and target sequence and availability of correct alignment is crucial. The comparative approach can model protein structure because a slight change in the amino-acid sequence may change its 3D structure, which is easily detectable [38]. Protein structure can be modeled because the protein in a family is more conserved than their prime sequences [39]. Thus, if the sequence similarity of two proteins is detected, their structural similarity is likely to be assumed. It should also be noted that some proteins show similarities many times. But actually, they have very little structure similar or an equal portion is non-detectable. In this scenario, the proteins are assumed to be identical to each other.

Each of these methods has some pros and cons. But if we compare both of these methods, then comparative modeling seems to predict the 3D structure of an unknown protein more reliable than *ab initio* protein structure prediction [33, 35].

The following are some important steps in protein modeling:

- To explore the most suitable proteins with known 3D structures that have a similar sequence to the target protein
- Selection of the template structures
- Alignment of the template sequences with the target protein sequence
- Based upon the template structure, build a model that best fit the target sequence
- Evaluate and validate the proposed model.

These important steps can be repeated again and again until a desired perfect model is achieved. SARS-CoV-2 has an important transmembrane spike (s) glycoprotein that facilitates the coronavirus entry into the host cells. Spike glycoprotein produces some sets of a glycoprotein called "homotrimers" that protrude out of the viral surface [40]. There are two sub-units of S-glycoprotein named S_1 and S_2. These sub-units are responsible for the attachment of viruses to host cells. After attachment, the viral membrane is fused with the host cell membrane. Different coronaviruses use different domains within the S_1 sub-unit for the entrance to the host cells. These domains are named S_A and S_B. SARS-CoV-2 and SARS-related coronaviruses enter the host cells *via* the interaction ACE2 by the domain S_B [41, 42]. Murine polyclonal antibodies may inhibit the entry of SARS-CoV-2 mediated by SB. It is expedited from the data that the vaccine having neutralizing antibodies could be a possible tool to combat coronavirus infections, including COVID-19 [43].

It was evident from the previous studies that a positive selective pressure builds on the spike glycoprotein, nucleocapsid, and ORF1ab, but there is no such evidence in SARS-CoV-2 until now. However, recent studies showed that the presence of pervasive episodic selection in 2 sites. The presence of Gln residue was found instead of Asn at the amino acid position of 380 of the Wuhan coronavirus sequence. Similarly, a Thr residue was found instead of Ala in the amino acid position of 140. These changes create negative pressure in 6 sites (14%) confirmed by FUBAR (Fast Unconstrained Bayesian Approximation) analysis.

Similarly, a remarkable pervasive episodic selection was found in the spike glycoprotein region because of the two different sites at 536 and 644 nucleotide positions compared to the reference sequence. There was Asn residue present instead of Asp acid at 536 positions of COVID-19, while a Thr residue was present at 644 positions instead of an Ala residue. A remarkable pervasive negative selection was confirmed by FUBAR analysis in 1065 sites that appropriately contributes to 8.7% [44].

There is some evidence for the positive selective pressure in the glycoprotein of SARS-CoV-2. Data have shown that an Asn residue was present in amino acid position 536 in SARS-CoV-2, while a Gln residue was present in Bat SARS-like coronavirus and Asp residue was found in SARS virus. The difference also exists at amino acid position 644. A Thr residue was present in SARS-CoV-2, while a Ser residue was present in Bat SARS-like coronavirus, and Ala residue was present in the SARS virus. Another study showed that there is variation in some key residues linked with the binding mechanism to the ACE2 receptor in SARS-CoV-2 receptor-binding domain. These include Asn501, Asn439, Gly485, Phe486 and Gln493, and SARS-CoV-2 numbering). Some missing residues in amino acid positions 455–457, 463–464, and 485–497 occurred in the bat-derived strains [45].

Some of the sites are also found that create positive selective pressure in the ORF1ab region. Significantly, amino acid position 501 is important in this regard. A Gln residue is present in SARS-CoV-2, while Thr residue is present in bat SARS-like coronavirus, whereas an Ala residue is present in the SARS-CoV-2 virus. The SARS-CoV-2 has a Ser residue at the amino acid position of 723. The Gly residue is present in the other two viruses of bat SARS-like virus and SARS virus. The SARS-CoV-2 has a pro residue at position 1010 of the amino acid sequence. A His residue is present in the bat SARS-like coronavirus, and an Ile residue is present in the SARS virus.

Regarding the residue position in 723, especially at 543 in the nsp3 protein, SARS-CoV-2 exhibited a Ser residue instead of Gly present in SARS coronavirus and the Bat SARS-like virus. In this scenario, it can be suggested that this replacement may enhance the firmness of the polypeptide chain in terms of a steric effect and the ability of the Ser side chain to make hydrogen bonds. Moreover, Serine residue has a special effect. It may act as a nucleophile in the known structures, or it might be active site for some enzymes, and it can be a site for the phosphorylation process. But one of the CADD approaches suggests that it is complicated for most of the solvent to identify this position.

Suppose we look into the detail of amino-acid position 1010 that contributes to 192 of the nsp3 protein. The common region of SARS virus and bat SARS-like coronavirus has a non-polar amino-acid a polar amino-acid, whereas a pro residue is present in SARS-CoV-2 at this position. This scenario expedites that the stiffness and steric bulge of pro leads to a change in the molecular shape of SARS-CoV-2 compared to the other two viruses.

In SARS-CoV-2, a mutation was observed near the polyprotein domain in nsp3, parallel to the presence of phosphatase in the SARS coronavirus (PDB code 2ACF). These are considered to have an important role in viral replication in the host cells [46]. Some of the CADD approaches like I-TASSER suggest that some of the solvents could partially reach these positions. Moreover, positive selective pressure in this region relates to some of the clinical importance of SARS-CoV-2 compared to bat SARS-like coronavirus and SARS virus. It is necessary to find the exact location of amino acid sequence change in SARS-CoV-2 by using modern CADD tools to predict the actual protein portion involved in viral entry and pathogenesis. It would be useful in the deep understanding of the SARS-Co--2 action and its virulence.

Furthermore, it is essential to identify the site of exact molecular evolution in SARS-CoV-2, which would be helpful in the drug development or preparation of a vaccine against this pandemic disease. One possible reason for the more contagious behavior of SARS-CoV-2 could be the structural similarity of the region where positive selective pressure exists, and the stability of the mutation occurred in the endosome-like protein domain of the nsp2 protein as compared to other coronaviruses. The other important destabilizing mutation that happened near the phosphatase domain of the nsp3 protein may provide a reason for slower viral replication of SARS-CoV-2 than the SARS virus. However, further detailed studies are required in this regard [47].

Fold and Function Assignment System

The nsp3 protein of SARS-CoV-2 has many functions and contains different domains. Many important functions such as interference with host immune response and cleavage of the viral polyprotein, replication, and transcription of viral genomic material are assisted by nsp3. The fold and function assignment system of bat coronavirus HKU9 revealed that a unique region called the "SARS-unique region" is present in the NMR structure of the protein. The detailed study of protein showed that a double-wing motif or frataxin fold (a1b fold) was present, which was supposed to bind with DNA or metal ions and interact with other proteins. The structure of the protein was very similar to the SARS coronavirus nsp3 protein. Moreover, biochemical and bioinformatics analyses identified a functional site that was conserved in a few *betacoronaviruses*. The presence of an active site supports the statement that the "SARS-unique" region is conserved only in some phylogenetic groups of coronaviruses and not related to the human SARS virus [48].

Protein Data Bank

In a study, some nucleoside analogs and HIV protease inhibitors were repurposed by the molecular docking approach to design the possible drug to treat COVID-19. RosettaCommons and AutoDock Vina evaluated docking scoring. The results showed that Remdesivir and Indinavir have the best docking scores and perfectly fit in the protein pockets. Contrary to this, the active form of remdesivir showed a perfect dock on the functional sites of the NTP binding motif. The detailed investigation revealed that Indinavir does not dock on the functional sites of protease; hence the efficacy of Indinavir is not good against COVID-19. However, further detailed clinical studies are required before issuing the final recommendation [49].

Pharmacophore Modeling

Pharmacophore modeling is an essential tool for CADD. It is a very versatile technique and can be used in various situations. This approach is mostly used for the rational drug designing of novel drug compounds. Pharmacophore was internationally accepted by the International Union of Pure and Applied Chemistry in 1977. It may be defined as "It is the ensemble of electronic and steric characteristics which are essential to secure the optimal supramolecular interactions to a specified biological target and to enhance or stop the biological action" [50].

The pharmacophore is considered one of the most common and largest characteristics of the molecular interaction of biological substances. Pharmacophore is a concept; it does not stand for an actual biological substance for interactions. Even though the definition of pharmacophore is very clear, some people have used this term to represent a drug molecule such as sulfonamides or prostaglandins or bioactive compounds such as flavones in medicinal chemistry [51].

In the early stage, the concept of pharmacophore was limited to some computer programs. Over time, it has become an important tool for CADD. Pharmacophore is related to any molecular recognition exhibited by any atom or any substance in a molecule. These molecular interactions may involve hydrogen bond acceptors or donors, anionic, cationic, hydrophobic or aromatic, or any other possible interactions [51].

Various molecules under investigation may be tested at the pharmacophore level. This practice is known as "pharmacophore fingerprints". Sometimes pharmacophore testing/fingerprints are limited to few characteristics in a 3D model. In this scenario, pharmacophore is referred to as a "query".

Pharmacophore Fingerprinting

Pharmacophore has the option to limit its functions to test the 3D or 2D molecule. If any 3D molecule undergoes pharmacophore fingerprinting, the software has the opportunity to change the setting [52, 53]. Pharmacophore fingerprinting is a unique way of testing that interprets a molecule in special data sets. In the process of pharmacophore fingerprinting, all of the possible available points are taken into consideration while testing a molecule [54]. In topological fingerprints, the distance between the various molecular features is measured and denoted as bonds. The result of the pharmacophore fingerprint is in the form of a string that shows various possible positions where the molecule may interact with other substances.

There are several different pharmacophore fingerprints available that are used according to the different situations. Some fingerprint is designed in a way that it can be used to predict the various molecular similarities among different molecules. Pharmacophore fingerprinting may also determine the similar features of active ligands that may help estimate the key contributing features of biological action.

Pharmacophore Model or Query

Some of the pharmacophore models are specially designed in a 3D pattern [55]. There are different ways to label various features. It may be a single feature or a combination of various similar features usually displayed as "AND", "NOT", and "OR" to merge multiple patterns of interaction in one label. There are some additional features usually used to describe the boundary of a receptor. These features are essential to screen a library of small molecules [56]. All the molecules show their low level of energy conformations in these libraries.

These conformations are used to create the pharmacophore query by adjusting the pharmacophore and relevant compound. The pharmacophore query consists of many spheres. If a molecule exactly fits in the sphere and fulfills the query features, it is known as a hit molecule. The pharmacophore query is not so simple it's a complex procedure. It is tough to find the hit molecule in the given libraries. Hence, partial matching may be used to decrease the complexity of the pharmacophore query. Only a few features that are most relevant to an activity are matched in such cases. These models are further aligned with the other tools of CADD, such as molecular docking simulations [57, 58].

Modeling Softwares

Some of the important modeling software used in the CADD approach are given below in Table **1**.

Table 1. Different modeling software in the CADD.

S.No.	Name of Modeling Software	Main Features	Uses
1.	MapCheck	To compare the dose or measure the fluency	Calculate the Pharmacokinetic parameters
2.	DDD Plus	To study the disintegration and Dissolution properties	Estimate the PK parameters
3.	GastroPlus	Estimate the *In-vivo* and *in-vitro* (IVIV) correlations of various preparations	Use in the pharmacokinetic studies
4.	Schrodinger	Ability to dock the Ligand-receptor binding	Molecular dynamics and interactions of ligand
5.	AutoDock	Estimate the interactions of the protein with ligand	Molecular dynamics and interactions of ligand

(Table 1) cont.....

S.No.	Name of Modeling Software	Main Features	Uses
6.	BioSuite	Powerful analysis of genome sequence	Molecular dynamics and interactions of ligand
7.	GOLD	Docking study of the ligand with proteins.	Molecular dynamics and interactions of ligand
8.	ArgusLab	Calculate the molecular docking and build the models of molecules	Structure-activity relationship (SAR) and molecular modeling
9.	Maestro	Analysis of the molecules models	Molecular modeling
10.	SYBYL-X Suite	Build the models on molecules and design the models relevant to ligands	Molecular modeling
11.	GRAMM	Docking of protein to protein and protein to a ligand	Structure-activity relationship (SAR) and molecular modeling
12.	PASS	Built and analyze the SAR models	Structure-activity relationship (SAR)
13.	Sanjeevini	Estimate the binding affinity of protein with ligands	Molecular modeling
14.	Discovery Studio® Visualizer	Predict the protein structure	Visualization and analysis of images
15.	Xenogen Living Image Software	Present and analyze the *in vivo* images	Visualization and analysis of images
16.	AMIDE (A Medical Image Data Examiner)	Analyze the images in molecular models	Visualization and analysis of images
17.	REST 2009 Software	Analyze the data of gene expressions	Analysis of large data sets
18.	QSARPro	Study the interactions of different proteins	Analysis of large data sets
19.	GeneSpring	Powerful capacity to identify the minor variation within the sample and rectify it.	Analysis of large data sets
20.	MARS (Multimodal Animal Rotation System)	To study the activity of enzymes and animal response. To track the nanoparticles and their delivery mechanism.	To study the behavior
21.	Ethowatcher	Critically examine the response of animals	To study the behavior

Monte Carlo Method

The Monte Carlo simulation technique is advantageous and is being used in a variety of computational methods. It is based on large numerical numbers for calculations. In the CADD, this technique is commonly employed to test the Boltzmann distribution and build a Markov Chain Monte Carlo [59], particularly with the Metropolis algorithm [60]. It can also be used to explore the bound structure conformations.

Modeling the protein-ligand complex can be possible using the all-atoms force field paradigm [61], resulting in a very high dimensional phase. In this case, it is tough to estimate a parameter. The building of the Monte Carlo simulation overcomes this difficulty if the relative probability is known [62]. In this scenario, Monte Carlo provides an alternation approach to calculate the molecular dynamics [63]. The routine simulation takes a very high cost for the computational evaluation of the model, and it takes a very long time for completion. The Monte Carlo method has resolved this issue. The use of the algorithm appropriately evaluates the data according to the need. It enables us to use the Monte Carlo method more efficiently in drug designing. However, the main challenge in the Monte Carlo method is to generate uncorrelated poses having a significant weight which usually produces ruggedness of the energy landscape. This energy can be measured by the force field. The possible cause of this difficulty might be ligand or protein flexibility.

The Stochastic Global Optimization Procedure

In the last few decades, stochastic global optimization procedure has gained much attention in drug designing. This procedure deals with any kind of issue having a discrete variable, non-differentiated functions, or continuous variables during the processing. It has also been applied in biochemical and environmental processes that show different algorithms.

Pseudo-Brownian Positional/Torsional

The molecular docking method usually predicts the interaction of two independent protein structures, which typically fail on a large set of data. The possible reasons for failure can be the complex methods, including determination of scoring functions, difficulty in simulating the data, and rearrangement of residues at binding sites. The pseudo-Brownian positional/torsional approach minimizes these problems by observing the interaction of side-chains and conserving the energy.

Protein-protein Docking

The most important phenomena in the majority of cellular reactions are PPI. It has been estimated that about 4 million protein interactions occur in the human body [65]. PPI forms the basic foundation of most biological processes. It also includes two important processes signal transduction and regulation of proteins. These processes dominate over the other processes in increasing the complexity of cells

[64]. These processes are fundamental. A mild error in these processes may result in immune diseases or increase the proliferation of cells [64].

For the computations studies of protein, the 3D structure of the protein is a prerequisite. The X-ray technology provides some insight into the protein, but this approach has few limitations. Hence, the best choice to determine the 3D picture of protein-protein complexes is the computational techniques [66, 67]. In these techniques, protein-protein docking (PPD) provides reliable data of the protein molecules.

Small molecule docking has been extensively used in modeling studies for a long time [68]. However, PPD is more complex than small molecular docking. Proteins are usually dynamic. It could be one of the possible reasons for the complexity of the PPD method. Typically, most of the proteins are not stable. They often fluctuate to a varying degree which increases the complexity for docking study the proteins. Determine the binding site in protein is also challenging.

PPD is still the most common method in docking studies despite these challenges [67]. There is an increasing trend in the publication of PPD studies. For docking of proteins, detailed information regarding the rotation and translation position of the binding molecules is required. This information can be collected by other CADD techniques [69].

It has been assumed that PPD can be performed by knowing the shape of the protein molecules and amino acid sequence [67]. Some other CADD techniques, such as Rigid-body docking, facilitate the PPD in locating proteins' fixed and transitory positions [70]. Typically, the PPI procedure involves the following important steps [71].

- To search for the appropriate stage when the protein-protein complex is made
- The sampling time involving the different scoring criteria of the protein complexes
- To refine the final solution based upon various scores.

The protein complex is scored according to its geometrical structure, Physico-chemical nature, hydrogen bonding interactions, and other important information needed for the docking procedure [70]. The majority of the PPD methods relied on the rigid-docking procedure in the past. Currently, the flexibility of the side-chain protein is also taken into consideration. This feature is very important in PPD experiments. The majority of experiments conducted in CAPRI failed due to the wrong measurement of protein conformational changes [67].

Drug-target Interaction

The identification of drug-target interaction (DTI) has a fundamental role in drug development. In general, drugs interact with one or more proteins as their target. However, discovering the novel drug interaction to their target is essential as the divergent behavior may result in some unwanted effects [72]. In recent years, scientists have tried to explore the DTI by conducting clinical experiments and observation. Conducting the clinical experiments is quite time-consuming, and the high attrition rate is the main hurdle in these experiments [73]. Hence, the CADD approaches to identify the DTI have gained much popularity in the last few decades.

Some large data about various DTIs have been discovered and placed in databases accessible to the public, offering them an excellent hands-on prediction of the drug-interaction model. Various databases used for DTIs have been developed and used for the public, such as Matador and SuperTarget, Therapeutic Target Database, Kyoto Encyclopedia of Genes, Genomes (KEGG), and DrugBank. These databases provide useful information for computational methods [74, 75].

Some of the CADD tools for DTIs are literature text mining methods, ligand-based methods, and docking simulation [76, 77]. But there are some restrictions/limitations for all of these three methods. The docking simulation method is successful only on a small scale because it needs a 3D profile of the target protein available only for a small portion of protein.

Recently, various commercially available anti-viral drugs are modeled through Molecule Transformer-Drug Target Interaction (MT-DTI) to predict the possible binding of these drugs to the viral protein of COVID-19. It was found that atazanavir, which is an antiretroviral drug used against HIV infection, showed the best inhibitory potency with Kd of 94.94 nM against 3C-like proteinase of COVID-19. The other drugs remdesivir, efavirenz, ritonavir, and dolutegravir, also showed good potential with Kd values of 113.13 nM, 199.17 nM, 204.05 nM, and 336.91 nM, respectively. Interestingly, some other drugs, such as darunavir, lopinavir, and ritonavir, are also designed to hit the COVID-19 protein. Data suggest that these drugs can bind with the COVID-19 replication complex with inhibitory potency of Kd below 1000 nM. Kaletra (lopinavir/ritonavir) was also found to have the potential to inhibit COVID-19. It was proposed to consider all anti-viral drugs selected by the MT-DTI model while developing therapies against COVID-19 [78].

Molecular Dynamic Simulation

In a study, 16 approved drugs by the FDA and large data sets of compounds consisting of about 1000 bioactive compounds from the Asinex Focused Covalent (AFCL) library were screened to target the 3CLpro protease SARS-CoV-2. The compounds showing remarkable better docking scores and stable interactions were selected. By applying the CADD approaches 621 potential compounds were identified having the ability to bind with SARS-CoV-2 3CLpro. A molecular dynamic (MD) simulation approach of 50 nanoseconds was applied to stabilize the binding between the SARS-CoV-2 3CLpro and identified bioactive compounds. These compounds may provide adequate control against COVID-19 after the conduction of further necessary studies [79].

The binding affinity of noscapine (23B)-molecular dynamic simulations examined protease of SARS-CoV-2 at various temperatures. Results showed that noscapine has an anti-viral effect. The first study explicit the anti-viral potential of noscapine compound based upon the molecular dynamic simulations [80]. In another study, the proposed anti-viral compound was investigated by molecular dynamic simulation and docking studies against COVID-19.

Binding Affinity

Recently, the binding mechanism of the novel SARS-CoV-2 spike protein to the host cell surface receptor (Glucose Regulated Protein 78 (GPR78) was predicted using the modern molecular modeling technique. The SARS spike protein was modeled in this experiment. CADD tools identified four regions that have similar sequences and functions to cyclic Pep42. The PPD approach was used to predict the best fit of the region in the GRP78 Substrate Binding Domain β (SBDβ). Data revealed that the receptor-binding domain and SBDβ of GRP78 have a critical role in identifying host cells' receptors. It is also speculated that SARS-CoV-2 was more likely to bind at region-IV (C480-C488) and in region III (C391-C525) and at the GRP78. Region IV was assumed to play the major factor which forces the GRP78 to bind with an estimated binding affinity of -9.8 kcal/mol. The predicted nine residues could provide important data to develop the specific therapy to combat COVID-19 [81].

Binding Free Energy Calculation

The stilbenoid analogs were repurposed by molecular docking and estimating the binding free energy and molecular dynamic simulation to search for the potential candidate for SARS-CoV-2 infection. Based upon the CADD approaches, four potential candidates with great affinity to spike protein of SARS-CoV-2 were selected. These compounds exhibited good affinity (> 7 kcal/mol). But the fifty nanoseconds molecular dynamic simulation showed the resveratrol firmly bound to viral proteins and ACE2 receptor complex. The net binding free energy calculated by MM-PBSA also confirmed that the resveratrol-viral protein complex was stable. It is expedited from the study that resveratrol can be a potential candidate for drug development against COVID-19 [82].

Method Validation

It is a very important step in computational techniques. All the techniques have specific criteria for their validity. For example, the compounds that undergo molecular docking are selected based on the best docking score. Similarly, pharmacophore modeling has a fingerprint for its validity.

CONCLUSION

The CADD approaches are very crucial in proposing the possible drug for the treatment of COVID-19. Computational methods offered some drugs (Clocortolone, Nelfinavir, Atazanavir, Indinavir, Lopinavir) to target nsp3 of SARS-CoV-2, which is the main protein for its pathogenicity. In addition, some of the antiviral drug (Remdesivir), antifungal drug (Itraconazole), anticoagulant drug (Dabigatran), drugs used to treat HIV/AIDS (Indinavir, Nelfinavir, Saquinavir, Lopinavir, Raltegravir Ritonavir, Darunavir, Dolutegravir, Efavirenz, and Atazanavir), CMV (Ganciclovir), HBV (Entecavir), HSV (Penciclovir) and HCV (Simeprevir, Ribavirin, Lomibuvir, Asunaprevir, and Grazoprevir) can provide some relief against COVID-19. There is a lack of direct clinical evidence for the efficacy of the majority of the drugs against COVID-19. However, clinical studies can conclude the most useful drug to inhibit SARS-CoV-2 progression in the future.

CONSENT FOR PUBLICATION

Not Applicable.

CONFLICT OF INTEREST

The author confirms that this chapter contents have no conflict of interest.

ACKNOWLEDGEMENT

Declared none.

REFERENCES

[1] Myers S, Baker A. Drug discovery--an operating model for a new era. Nat Biotechnol 2001; 19(8): 727-30.

[http://dx.doi.org/10.1038/90765] [PMID: 11479559]

[2] Moses H III, Dorsey ER, Matheson DH, Thier SO. Financial anatomy of biomedical research. JAMA 2005; 294(11): 1333-42.
[http://dx.doi.org/10.1001/jama.294.11.1333] [PMID: 16174691]

[3] Shekhar C. In silico pharmacology: computer-aided methods could transform drug development. Chem Biol 2008; 15(5): 413-4.
[http://dx.doi.org/10.1016/j.chembiol.2008.05.001] [PMID: 18482690]

[4] Song CM, Lim SJ, Tong JC. Recent advances in computer-aided drug design. Brief Bioinform 2009; 10(5): 579-91.
[http://dx.doi.org/10.1093/bib/bbp023] [PMID: 19433475]

[5] Jorgensen WL. The many roles of computation in drug discovery. Science 2004; 303(5665): 1813-8.
[http://dx.doi.org/10.1126/science.1096361] [PMID: 15031495]

[6] Zhang S. Computer-aided drug discovery and development Drug Des Discov. Springer 2011; pp. 23-38.

[7] Tan JJ, Cong XJ, Hu LM, Wang CX, Jia L, Liang XJ. Therapeutic strategies underpinning the development of novel techniques for the treatment of HIV infection. Drug Discov Today 2010; 15(5-6): 186-97.
[http://dx.doi.org/10.1016/j.drudis.2010.01.004] [PMID: 20096804]

[8] Acharya C, Coop A, E, Polli J, D, MacKerell A. Recent advances in ligand-based drug design: relevance and utility of the conformationally sampled pharmacophore approach. Curr Comput Aided Drug Des 2011; 7(1): 10-22.
[http://dx.doi.org/10.2174/157340911793743547]

[9] Lauro G, Terracciano S, Cantone V, *et al.* A Combinatorial Virtual Screening Approach Driving the Synthesis of 2,4-Thiazolidinedione-Based Molecules as New Dual mPGES-1/5-LO Inhibitors. ChemMedChem 2020; 15(6): 481-9.
[http://dx.doi.org/10.1002/cmdc.201900694] [PMID: 32022480]

[10] Kouman KC, Keita M, Kre N'Guessan R, *et al.* Structure-based design and in silico screening of virtual combinatorial library of benzamides inhibiting 2-trans enoyl-acyl carrier protein reductase of Mycobacterium tuberculosis with favorable predicted pharmacokinetic profiles. Int J Mol Sci 2019; 20(19): 4730.
[http://dx.doi.org/10.3390/ijms20194730] [PMID: 31554227]

[11] Ahmed A, Choo H, Cho YS, Park W-K, Pae AN. Identification of novel serotonin 2C receptor ligands by sequential virtual screening. Bioorg Med Chem 2009; 17(13): 4559-68.
[http://dx.doi.org/10.1016/j.bmc.2009.05.003] [PMID: 19464901]

[12] Hilgenfeld R. From SARS to MERS: crystallographic studies on coronaviral proteases enable antiviral drug design. FEBS J 2014; 281(18): 4085-96.
[http://dx.doi.org/10.1111/febs.12936] [PMID: 25039866]

[13] Kandeel M, Altaher A, Alnazawi M. Molecular dynamics and inhibition of mers cov papain-like protease by small molecule imidazole and aminopurine derivatives. Lett Drug Des Discov 2019; 16(5): 584-91.
[http://dx.doi.org/10.2174/1570180815666180918161922]

[14] Zumla A, Chan JF, Azhar EI, Hui DS, Yuen K-Y. Coronaviruses - drug discovery and therapeutic options. Nat Rev Drug Discov 2016; 15(5): 327-47.
[http://dx.doi.org/10.1038/nrd.2015.37] [PMID: 26868298]

[15] Kandeel M, Al-Nazawi M. Virtual screening and repurposing of FDA approved drugs against COVID-19 main protease. Life Sci 2020; 251: 117627.
[http://dx.doi.org/10.1016/j.lfs.2020.117627] [PMID: 32251634]

[16] Gentile D, Patamia V, Scala A, Sciortino MT, Piperno A, Rescifina A. Putative inhibitors of SARS-

CoV-2 main protease from a library of marine natural products: A virtual screening and molecular modeling study. Mar Drugs 2020; 18(4): 225.
[http://dx.doi.org/10.3390/md18040225] [PMID: 32340389]

[17] Wang J, Ge Y, Xie X-Q. Development and testing of druglike screening libraries. J Chem Inf Model 2019; 59(1): 53-65.
[http://dx.doi.org/10.1021/acs.jcim.8b00537] [PMID: 30563329]

[18] Friesner RA, Banks JL, Murphy RB, *et al.* Glide: a new approach for rapid, accurate docking and scoring. 1. Method and assessment of docking accuracy. J Med Chem 2004; 47(7): 1739-49.
[http://dx.doi.org/10.1021/jm0306430] [PMID: 15027865]

[19] Wang J, Morin P, Wang W, Kollman PA. Use of MM-PBSA in reproducing the binding free energies to HIV-1 RT of TIBO derivatives and predicting the binding mode to HIV-1 RT of efavirenz by docking and MM-PBSA. J Am Chem Soc 2001; 123(22): 5221-30.
[http://dx.doi.org/10.1021/ja003834q] [PMID: 11457384]

[20] Wang J, Kang X, Kuntz ID, Kollman PA. Hierarchical database screenings for HIV-1 reverse transcriptase using a pharmacophore model, rigid docking, solvation docking, and MM-PB/SA. J Med Chem 2005; 48(7): 2432-44.
[http://dx.doi.org/10.1021/jm049606e] [PMID: 15801834]

[21] Zhou Y, Hou Y, Shen J, Huang Y, Martin W, Cheng F. Network-based drug repurposing for novel coronavirus 2019-nCoV/SARS-CoV-2. Cell Discov 2020; 6(1): 14.
[http://dx.doi.org/10.1038/s41421-020-0153-3] [PMID: 33723226]

[22] Pant S, Singh M, Ravichandiran V, Murty U, Srivastava HK. Peptide-like and small-molecule inhibitors against Covid-19. J Biomol Struct Dyn 2020; 1-10.
[PMID: 32306822]

[23] ul Qamar MT, Alqahtani SM, Alamri MA, Chen L-L. Structural basis of SARS-CoV-2 3CLpro and anti-COVID-19 drug discovery from medicinal plants. J Pharm Anal 2020.

[24] Lengauer T, Rarey M. Computational methods for biomolecular docking. Curr Opin Struct Biol 1996; 6(3): 402-6.
[http://dx.doi.org/10.1016/S0959-440X(96)80061-3] [PMID: 8804827]

[25] Gray JJ, Moughon S, Wang C, *et al.* Protein-protein docking with simultaneous optimization of rigid-body displacement and side-chain conformations. J Mol Biol 2003; 331(1): 281-99.
[http://dx.doi.org/10.1016/S0022-2836(03)00670-3] [PMID: 12875852]

[26] Van Dijk M, Bonvin AM. A protein–DNA docking benchmark. Nucleic Acids Res 2008; 26(14): e88.
[http://dx.doi.org/10.1093/nar/gkn386]

[27] Hui DS. IAE, Madani T, Ntoumi F, Koch R, Dar O. The continuing 2019-nCoV epidemicthreatof novel coronaviruses to global health: the latest 2019 novel coronavirus outbreak in Wuhan, China. Int J Infect Dis 2020; 91: 264-6.
[http://dx.doi.org/10.1016/j.ijid.2020.01.009] [PMID: 31953166]

[28] Xu X, Chen P, Wang J, *et al.* Evolution of the novel coronavirus from the ongoing Wuhan outbreak and modeling of its spike protein for risk of human transmission. Sci China Life Sci 2020; 63(3): 457-60.
[http://dx.doi.org/10.1007/s11427-020-1637-5] [PMID: 32009228]

[29] Liu X, Zhang B, Jin Z, Yang H, Rao Z. The crytal structure of 2019-nCoV main protease in complex with an inhibitor N3. RCSB PDB 2020.

[30] Anand K, Ziebuhr J, Wadhwani P, Mesters JR, Hilgenfeld R. Coronavirus main proteinase (3CLpro) structure: basis for design of anti-SARS drugs. Science 2003; 300(5626): 1763-7.
[http://dx.doi.org/10.1126/science.1085658] [PMID: 12746549]

[31] Bacha U, Barrila J, Velazquez-Campoy A, Leavitt SA, Freire E. Identification of novel inhibitors of the SARS coronavirus main protease 3CLpro. Biochemistry 2004; 43(17): 4906-12.

[http://dx.doi.org/10.1021/bi0361766] [PMID: 15109248]

[32] Fiser A, Feig M, Brooks CL III, Sali A. Evolution and physics in comparative protein structure modeling. Acc Chem Res 2002; 35(6): 413-21.
[http://dx.doi.org/10.1021/ar010061h] [PMID: 12069626]

[33] Bonneau R, Baker D. Ab initio protein structure prediction: progress and prospects. Annu Rev Biophys Biomol Struct 2001; 30(1): 173-89.
[http://dx.doi.org/10.1146/annurev.biophys.30.1.173] [PMID: 11340057]

[34] Domingues FS, Lackner P, Andreeva A, Sippl MJ. Structure-based evaluation of sequence comparison and fold recognition alignment accuracy. J Mol Biol 2000; 297(4): 1003-13.
[http://dx.doi.org/10.1006/jmbi.2000.3615] [PMID: 10736233]

[35] Marti-Renom MA, Madhusudhan MS, Fiser A, Rost B, Sali A. Reliability of assessment of protein structure prediction methods. Structure 2002; 10(3): 435-40.
[http://dx.doi.org/10.1016/S0969-2126(02)00731-1] [PMID: 12005441]

[36] Sánchez R, Šali A. Advances in comparative protein-structure modelling. Curr Opin Struct Biol 1997; 7(2): 206-14.
[http://dx.doi.org/10.1016/S0959-440X(97)80027-9] [PMID: 9094331]

[37] Fiser A, Sali A. MODELLER: generation and refinement of homology models. Methods Enzymol 2001; 567-89.
[PMID: 14696385]

[38] Chothia C, Lesk AM. The relation between the divergence of sequence and structure in proteins. EMBO J 1986; 5(4): 823-6.
[http://dx.doi.org/10.1002/j.1460-2075.1986.tb04288.x] [PMID: 3709526]

[39] Lesk AM, Chothia C. How different amino acid sequences determine similar protein structures: the structure and evolutionary dynamics of the globins. J Mol Biol 1980; 136(3): 225-70.
[http://dx.doi.org/10.1016/0022-2836(80)90373-3] [PMID: 7373651]

[40] Bartlam M, Yang H, Rao Z. Structural insights into SARS coronavirus proteins. Curr Opin Struct Biol 2005; 15(6): 664-72.
[http://dx.doi.org/10.1016/j.sbi.2005.10.004] [PMID: 16263266]

[41] Ge X-Y, Li J-L, Yang X-L, *et al.* Isolation and characterization of a bat SARS-like coronavirus that uses the ACE2 receptor. Nature 2013; 503(7477): 535-8.
[http://dx.doi.org/10.1038/nature12711] [PMID: 24172901]

[42] Li F, Li W, Farzan M, Harrison SC. Structure of SARS coronavirus spike receptor-binding domain complexed with receptor. Science 2005; 309(5742): 1864-8.
[http://dx.doi.org/10.1126/science.1116480] [PMID: 16166518]

[43] Walls AC, Park Y-J, Tortorici MA, Wall A, McGuire AT, Veesler D. Structure, function, and antigenicity of the SARS-CoV-2 spike glycoprotein. Cell 2020; 181(2): 281-292.e6.
[http://dx.doi.org/10.1016/j.cell.2020.11.032]

[44] Benvenuto D, Giovanetti M, Ciccozzi A, Spoto S, Angeletti S, Ciccozzi M. The 2019-new coronavirus epidemic: Evidence for virus evolution. J Med Virol 2020; 92(4): 455-9.
[http://dx.doi.org/10.1002/jmv.25688] [PMID: 31994738]

[45] Lu R, Zhao X, Li J, *et al.* Genomic characterisation and epidemiology of 2019 novel coronavirus: implications for virus origins and receptor binding. Lancet 2020; 395(10224): 565-74.
[http://dx.doi.org/10.1016/S0140-6736(20)30251-8] [PMID: 32007145]

[46] Saikatendu KS, Joseph JS, Subramanian V, *et al.* Structural basis of severe acute respiratory syndrome coronavirus ADP-ribose-1″-phosphate dephosphorylation by a conserved domain of nsP3. Structure 2005; 13(11): 1665-75.
[http://dx.doi.org/10.1016/j.str.2005.07.022] [PMID: 16271890]

[47] Angeletti S, Benvenuto D, Bianchi M, Giovanetti M, Pascarella S, Ciccozzi M. COVID-2019: The role of the nsp2 and nsp3 in its pathogenesis. J Med Virol 2020; 92(6): 584-8. [http://dx.doi.org/10.1002/jmv.25719] [PMID: 32083328]

[48] Hammond RG, Tan X, Johnson MA. SARS-unique fold in the Rousettus bat coronavirus HKU9. Protein Sci 2017; 26(9): 1726-37. [http://dx.doi.org/10.1002/pro.3208] [PMID: 28580734]

[49] Chang Y-C, Tung Y-A, Lee K-H, Chen T-F, Hsiao Y-C, Chang H-C, *et al.* Potential therapeutic agents for COVID-19 based on the analysis of protease and RNA polymerase docking 2020.

[50] Wermuth C-G, Ganellin C, Lindberg P, Mitscher L. Glossary of terms used in medicinal chemistry (IUPAC Recommendations 1998). Pure Appl Chem 1998; 70(5): 1129-43. [http://dx.doi.org/10.1351/pac199870051129]

[51] Gund P. Evolution of the Pharmacophore Concept in 2000.

[52] McGregor MJ, Muskal SM. Pharmacophore fingerprinting. 1. Application to QSAR and focused library design. J Chem Inf Comput Sci 1999; 39(3): 569-74. [http://dx.doi.org/10.1021/ci980159j] [PMID: 10361729]

[53] McGregor MJ, Muskal SM. Pharmacophore fingerprinting. 2. Application to primary library design. J Chem Inf Comput Sci 2000; 40(1): 117-25. [http://dx.doi.org/10.1021/ci990313h] [PMID: 10661558]

[54] Mason JS, Morize I, Menard PR, Cheney DL, Hulme C, Labaudiniere RF. New 4-point pharmacophore method for molecular similarity and diversity applications: overview of the method and applications, including a novel approach to the design of combinatorial libraries containing privileged substructures. J Med Chem 1999; 42(17): 3251-64. [http://dx.doi.org/10.1021/jm9806998] [PMID: 10464012]

[55] Geppert TD, Lipsky PE. Antigen presentation at the inflammatory site. Crit Rev Immunol 1989; 9(4): 313-62. [PMID: 2679663]

[56] Sheridan RP, Rusinko A III, Nilakantan R, Venkataraghavan R. Searching for pharmacophores in large coordinate data bases and its use in drug design. Proc Natl Acad Sci USA 1989; 86(20): 8165-9. [http://dx.doi.org/10.1073/pnas.86.20.8165] [PMID: 2813386]

[57] Jones G, Willett P, Glen RC. A genetic algorithm for flexible molecular overlay and pharmacophore elucidation. J Comput Aided Mol Des 1995; 9(6): 532-49. [http://dx.doi.org/10.1007/BF00124324] [PMID: 8789195]

[58] Wolber G, Seidel T, Bendix F, Langer T. Molecule-pharmacophore superpositioning and pattern matching in computational drug design. Drug Discov Today 2008; 13(1-2): 23-9. [http://dx.doi.org/10.1016/j.drudis.2007.09.007] [PMID: 18190860]

[59] Hastings WK. Monte carlo sampling methods using markov chains and their applications. Biometrika 1970; 57(1): 97-109. [http://dx.doi.org/10.1093/biomet/57.1.97]

[60] Metropolis N, Rosenbluth AW, Rosenbluth MN, Teller AH, Teller E. Equation of state calculations by fast computing machines. J Chem Phys 1953; 21(6): 1087-92. [http://dx.doi.org/10.1063/1.1699114]

[61] Ponder JW, Case DA. Force fields for protein simulations Advances in protein chemistry. Elsevier 2003; pp. 27-85.

[62] Frenkel D, Smit B. Understanding molecular simulation: From algorithms to applications. Elsevier (formerly published by Academic Press), 2002; p. 1-638.

[63] Paquet E, Viktor HL. Molecular dynamics, monte carlo simulations, and langevin dynamics: a computational review. Biomed Res Int 2015; 183918.

[http://dx.doi.org/10.1155/2015/183918]

[64] Andreani J, Guerois R. Evolution of protein interactions: from interactomes to interfaces. Arch Biochem Biophys 2014; 554: 65-75. [http://dx.doi.org/10.1016/j.abb.2014.05.010] [PMID: 24853495]

[65] Petta I, Lievens S, Libert C, Tavernier J, De Bosscher K. Modulation of protein–protein interactions for the development of novel therapeutics. Mol Ther 2016; 24(4): 707-18. [http://dx.doi.org/10.1038/mt.2015.214] [PMID: 26675501]

[66] Rodrigues JP, Bonvin AM. Integrative computational modeling of protein interactions. FEBS J 2014; 281(8): 1988-2003. [http://dx.doi.org/10.1111/febs.12771] [PMID: 24588898]

[67] Kaczor AA, Selent J, Poso A. Structure-based molecular modeling approaches to GPCR oligomerization Methods in cell biology. Elsevier 2013; pp. 91-104.

[68] Kuntz ID, Blaney JM, Oatley SJ, Langridge R, Ferrin TE. A geometric approach to macromolecule-ligand interactions. J Mol Biol 1982; 161(2): 269-88. [http://dx.doi.org/10.1016/0022-2836(82)90153-X] [PMID: 7154081]

[69] Park H, Lee H, Seok C. High-resolution protein-protein docking by global optimization: recent advances and future challenges. Curr Opin Struct Biol 2015; 35: 24-31. [http://dx.doi.org/10.1016/j.sbi.2015.08.001] [PMID: 26295792]

[70] Kaczor AA, Selent J, Sanz F, Pastor M. Modeling complexes of transmembrane proteins: systematic analysis of protein-protein docking tools. Mol Inform 2013; 32(8): 717-33. [http://dx.doi.org/10.1002/minf.201200150] [PMID: 27480064]

[71] Zacharias M. Accounting for conformational changes during protein-protein docking. Curr Opin Struct Biol 2010; 20(2): 180-6. [http://dx.doi.org/10.1016/j.sbi.2010.02.001] [PMID: 20194014]

[72] Ban T, Ohue M, Akiyama Y. Multiple grid arrangement improves ligand docking with unknown binding sites: Application to the inverse docking problem. Computational biology and chemistry 2018; 73: 139-46. [http://dx.doi.org/10.1016/j.compbiolchem.2018.02.008]

[73] Kapetanovic IM. Computer-aided drug discovery and development (CADDD): in silico-chemic--biological approach. Chem Biol Interact 2008; 171(2): 165-76. [http://dx.doi.org/10.1016/j.cbi.2006.12.006] [PMID: 17229415]

[74] Wu L, Shen Y, Li M, Wu F-X. Network output controllability-based method for drug target identification. IEEE T NANOBIOSCI 2015; 14(2): 184-91. [http://dx.doi.org/10.1109/TNB.2015.2391175] [PMID: 25643411]

[75] Wishart DS, Knox C, Guo AC, *et al.* DrugBank: a knowledgebase for drugs, drug actions and drug targets. Nucleic Acids Res 2008; 36(Database issue) (Suppl. 1): D901-6. [http://dx.doi.org/10.1093/nar/gkm958] [PMID: 18048412]

[76] Cheng AC, Coleman RG, Smyth KT, *et al.* Structure-based maximal affinity model predicts small-molecule druggability. Nat Biotechnol 2007; 25(1): 71-5. [http://dx.doi.org/10.1038/nbt1273] [PMID: 17211405]

[77] Keiser MJ, Roth BL, Armbruster BN, Ernsberger P, Irwin JJ, Shoichet BK. Relating protein pharmacology by ligand chemistry. Nat Biotechnol 2007; 25(2): 197-206. [http://dx.doi.org/10.1038/nbt1284] [PMID: 17287757]

[78] Beck BR, Shin B, Choi Y, Park S, Kang K. Predicting commercially available anti-viral drugs that may act on the novel coronavirus (SARS-CoV-2) through a drug-target interaction deep learning model. Comput Struct Biotechnol J. Comput Struct Biotec 2020; 18: pp. 784-90.

[79] Alamri MA. Pharmacoinformatics and molecular dynamic simulation studies reveal potential

inhibitors of SARS-CoV-2 main protease 3CLpro. J Biomol Struct Dyn 2020; 39(13): 4936-4948.

[80] Kumar D, Kumari K, Jayaraj A, Kumar V, Kumar RV, Dass SK, *et al.* Understanding the binding affinity of noscapines with protease of SARS-CoV-2 for COVID-19 using MD simulations at different temperatures. J Biomol Struct Dyn 2020; 1-14.
[http://dx.doi.org/10.1080/07391102.2020.1752310] [PMID: 32362235]

[81] Ibrahim IM, Abdelmalek DH, Elshahat ME, Elfiky AA. COVID-19 spike-host cell receptor GRP78 binding site prediction. J Infect 2020; 80(5): 554-62.
[http://dx.doi.org/10.1016/j.jinf.2020.02.026] [PMID: 32169481]

[82] Wahedi HM, Ahmad S, Abbasi SW. Stilbene-based natural compounds as promising drug candidates against COVID-19. J Biomol Struct Dyn 2020 (just-accepted): 1-16.

CHAPTER 13

Vaccine Development, Advantages, and Disadvantages of Group Immunity and Future Perspective for COVID-19

Abdullah [1], **Maqsood ur Rehman**[1], **Fazlullah Khan**[2,*] and **Tapan Behl**[3]

[1] *Department of Pharmacy University of Malakand, Chakdara Dir Lower, Pakistan*

[2] *Department of Allied Health Sciences, Bashir Institute of Health Sciences, Bharakahu, Islamabad, Pakistan*

[3] *Chitkara College of Pharmacy, Chitkara University, Punjab, India*

Abstract: Since its outbreak in late 2019, SARS-CoV-2 has infected millions of people and caused 432, 204 deaths across the globe up to June 14, 2020 (WHO website). SARS-CoV-2 has a high transmission, prolonged incubation time, and an increased prevalence of asymptomatic infection. All over the world, the authorities are insisting on non-pharmaceutical interventions such as social distancing, imposing lockdowns, social isolation, and provision of personal protective equipment (PPEs) to the hospital and other essential departments. However, these measures have only slowed down the virus and cannot prevent rebounds on easing the restrictions. Moreover, the hype about the off-label use of drugs is on the rise. However, the efficacy and the risk of adverse effects have yet to be explored in clinical trials. Therefore, the only way to confer immunity and control the pandemic, the development of vaccines, is currently the research focus. The genetic sequencing of SARS-Cov-2 was done quickly, only in one month. To develop vaccines at pandemic speed, the scientific community faces the challenge of proof of clinical safety and efficacy. Moreover, the previous work is done, and scientists are utilizing the experience of SAR-CoV and MERS and the technologies thereof for COVID-19. Several manufacturers have announced their program and progress on vaccine development. Some vaccines have cleared phase I, and phase II clinical trials, while few are in phase III.

Keywords: Clinical trials, Coronavirus, COVID-19 vaccines, Group immunity, Herd immunity, Vaccine candidate.

* **Corresponding author Fazlullah Khan:** Department of Allied Health Sciences, Bashir Institute of Health Sciences, Bharakahu, Islamabad, Pakistan; Tel.: +92 346 9433 155; E-mail: fazlullahdr@gmail.com

Kamal Niaz & Muhammad Farrukh Nisar (Eds.)

INTRODUCTION

Historically, vaccination is the most efficient countermeasure against infections, as the administration of pathogen-resembling agents increases the immune response against the invader. Vaccine technology continuously progressed in emerging viral threats to promote immune response [1, 2]. The development of vaccines is more time-consuming and complicated, which is different from the conventional medicine development process. Vaccine development usually takes 12-15 years [3]. Conventional medicines are used to treat disease whose symptoms have appeared, while vaccines are being used for a disease, the symptoms of which are yet to occur [4]. Clinical trials evaluate the effectiveness of vaccines and determine their ability to prevent disease with minimum adverse effects [5].

COVID-19 vaccines are initially tested in mice/rabbits for assessment of safety. Testing in humans is initiated after the animals do not exhibit signs of disease after administering the vaccine. The number of subjects is gradually increased with advancing stages of clinical trials to detect rare adverse effects. Before the approval of general-purpose vaccines, thousands of vaccinated people are followed for several months [6]. If the vaccine results in malfunctioning of the immune system or causes severe inflammation, the vaccine may not be suitable for widespread use. Delay in vaccine development is inevitable when such adverse effects are detected [7].

The term "herd immunity" was introduced almost a century ago and is now widely used after increasing vaccines for the eradication of disease [8]. It is also known as group immunity or community immunity. Herd immunity is achieved when a large portion of the population is immune to a specific disease, protecting the susceptible individuals indirectly. The higher the portion of the population that is immune to a disease, the lower the chance for a susceptible individual to contact an infectious person. If many people (herd) are immune, the circulation of infection in the community will stop. Herd immunity should be in more than 80% of individuals to confer protection upon susceptible individuals [9]. This percentage is different for different pathogens depending on the contagiousness of pathogens. Higher the contagiousness of pathogen, a more significant portion of the population must be immune to provide herd immunity. For example, in SARS-CoV-2, the percentage of the people needed for herd immunity is 70% [8]. If the fraction of susceptible individuals in a population is too few, then the pathogen cannot successfully spread, and its prevalence will decline. Herd immunity threshold is the point at which the proportion of susceptible individuals falls below the threshold required for transmission [10]. Sensitive individuals take benefit from indirect protection from infection above the herd immunity threshold. The benefits of herd immunity imply various segments of the population. For example, it is useful to protect immuno compromised individuals who cannot be vaccinated. It includes elders who cannot exhibit an optimal immune response to vaccines, children too young to be vaccinated, individuals having no access to mass immunization, and people who do not get vaccinated [10].

For COVID-19 vaccine efficacy, immune deficiency is a risk factor, especially in elders whose immune system has already been weakened by many factors. Moreover, obesity also results in the weakening of the immune system. It occurs due to lower IgG levels and a higher level of IL-6. Respiratory infections and infections caused by parasites also affect the immune response to COVID-19 vaccines [11]. Research on SARS-CoV and MERS has helped scientists to unveil the mechanism of protection offered by the immune system against the disease and the human body's response to coronaviruses. In pandemic situations, hundreds of millions of vaccine doses are required, which, if already production lines are available, are manufactured in about six months. A new vaccine needs several quality control checks because the unique production process is involved [12]. This chapter aims to summarize the development of vaccines for COVID-19 and the advantages and disadvantages of group immunity.

Clinical-Phase Vaccine Candidates for COVID-19

Several strategies are adopted for COVID-19 vaccine development; most of these target S proteins as the primary inducer of neutralizing antibodies [13]. The S protein molecule has S1 and S2 subunits. Subunit S1 contains a receptor-binding domain (RBD) which interacts with the host cell receptor (ACE2). The S protein plays a crucial role in inducing protective immunity during infection with SARS-CoV by eliciting T-cell responses and neutralizing antibodies. In contrast, the subunit S2 facilitates the fusion of the virus with the host cell membrane to release the viral RNA into the cytoplasm for replication [13]. Hence, vaccines based on S-protein should induce antibodies that block virus genome uncoating as well asnd viral receptor binding. Thus, the whole S glycoprotein or its appropriate parts are considered the key candidates for the vaccine composition of CoVID-19 [14].

Up till now, no vaccine is licensed to prevent human respiratory infection. About 10 COVID-19 vaccine candidates are in different stages of development, as shown in Table **1** [15]. The main criterion for a vaccine is safety, efficacy, and duration of immunity. The pandemic vaccine needs high production capacity and rapid development. This limits their rapid deployment during pandemics. Furthermore, live attenuated coronavirus vaccines are produced by reverse genetics from infectious virus clones by deleting multiple key virulence determinants to prevent reversion. It remains the most immunologically robust, inducing systemic, mucosal, cell-mediated, and humoral immunity and broader cross-protection [15 - 17].

Table 1. COVID-19 candidate vaccines – June 9 2020 [27].

S.No.	Platform	Type of Candidate Vaccine	Developer	Stage of Development
1	Inactivated	Inactivated + alum	Sinovac	Phase 3 NCT04456595 Phase 1/2 NCT04383574
2	Non-Replicating Viral Vector	ChAdOx1-S	University of Oxford/AstraZeneca	Phase 3 ISRCTN89951424 Phase2b/3 2020-001228-32
3	Non-Replicating Viral Vector	Adenovirus Type 5 Vector	CanSino Biological Inc./Beijing Institute of Biotechnology	Phase 2 ChiCTR2000031781 Phase 1 ChiCTR2000030906
4	RNA	LNP-encapsulated mRNA	Moderna/NIAID	Phase 2 NCT044056 Phase 1 NCT042831
5	DNA	DNA plasmid vaccine with electroporation	Inovio Pharmaceuticals/ International Vaccine Institute	Phase 1/2 NCT04447781 NCT04336410
6	DNA	DNA plasmid vaccine	Cadila Healthcare Limited	Phase 1/2 CTRI/2020/07/026352
7	Inactivated	Inactivated	Wuhan Institute of Biological Products/Sinopharm	Phase 1/2 ChiCTR2000031809
8	Inactivated	Inactivated	Beijing Institute of Biological Products/Sinopharm	Phase 1/2 ChiCTR2000032459
9	Protein subunit	Full-length recombinant SARS CoV-2 glycoprotein nanoparticle vaccine adjuvanted with Matrix M	Novavax	Phase 1/2 NCT04368988
10	RNA	3 LNP-mRNAs	BioNTech/Fosun Pharma/Pfizer	Phase 1/2 2020-00103--36 NCT04368728

(Table 1) cont.....

S.No.	Platform	Type of Candidate Vaccine	Developer	Stage of Development
11	DNA	DNA Vaccine (GX-19)	Genexine Consortium	Phase 1 NCT04445389
12	DNA	DNA plasmid vaccine + Adjuvant	Osaka University/ AnGes/ Takara Bio	Phase 1 JapicCTI-205328
13	Inactivated	Inactivated	Institute of Medical Biology, Chinese Academy of Medical Sciences	Phase 1 NCT04412538
14	Non-Replicating Viral Vector	Adeno-based	Gamaleya Research Institute	Phase 1 NCT04436471 NCT04437875
15	Protein subunit	Native like Trimeric subunit Spike Protein vaccine	Clover Biopharmaceuticals Inc./GSK/Dynavax	Phase 1 NCT04405908
16	Protein subunit	The adjuvanted recombinant protein (RBD-Dimer)	Anhui Zhifei Longcom Biopharmaceutical/ Institute of Microbiology, Chinese Academy of Sciences	Phase 1 NCT04445194
17	Protein subunit	Recombinant spike protein with Advax™ adjuvant	Vaxine Pty Ltd/Medytox	Phase 1 NCT04453852
18	RNA	LNP-nCoVsaRNA	Imperial College London	Phase 1 ISRCTN17072692
19	RNA	mRNA	Curevac	Phase 1 NCT04449276
20	RNA	mRNA	People's Liberation Army (PLA) Academy of Military Sciences/Walvax Biotech.	Phase 1 ChiCTR2000034112
21	VLP	Plant-derived VLP	Medicago Inc./ Université Laval	Phase 1 NCT04450004

A clinical trial for a new DNA vaccine against coronavirus (ChAdOx1) aimed against MERS, has started [18]. This vaccine is based on the spike protein of SARS-CoV-2 and the adenovirus as a vaccine vector [19]. It has been modified such that the genetic code sends instructions for spike protein production that allows the production of this protein by adenovirus after vaccination. Thus, antibodies are produced against spike protein [20]. The University of Oxford, UK is striving to develop a chimpanzee adenovirus vector (ChAdOx1 nCoV-19) based COVID-19 vaccine. It encodes the spike protein of SARS-CoV-2. It is tested in phase II and III trials for tolerability, safety, reactogenicity, and immunogenicity profile. ChAdOx1 is a non-replication vaccine vector and stimulates both sides of the adaptive immune response, including cytotoxic T-cells and humoral response. It has exhibited efficacy in several clinical trials, including those for Zika, Chikungunya, and MERS, and is also being tested as a cancer vaccine platform [21].

Traditionally, inactivated purified viruses have been used to develop vaccines that are safe and effective for the prevention of diseases caused by polio and influenza virus [22, 23]. This technology is being utilized by the Institute of Medical Biology, the Chinese Academy of Medical Sciences, and the Beijing Institute of Biological Products to develop vaccines for COVID-19.

Protein subunit vaccines are obtained either by recombinant DNA technology or by conventional cultivation methods. It contains only certain antigenic determinants of pathogenic microorganisms [24]. The antigenic determinants enhance the efficiency of immune response, and the risk of side effects is reduced by the presence of a small number of pathogens. The antigens are conjugated with protein molecules to obtain vaccines of strong immunogenicity [25]. DNA vaccines have the advantage of high stability and stimulating both humoral and cellular immunity. Its other benefits are that it confers long-term immunity, and the plasmid can be manufactured in large amounts [26].

Diversity of Technology

Scientists across the globe are struggling hard to search for potential techniques to develop efficient vaccines against COVID-19. Neutralizing antibody production against the spike protein (S) and the blockade of ACE2 receptor is the key target for the majority of COVID-19 vaccine candidates [28, 29]. The prominent feature of COVID 19 vaccine development is the diversity of platforms under investigation.

The conventional approach to developing COVID-19 vaccines may be the application of attenuated or inactivated strains of SARS-CoV-2. Still, these have disadvantages, including a long duration for sufficient material production, the risk of re-acquired virulence, and adverse effects [30, 31]. A safer and quicker method is subunit vaccines based on individual proteins, which may be administered in combination with adjuvant or VLPs. Currently, it is used for the development of vaccines against SARS-CoV-2. All the structural proteins of SARS-CoV-2 are immunogenic and can produce CD4+/CD8+ T cell responses [32]. However, studies have indicated that antibodies against N protein do not provide protective immunity while E and M proteins provide a weak protective response [33]. The virus-like particles (VLPs) lack the viral genome. It may be an alternative platform of inactivated or attenuated vaccines as it has no reactogenicity and reversion to pathogenic forms [34, 35].

Nucleic Acid (DNA and RNA)

Several platforms are under extensive research to develop COVID 19 vaccines. Out of these, nucleic acid-based platforms have the most significant potential because these require a synthetic process and do not need fermentation or culture [36]. That's why even just after 2 months of SARS-COV2 sequence identification, Moderna started testing its mRNA-based vaccine mRNA-1273. The mRNA vaccines are directly administered into the cells to produce antigens *in vivo*. Once translated, the antigens are transported extracellularly for antibody recognition and presentation to T cells and immune response [36, 37]. It has the advantage that as the antigen is produced *in vivo*. The natural immune response is achieved. However, it has the disadvantage of being unstable and inefficient *in vivo* delivery of mRNA [38].

Similarly, DNA vaccines are administered extracellularly to express antigens *in vivo*. DNA-base vaccines are more stable and induce more prolonged antigen expression. Therefore, it confers a long-lasting immune response compared to RNA vaccines [39].

Virus-like Particle

It consists of the structural proteins of the virus assembled to form a particle. These are non-infectious and large but still heterogeneous antigenically. It combines the best traits of whole virus vaccines and subunit vaccines. Structurally, virus-like particles resemble infectious viruses; therefore, they can induce potent cellular and humoral response without adjuvant use [40]. The particulate nature of virus-like particles makes them capable of inducing potent T cell-mediated immune responses by interaction with antigen-presenting cells, particularly the dendritic cells. Due to their enhanced efficacy compared to subunit vaccines, the virus-like particle garners high scientific interest as vaccine candidates [41]. The high pathogenic nature and contagiousness bring great difficulties in SARS-CoV-2 related research. Therefore, VLPs provide a better alternative to study SARS-CoV-2 vaccine efficacy in the lack of suitable animal models [42].

Peptide

No peptide vaccine has yet been approved for use in humans. The first peptide vaccine was designed for canines. Several studies have exhibited that peptide vaccines are pretty effective, especially in cancerous tumors. It has been reported that traditional vaccines require more time and money than peptide vaccines [43].

The pathogen-derived antigens (spike protein in case of COVID-19) are used to elicit an immune response. The spike glycoprotein induces the highest neutralizing antibody titers. It is a promising candidate for the development of vaccines [44, 45]. But the peptide vaccines developed for SARS and MERS were partially effective in protecting viral challenges in animals. They were unable to elicit an immune response that occurred in natural infections. One of the many reasons for this failure could be that peptides are just a portion of the virus [46].

The advantages of peptide vaccines are their easy manufacturing process and storage, while the demerits are limited global production capacity, require adjuvants, and poor immunogenicity [47]. Nevertheless, Most of the peptide vaccine candidates are based on spike protein with the addition of an adjuvant to improve immunogenicity. For instance, Innovax plans to study several truncated spike proteins in pre-clinical trials to select a lead candidate from the resulting immunogenicity data that will further be evaluated with oil in water adjuvant [47].

Live Attenuated Virus

These vaccines are the most immunogenic but carry the risk of becoming pathogenic after mutation. Moreover, the inactivation of the whole virus is carried out *via* different chemical and physical means that turn the virus “dead”. Yet, its immunogenicity is intact. In this technique, a modified live SARS-CoV-2 virus having reduced virulence (*e.g.,* mutated E protein or codon deoptimization) is used [48]. Its advantage includes all of the virus's natural components such as nucleic acids, proteins, glycans, and lipids, thereby eliciting a potent immune response and outperforming other vaccine development strategies. It may require just a single dose and are self-replicating [49].

Viral Vector (replicating and non-replicating

Engineered non-pathogenic viruses carry the genetic material of another virus and deliver it into cells to produce antigen *in vivo*. The adenovirus and measles virus is commonly used vectors. Like nucleic acid vaccines, viral vector technology may be modified to express the antigen of choice. Moreover, this technology delivers the genome intracellular, doesn’t rely on adjuvant, and can induce a robust T-cell response [50].

Adenoviruses are the most commonly employed vectors for vaccine development. Its molecular biology and virology have been investigated for many years as a tool for gene therapy applications, thus, providing sufficient knowledge for vaccine development [51]. The deletion makes adenovirus non-replicating of genes from the area responsible for replication (E1 region). Furthermore, to increase space for the foreign genes, the E3 region genes are also deleted. The most extensively exploited adenovirus used as a non-replication vector is adenovirus 5. The replicating adenovirus has its E1 region intact, which has the advantage of dose sparing i-e little amount is required because the vaccine vector replicates *in vivo*. Adenovirus 4 and 7 are commonly used as replication-competent vectors [52].

COVID-19 vaccine (ChAdOx1 nCoV-19) encoding the SARS-CoV-2 Spike protein, being developed by the University of Oxford, UK, is based on a chimpanzee adenovirus vector [53]. ChAdOx1 is a non-replication vaccine vector and stimulates both wings of an adaptive immune response, including cytotoxic T-cells and humoral response, has demonstrated efficacy in various clinical trials [54]. Viral vectors-based vaccines exhibit long-term stability and a high degree of protein expression and thereby induce a strong immune response [55].

Recombinant Protein

Although all the four structural proteins of SARS-CoV-2 such as spike, nucleoprotein (N-protein), membrane protein (M-protein), and envelope (E-protein), can be the targets for vaccine development. The high immunogenicity of the S protein makes it the best candidate for the development of the vaccine [48]. Moreover, the S vaccines preclude the interaction between SARS-CoV-2 and ACE2 and thus prevent/bring to halt COVID-19. SARS CoV2 proteins (S protein) are administered to the host to elicit an immune response. An adjuvant is also co-administered to increase immunogenicity. Recombinant protein vaccine candidates can benefit from the already existing large-scale production because such vaccines have already been licensed for other diseases [56].

Monoclonal Antibodies (mAbs)

Passive immunization with mAbs causes a reduction in virus replication and spread. It has been demonstrated in several studies that these antibodies are effective in the treatment/prevention of highly pathogenic viral diseases *via* neutralization of structural proteins of the virus [57, 58]. *In vivo* and *in vitro* studies evaluating the use of mAbs against SARS and MERS blocked the replication of viruses and improved the clinical condition of patients. Moreover, the inhibition of the virus was explained with the use of antibodies against MERS-CoV glycoprotein S after 24 hours of infection in a humanized dipeptidyl peptidase 4 (DPP4) receptor mouse model [58].

Inactivated Virus

Purified inactivated viruses have been traditionally used for the development of vaccines. Such vaccines are safer and effective in preventing infections caused by influenza and poliovirus [22, 23]. In a study carried out in China, the SARS-Co--2 vaccine candidate has resulted in neutralizing antibodies in non-human primates, rats, and mice. A clinical trial (Phase 1/2) is in progress on 744 humans participants [23]. Inactivated virus vaccines have the advantage of the requirement of single-dose; have a broad and potent immune response. However, it has some disadvantages like these are less immunogenic as compared to the attenuated vaccines. It has to be supplied in dry form to make the structure more stable, requires a separate solvent supply, and be transported in a cold chain. These steps increase the production cost of the vaccine [58].

Clinical Trials in Terms of Vaccine Development

Clinical trials are research studies on human volunteers to evaluate the safety and efficacy of treatment products or preventative measures such as medicines or medical devices, and vaccines. It provides deeper insight into vaccines that can help prevent diseases. Clinical trials are a critical step to get approval from regulatory bodies of vaccines or medicines and medical devices [45]. An individual novel vaccine must be assessed for its immunogenicity, safety, and effectiveness before it is licensed for human use. After discovery, every novel vaccine endures an extravagant development process. The vaccines must pass some clinical trials before launching for human use, including toxicity, an immunogenetic response in adults, chances of acceptance by the community, possible impact on public health, cost-effectiveness, and benefit to risk ratio.

Looking to this fast drive of COVID-19 vaccine candidates into human trials, the time it takes to develop vaccines for this evolving pathogenic microorganism is reducing compared with other vaccine candidates of the past. They are generally used as traditional infantile vaccines. Lately, a DNA-based vaccine candidate for the novel SARS or original SARS, *i.e.,* SARS-CoV-1, was developed in one. A half-year vaccine for H-5 influenza A in almost one year (approximately 11 months) in Indonesia in 2006, another vaccine candidate for H-1 influenza A took just four months to develop at California USA in 2009. Similarly, a vaccine candidate used against the Zika virus was developed in just three and half months [59]. These accomplishments have been carried out by modern skills, innovative technologies, and advanced approaches that have allowed for the rapid identification and sequencing of new and emerging pathogenic viruses and the latest technologies for vaccine candidate delivery [59]. For the past 15 years, the HIV vaccine arena has founded the development and usage of recombinant DNA or recombinant antibody technology. It is novel animal models (*in-vivo* studies), cutting-edge computational methods, and advanced vaccine delivery methods with new approaches to fast-track HIV vaccine immunogen development, design, and delivery [60 - 63]. The timeline for a COVID-19 vaccine candidate will probably be much faster. It is even much easier than for other vaccine candidates of the past. Investigators, researchers, and scientists have worked to assimilate these iterative aspects and approaches for vaccine development and antibody countermeasure development and apply them to a quick response to the COVID-19 pandemic.

Clinical trials are needed to be designed based on some parameters to get the required data: • Product to be investigated • Methods by which the trial will be conducted •Goals or endpoints • The population to be studied • Double Blinding [64]. Randomization is a method in which study participants are placed in different treatment groups based on chance. Different treatments in similar groups are comparably tested by researchers using randomization [65].

Several organizations, including BioNTech/Fosun, Moderna/NIAID, and Pharma/Pfizer, are now developing vaccines/medicine to prevent COVID-19. These candidates use several mRNAs with lipid nanoparticles or DNA. For example, "Inovio" vaccines, nanoparticles, attenuated viruses, proteins, and viral vectors carrying SARS-CoV-2 viral genes as vaccine goes through immunogenicity and safety trials. A lesser number of vaccine candidates will be tested in phase III clinical trials or efficacy trials to determine its effectiveness and safety. On the other hand, presently, with Phase I and Phase II clinical trials, it is significant to develop the capacity for large-scale vaccine production in a successful efficacy trial [66, 67]. It is possible that genetic immunization techniques such as mRNA in LNPs or DNA can be manufactured quickly as compared to viral vectors or proteins and may be more economical [68].

Preclinical Research

Identification of vaccine candidates is made through pre-clinical evaluations, which may involve selecting proper antigens to elicit an immune response and high throughput screening [69]. Appropriate drug formulations (*i.e.,* injection, tablet, *etc.*) and approximate dose ranges are determined during the pre-clinical stages. Before moving to the phase one trials, the vaccine candidate may be first tested in laboratory animals in pre-clinical research. For testing of adverse effects and immunogenicity, the oral polio vaccine has been first tested in non-human primates and monkeys [70]. Determination of the immunological response to the vaccine and its safety, such as toxicity, are necessary components of the pre-clinical stage [71]. Conventional drug trials focus on pharmacokinetics and pharmacodynamics. It is mandatory to determine the interactions with the immune system and toxic effects at all possible dosage levels during vaccine trail [72].

The vaccines were not always as pure as possible to prevent adverse effects due to a lack of regulations on pharmaceutical manufacturers. Vaccine trials and manufacturing must be handled cautiously to avoid infecting the recipients or causing adverse effects. Since the Cutter Incident, the public has not gained the same confidence level in science and vaccines, which risks public health for everyone [73].

Structural determination of the principal targets of antibodies to counteract, *e.g.,* the spike protein in SARS-CoV-2, Env in HIV, and hemagglutinin in influenza A, has provided a valued atomic-level image develop strategies for the vaccine (s). Especially, cryo-electron microscopy has enabled the rapid solution of the structure of the SARS-CoV-2 spike protein [74, 75]. The supercomputer combines different fields and aspects, including computational biology, structural biology analysis of viral pathogens cartels structural, biophysical, and biochemical approaches to comprehend the interactions of pathogenic virus or other microorganisms with the human immune system [76 - 79]. It can be implemented for the production of the COVID-19 vaccine, as shown in Fig. (**1**). To accelerate structure-based vaccine design for COVID-19, recently, structural biologists spun to apply technology developed for respiratory syncytial virus (RSV) or HIV-1 envelope structural biology [74, 75, 80, 81]. Presently, recognized pipelines for high-resolution cryo-EM determination of the structure of the SARS-CoV-2 spike are unified with the computational teams with the help of a supercomputer, consequently providing atomic-level feedback to SARS-CoV-2 (COVID-19) vaccine designs.

HIV-1 antibody discovery in the recent past has provided patterns for HIV-1 vaccine candidate design and development, which aimed to provoke broadly reactive neutralizing antibodies [82, 83]. It has become clearer that an effective vaccine will likely require multiple immunogens administered in a specific order. It has facilitated proper antibody development to multiple neutralizing targets on HIV from the contemporary literature available for the ontogeny of HIV neutralizing antibodies [62]. Expectantly, the development of SARS-CoV-2 neutralizing antibodies against COVID-19 disease will necessitate a much simpler vaccination regimen like that of the vaccine developed against the Zika virus, where only a single immunization with a single antigen was enough to induce protective neutralization of antibodies [84]. This kind of vaccine would be suitable for fast-track development, large-scale manufacturing with global administration to mankind.

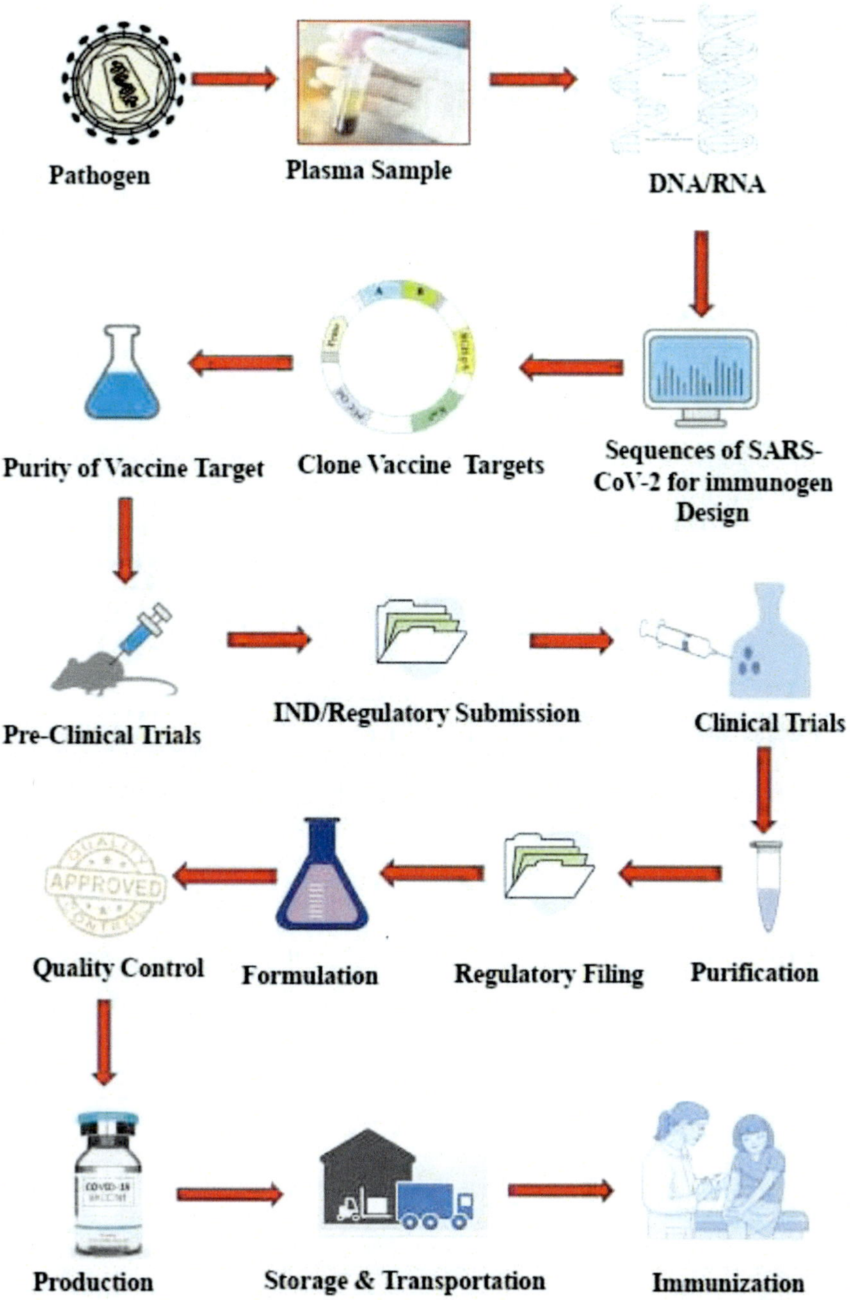

Fig. (1). Schematic Diagram of vaccine Development for COVID-19 supercomputers assisted research on COVID-19 vaccine.

Non-Specific Vaccine

There is evidence of the effectiveness of the BCG vaccine in respiratory infections, but the duration and magnitude of these non-specific effects are unknown at present. Therefore, implications on practice and policy on the BCG vaccine cannot be determined [96]. The WHO has explained that evidence-based recommendations currently do not justify changes to the current global immunization policy [96]. There is systematic review evidence with low to moderate risk of bias that BCG vaccination prevents respiratory infections (influenza and pneumonia) in elders and children. BCG vaccine modifies humoral responses to influenza and pneumococcal vaccines. More extensive research is required to study the duration and magnitude of the non-specific effects of the BCG vaccine on mortality of any cause before considering implications for policy and practice. At present, there is no evidence that the BCG vaccine provides protection against COVID-19, and caution should be exercised when interpreting and studying their correlation. It is too early to jump to immature conclusions being still during the COVID-19 pandemic, where COVID-19 cases/deaths may still increase over time in some BCG-using countries. Good evidence should be obtained from prospective randomized trials before reflecting on practice and policy [97].

Group Immunity

Protection from the disease in a group, due to a large enough proportion of the population having immunity to prevent the disease from spreading from person to person" [98]. When the majority of people in the community are immune to an infectious disease, let leads to provides in-direct defense (herd immunity). It is also called herd protection, *e.g.,* if 75- 80% of people in the community are immune to a specific virus, 4 out of 5 people who meet or contact with someone having the disease would not get ill and so would not be able to spread the disease further. In this fashion, the spreading of infectious diseases can be kept under control. Depending on how transmissible it is, typically, 70%-90% of people require immunity to attain herd immunity. There are several diseases (Measles, mumps, polio, and chickenpox, *etc.*) that were once very common, but now these diseases are sporadic across the globe. This reduction or even eradication of these infectious diseases was possible because of the development of the vaccine. It provided herd immunity against these diseases. Sometimes outbreaks can be observed for vaccine-preventable conditions, particularly in lowered vaccine coverage communities due to lake of because of herd immunity.

Infectious diseases have no vaccine. Even if most people have attained immunity because of the previous infection, the disease can still spread among the communities, especially the children and the people with poor or less developed immune systems. This was observed in the past for several diseases before vaccines were developed for them.

COVID-19 is also similar to other coronaviruses that are presently spread in the whole world. Due to mutation with time, antibodies from a prior infection can give protection for a short period only. Therefore, we can expect that all those who get infected and recovered from COVID-19 would be immune for few months to few years, but most possibly not to be immune for their whole lives.

Herd Immunity and COVID-19

There are only two ways to get herd immunity: 1. Majority of the population, *i.e.,* 80%, either get an infection and then recovered, as discussed earlier, or 2. The vaccine can protect them. According to the literature available on coronavirus infection, we require at least 70% of the population to be immune to get herd protection. If social distances and other means of contact are not reduced, the disease can spread within a few months. According to Imperial College London, this would defiantly devastate the hospitals and leads to a high mortality rate. In the finest case, we can uphold current levels of disease or can decrease the level until the availability of a vaccine [99]. According to the instruction, this is only possible to follow SOPs by keeping physical distancing for a prolonged period, probable for one year or even longer. Sometimes people exposed themselves intentionally to achieve immunity. This was done before the development of varicella vaccines. This approach might be reasonable for less severe diseases. But this method can not be applied in SARS-CoV-2 as it carries a much higher risk of severe disease and even death. Scientists are striving furiously to develop an effective vaccine. Meanwhile, as most of the population is not infected by SARS-CoV-2, some preventive measures are required to prevent explosive outbreaks like those we have seen in places like New York City [99].

Advantages and Disadvantages of Herd Immunity

There are lots of people who only depend on herd immunity to protect themselves from COVID-19. These people are mainly susceptible to diseases. The following are groups of people who need herd immunity: people living without the spleen as they have no completely functional immune system; Patients who have cancer and are under chemotherapy treatment; patients who have HIV/AIDS; neonates and old age people. The main advantages of herd immunity include the complete elimination of infection, reducing the hazard of disease for those who can't take vaccines due to contraindication, and last the people who refused to take vaccines [99]. On the other hand, herd immunity has some disadvantages: herd immunity applies only to contagious diseases and raises the average age of infection among those infected (*e.g.*, polio, rubella, and varicella), *etc.*

FUTURE PERSPECTIVE OF VACCINE DEVELOPMENT

Usually, herd immunity is not achieved in one or two years to prevent the spread of disease, and vaccine development may take a decade or more based on its ability to prevent disease in tens of thousands of people [100]. Therefore, based on the emergency of the COVID-19 pandemic, the FDA may accelerate the standard process of vaccine approval and grant approval for the emergency use of vaccines. In such a situation, when the vaccine has exhibited safety and efficacy to get an immune response in a high percentage of people. The authorities may prioritize high-risk individuals such as health care professionals/workers who will serve as a test case to determine how well the vaccine protects people from COVID-19 [101]. Moreover, mass immunization up to about 70% of the population may take years. Moreover, to provide vaccines to the general public, the biopharmaceutical industry will need a herculean manufacturing effort.

The development of vaccines for human use can take years, particularly when new technologies are being used which have not been extensively tested for safety or scaled up for mass production. As no coronavirus vaccines are available and no large-scale manufacturing capacity exists for these vaccines, there is a need to build processes and capacities. It can be tedious and time-consuming for the first time [102].

CONCLUSION

Scientists started developing vaccines for recent outbreaks of coronavirus (SARS-CoV, 2002 and MERS, 2012) but were not materialized for many reasons. COVID-19 outbreak is more severe and broad, and according to some researchers, the disease may become seasonal and endemic. Therefore, many companies and researchers are working to develop a vaccine against SARS-CoV-2 throughout the world. A varied range of technological platforms is being evaluated for vaccine development, including live attenuated virus, inactivated virus, nucleic acids (RNA and DNA), peptides, virus-like particles, recombinant proteins, monoclonal antibodies, and viral vectors. As there is no treatment available to cope with COVID-19, the social distancing and lockdown harm the economy of the world. Therefore, there is a dire need for vaccines across the globe. The speed of research is unprecedented, and it is hoped to get the vaccine soon.

CONSENT FOR PUBLICATION

Not Applicable.

CONFLICT OF INTEREST

The authors confirm that this chapter contents have no conflict of interest.

ACKNOWLEDGEMENT

Declared none.

REFERENCES

[1] Moon JJ, Suh H, Li AV, Ockenhouse CF, Yadava A, Irvine DJ. Enhancing humoral responses to a malaria antigen with nanoparticle vaccines that expand Tfh cells and promote germinal center induction. Proc Natl Acad Sci USA 2012; 109(4): 1080-5. [http://dx.doi.org/10.1073/pnas.1112648109] [PMID: 22247289]

[2] Bachmann MF, Jennings GT. Vaccine delivery: a matter of size, geometry, kinetics and molecular patterns. Nat Rev Immunol 2010; 10(11): 787-96. [http://dx.doi.org/10.1038/nri2868] [PMID: 20948547]

[3] Han S. Clinical vaccine development. Clin Exp Vaccine Res 2015; 4(1): 46-53. [http://dx.doi.org/10.7774/cevr.2015.4.1.46] [PMID: 25648742]

[4] Kamal AM, Mitrut P, Docea AO, *et al.* Double therapy with pegylated Interferon and Ribavirin for chronic hepatitis C. A pharmacogenenetic guide for predicting adverse events. Farmacia 2017; 65: 877-84.

[5] Black S. The costs and effectiveness of large Phase III pre-licensure vaccine clinical trials. Expert Rev Vaccines 2015; 14(12): 1543-8. [http://dx.doi.org/10.1586/14760584.2015.1091733] [PMID: 26414015]

[6] DeStefano F, Bodenstab HM, Offit PA. Principal controversies in vaccine safety in the United States. Clin Infect Dis 2019; 69(4): 726-31. [http://dx.doi.org/10.1093/cid/ciz135] [PMID: 30753348]

[7] Peeples L. News Feature: Avoiding pitfalls in the pursuit of a COVID-19 vaccine. Proc Natl Acad Sci USA 2020; 117(15): 8218-21. [http://dx.doi.org/10.1073/pnas.2005456117] [PMID: 32229574]

[8] Topley WW, Wilson GS. The spread of bacterial infection: the problem of herd immunity. J Hyg (Lond) 1923; 21(3): 243-9. [http://dx.doi.org/10.1017/S0022172400031478] [PMID: 20474777]

[9] Kim TH, Johnstone J, Loeb M. Vaccine herd effect. Scand J Infect Dis 2011; 43(9): 683-9. [http://dx.doi.org/10.3109/00365548.2011.582247] [PMID: 21604922]

[10] Anderson RM, May RM. Vaccination and herd immunity to infectious diseases. Nature 1985; 318(6044): 323-9. [http://dx.doi.org/10.1038/318323a0] [PMID: 3906406]

[11] Eliakim A, Schwindt C, Zaldivar F, Casali P, Cooper DM. Reduced tetanus antibody titers in overweight children. Autoimmunity 2006; 39(2): 137-41. [http://dx.doi.org/10.1080/08916930600597326] [PMID: 16698670]

[12] Skalny AV, Rink L, Ajsuvakova OP, *et al.* Zinc and respiratory tract infections: Perspectives for COVID-19 (Review). Int J Mol Med. 2020 46(1): 17-26.

[13] Zhou P, Yang XL, Wang XG, *et al.* A pneumonia outbreak associated with a new coronavirus of probable bat origin. Nature 2020; 579(7798): 270-3. [http://dx.doi.org/10.1038/s41586-020-2012-7] [PMID: 32015507]

[14] Rauch S, Jasny E, Schmidt KE, Petsch B. New vaccine technologies to combat outbreak situations. Front Immunol 2018; 9: 1963. [http://dx.doi.org/10.3389/fimmu.2018.01963] [PMID: 30283434]

[15] Du L, He Y, Zhou Y, Liu S, Zheng BJ, Jiang S. The spike protein of SARS-CoV--a target for vaccine and therapeutic development. Nat Rev Microbiol 2009; 7(3): 226-36. [http://dx.doi.org/10.1038/nrmicro2090] [PMID: 19198616]

[16] Coronavirus disease (COVID-2019) R & D. Available at: https://www.who. int/blueprint/priority-diseases/key-action/novel-coronavirus/en/

[17] Enjuanes L, Dediego ML, Alvarez E, Deming D, Sheahan T, Baric R. Vaccines to prevent severe acute respiratory syndrome coronavirus-induced disease. Virus Res 2008; 133(1): 45-62. [http://dx.doi.org/10.1016/j.virusres.2007.01.021] [PMID: 17416434]

[18] Thanh LT, Andreadakis Z, Kumar A, *et al.* The COVID-19 vaccine development landscape. Nat Rev Drug Discov 2020. Epub ahead of print

[19] U.S. National Library of Medicine, ClinicalTrials.gov: A Study of a Candidate COVID 19 Vaccine (COV001). https://clinicaltrials.gov/ct2/show/NCT04324606

[20] Clinical Trials Arena. University of oxford starts enrolment for Covid-19 vaccine trial https://www.clinicaltrialsarena.com/news/oxford-university-covid-19-vaccine-trial/

[21] https://www.vaccitech.co.uk/technology/

[22] Murdin AD, Barreto L, Plotkin S. Inactivated poliovirus vaccine: past and present experience. Vaccine 1996; 14(8): 735-46. [http://dx.doi.org/10.1016/0264-410X(95)00211-I] [PMID: 8817819]

[23] Vellozzi C, Burwen DR, Dobardzic A, Ball R, Walton K, Haber P. Safety of trivalent inactivated influenza vaccines in adults: background for pandemic influenza vaccine safety monitoring. Vaccine 2009; 27(15): 2114-20. [http://dx.doi.org/10.1016/j.vaccine.2009.01.125] [PMID: 19356614]

[24] Zhang N, Tang J, Lu L, Jiang S, Du L. Receptor-binding domain-based subunit vaccines against MERS-CoV. Virus Res 2015; 202: 151-9. [http://dx.doi.org/10.1016/j.virusres.2014.11.013] [PMID: 25445336]

[25] Lee NH, Lee JA, Park SY, Song CS, Choi IS, Lee JB. A review of vaccine development and research for industry animals in Korea. Clin Exp Vaccine Res 2012; 1(1): 18-34. [http://dx.doi.org/10.7774/cevr.2012.1.1.18] [PMID: 23596575]

[26] Hobernik D, Bros M. DNA vaccines-how far from clinical use? Int J Mol Sci 2018; 19(11): E3605. [http://dx.doi.org/10.3390/ijms19113605] [PMID: 30445702]

[27] https://www.who.int/publications/m/item/draft-landscape-of-covid-19-candidate-vaccines

[28] Agrawal AS, Tao X, Algaissi A, *et al.* Immunization with inactivated Middle East Respiratory Syndrome coronavirus vaccine leads to lung immunopathology on challenge with live virus. Hum Vaccin Immunother 2016; 12(9): 2351-6. [http://dx.doi.org/10.1080/21645515.2016.1177688] [PMID: 27269431]

[29] Amanat F, Krammer F. SARS-CoV-2 Vaccines: Status Report. Immunity 2020; 52(4): 583-9. [http://dx.doi.org/10.1016/j.immuni.2020.03.007] [PMID: 32259480]

[30] Jiang S, He Y, Liu S. SARS vaccine development. Emerg Infect Dis 2005; 11(7): 1016-20. [http://dx.doi.org/10.3201/eid1107.050219] [PMID: 16022774]

[31] Regla-Nava JA, Nieto-Torres JL, Jimenez-Guardeño JM, *et al.* Severe acute respiratory syndrome

coronaviruses with mutations in the E protein are attenuated and promising vaccine candidates. J Virol 2015; 89(7): 3870-87.
[http://dx.doi.org/10.1128/JVI.03566-14] [PMID: 25609816]

[32] Shang W, *et al.* The outbreak of SARS-CoV-2 pneumonia calls for viral vaccines. NPJ Vaccines 2020; 5: 18.
[http://dx.doi.org/10.1038/s41541-020-0170-0]

[33] Gralinski LE, Menachery VD. Return of the coronavirus: 2019-nCoV. Viruses 2020; 12(2): 135.
[http://dx.doi.org/10.3390/v12020135] [PMID: 31991541]

[34] Chansaenroj J, Chuchaona W, Thanusuwannasak T, *et al.* Prevalence of poliovirus vaccine strains in randomized stool samples from 2010 to 2018: encompassing transition from the trivalent to bivalent oral poliovirus vaccine. Virusdisease 2019; 30(2): 201-6.
[http://dx.doi.org/10.1007/s13337-019-00515-8] [PMID: 31179357]

[35] Chabeda A, van Zyl AR, Rybicki EP, Hitzeroth II. Substitution of human papillomavirus type 16 L2 neutralizing epitopes into L1 surface loops: The effect on virus-like particle assembly and immunogenicity. Front Plant Sci 2019; 10: 779.
[http://dx.doi.org/10.3389/fpls.2019.00779] [PMID: 31281327]

[36] Diken M, Kreiter S, Selmi A, *et al.* Selective uptake of naked vaccine RNA by dendritic cells is driven by macropinocytosis and abrogated upon DC maturation. Gene Ther 2011; 18(7): 702-8.
[http://dx.doi.org/10.1038/gt.2011.17] [PMID: 21368901]

[37] Kreiter S, Selmi A, Diken M, *et al.* Intranodal vaccination with naked antigen-encoding RNA elicits potent prophylactic and therapeutic antitumoral immunity. Cancer Res 2010; 70(22): 9031-40.
[http://dx.doi.org/10.1158/0008-5472.CAN-10-0699] [PMID: 21045153]

[38] Pardi N, Hogan MJ, Porter FW, Weissman D. mRNA vaccines - a new era in vaccinology. Nat Rev Drug Discov 2018; 17(4): 261-79.
[http://dx.doi.org/10.1038/nrd.2017.243] [PMID: 29326426]

[39] Armengol G, Ruiz LM, Orduz S. The injection of plasmid DNA in mouse muscle results in lifelong persistence of DNA, gene expression, and humoral response. Mol Biotechnol 2004; 27(2): 109-18.
[http://dx.doi.org/10.1385/MB:27:2:109] [PMID: 15208453]

[40] Donaldson B, Lateef Z, Walker GF, Young SL, Ward VK. Virus-like particle vaccines: immunology and formulation for clinical translation. Expert Rev Vaccines 2018; 17(9): 833-49.
[http://dx.doi.org/10.1080/14760584.2018.1516552] [PMID: 30173619]

[41] Qiang C, Huafang L. Plant-derived virus-like particles as vaccines, Human Vaccines & Immunotherapeutics. 2013.9:1, 26-49.

[42] Zhang J, Zeng H, Gu J, Li H, Zheng L, Zou Q. Progress and prospects on vaccine development against SARS-CoV-2. Vaccines (Basel) 2020; 8(2): 153.
[http://dx.doi.org/10.3390/vaccines8020153] [PMID: 32235387]

[43] Ghosh A, Chattopadhyay S, Chawla-Sarkar M, Nandy P, Nandy A. In-Silico Study of Rotavirus VP. Surface Accessible Conserved Regions for Antiviral Drug/Vaccine Design. PLoS One 2012; 7: 7.
[http://dx.doi.org/10.1371/journal.pone.0040749]

[44] Prompetchara E, Ketloy C, Palaga T. Immune responses in COVID-19 and potential vaccines: Lessons learned from SARS and MERS epidemic. Asian Pac J Allergy Immunol 2020; 38(1): 1-9.
[PMID: 32105090]

[45] Lurie N, Saville M, Hatchett R, Halton J. Developing Covid-19 Vaccines at Pandemic Speed. N Engl J Med 2020; 382(21): 1969-73.
[http://dx.doi.org/10.1056/NEJMp2005630] [PMID: 32227757]

[46] Lai CC, Shih TP, Ko WC, Tang HJ, Hsueh PR. Severe acute respiratory syndrome coronavirus 2 (SARS-CoV-2) and coronavirus disease-2019 (COVID-19): The epidemic and the challenges. Int J Antimicrob Agents 2020; 55(3): 105924.

[http://dx.doi.org/10.1016/j.ijantimicag.2020.105924] [PMID: 32081636]

[47] Garçon N, Vaughn DW, Didierlaurent AM. Development and evaluation of AS03, an Adjuvant System containing α-tocopherol and squalene in an oil-in-water emulsion. Expert Rev Vaccines 2012; 11(3): 349-66.
[http://dx.doi.org/10.1586/erv.11.192] [PMID: 22380826]

[48] Prompetchara E, Ketloy C, Palaga T. Immune responses in COVID-19 and potential vaccines: Lessons learned from SARS and MERS epidemic. Asian Pac J Allergy Immunol 2020; 38(1): 1-9.
[PMID: 32105090]

[49] Minor PD. Live attenuated vaccines: Historical successes and current challenges. Virology. 2015, 03-32 .

[50] Himani B, Anjeanette R, Leatrice V, *et al.* Severe acute respiratory syndrome coronavirus spike protein expressed by attenuated vaccinia virus protectively immunizes mice 2004.

[51] Robert-Guroff M, Nabel GJ, Shiver JW. Replication-defective and competent adenovirus recombinants as vaccine vectors. In: Levine MM, Ed. New Generation Vaccines. 4th ed., Informa Healthcare 2007.

[52] Robert-Guroff M. Replicating and non-replicating viral vectors for vaccine development. Curr Opin Biotechnol 2007; 18(6): 546-56.
[http://dx.doi.org/10.1016/j.copbio.2007.10.010] [PMID: 18063357]

[53] Dicks MD, Spencer AJ, Edwards NJ, *et al.* A novel chimpanzee adenovirus vector with low human seroprevalence: improved systems for vector derivation and comparative immunogenicity. PLoS One 2012; 7(7): e40385.
[http://dx.doi.org/10.1371/journal.pone.0040385] [PMID: 22808149]

[54] https://www.vaccitech.co.uk/technology/

[55] Thanh Le T, Andreadakis Z, Kumar A, *et al.* The COVID-19 vaccine development landscape. Nat Rev Drug Discov 2020; 19(5): 305-6.
[http://dx.doi.org/10.1038/d41573-020-00073-5] [PMID: 32273591]

[56] DeDiego ML, Alvarez E, Almazán F, *et al.* A severe acute respiratory syndrome coronavirus that lacks the E gene is attenuated *in vitro* and *in vivo*. J Virol 2007; 81(4): 1701-13.
[http://dx.doi.org/10.1128/JVI.01467-06] [PMID: 17108030]

[57] Totura AL, Bavari S. Broad-spectrum coronavirus antiviral drug discovery. Expert Opin Drug Discov 2019; 14(4): 397-412.
[http://dx.doi.org/10.1080/17460441.2019.1581171] [PMID: 30849247]

[58] Babcook JS, Prabhakar BS, Coughlin M. inventors; Amgen Inc., assignee. Antibodies to SARS coronavirus. World Organization patent WO 2008060331. 2008 May 22.

[59] Singh K, Mehta S. The clinical development process for a novel preventive vaccine: An overview. J Postgrad Med 2016; 62(1): 4-11.
[http://dx.doi.org/10.4103/0022-3859.173187] [PMID: 26732191]

[60] Burton DR, Ahmed R, Barouch DH, *et al.* A blueprint for HIV vaccine discovery. Cell Host Microbe 2012; 12(4): 396-407.
[http://dx.doi.org/10.1016/j.chom.2012.09.008] [PMID: 23084910]

[61] Caskey M, Schoofs T, Gruell H, *et al.* Antibody 10-1074 suppresses viremia in HIV-1-infected individuals. Nat Med 2017; 23(2): 185-91.
[http://dx.doi.org/10.1038/nm.4268] [PMID: 28092665]

[62] Haynes BF, Burton DR, Mascola JR. Multiple roles for HIV broadly neutralizing antibodies. Sci Transl Med 2019; 11(516): eaaz2686.
[http://dx.doi.org/10.1126/scitranslmed.aaz2686] [PMID: 31666399]

[63] Haynes BF, Gilbert PB, McElrath MJ, *et al.* Immune-correlates analysis of an HIV-1 vaccine efficacy

trial. N Engl J Med 2012; 366(14): 1275-86.
[http://dx.doi.org/10.1056/NEJMoa1113425] [PMID: 22475592]

[64] Kobayashi K, Atwood A. Takeda's Dengue Vaccine Candidate Meets Primary Endpoint in Pivotal Phase 3 Efficacy Trial.

[65] Martien N, Nelligan J. The Sourcebook for Clinical Research: A Practical Guide for Study Conduct. Academic Press 2018.

[66] Corey L, Mascola JR, Fauci AS, Collins FS. A strategic approach to COVID-19 vaccine R&D. Science 2020; 368(6494): 948-50.
[http://dx.doi.org/10.1126/science.abc5312] [PMID: 32393526]

[67] Graham BS. Rapid COVID-19 vaccine development. Science 2020; 368(6494): 945-6.
[http://dx.doi.org/10.1126/science.abb8923] [PMID: 32385100]

[68] Richner JM, *et al.* Modified mRNA vaccines protect against Zika virus infection 2017.

[69] Rogers KM. Immunization noncompliance: Gauging the cause, effect, and management in the school setting. NASN Sch Nurse 2019; 34(3): 140-4.
[http://dx.doi.org/10.1177/1942602X18799868] [PMID: 30336072]

[70] Singh K, Mehta S. The clinical development process for a novel preventive vaccine: An overview. J Postgrad Med 2016; 62(1): 4-11.
[http://dx.doi.org/10.4103/0022-3859.173187] [PMID: 26732191]

[71] Burton DR, Ahmed R, Barouch DH, *et al.* A blueprint for HIV vaccine discovery. Cell Host Microbe 2012; 12(4): 396-407.
[http://dx.doi.org/10.1016/j.chom.2012.09.008] [PMID: 23084910]

[72] Caskey M, Schoofs T, Gruell H, *et al.* Antibody 10-1074 suppresses viremia in HIV-1-infected individuals. Nat Med 2017; 23(2): 185-91.
[http://dx.doi.org/10.1038/nm.4268] [PMID: 28092665]

[73] Haynes BF, Burton DR, Mascola JR. Multiple roles for HIV broadly neutralizing antibodies. Sci Transl Med 2019; 11(516): 516.
[http://dx.doi.org/10.1126/scitranslmed.aaz2686] [PMID: 31666399]

[74] Haynes BF, Gilbert PB, McElrath MJ, *et al.* Immune-correlates analysis of an HIV-1 vaccine efficacy trial. N Engl J Med 2012; 366(14): 1275-86.
[http://dx.doi.org/10.1056/NEJMoa1113425] [PMID: 22475592]

[75] BM East. Takeda's dengue vaccine candidate meets primary endpoint in pivotal phase 3 efficacy trial.

[76] Martien N, Nelligan J. The sourcebook for clinical research: a practical guide for study conduct. Academic Press 2018.

[77] Corey L, Mascola JR, Fauci AS, Collins FS. A strategic approach to COVID-19 vaccine R&D. Science 2020; 368(6494): 948-50.
[http://dx.doi.org/10.1126/science.abc5312] [PMID: 32393526]

[78] Graham BS. Rapid COVID-19 vaccine development. Science 2020; 368(6494): 945-6.
[http://dx.doi.org/10.1126/science.abb8923] [PMID: 32385100]

[79] Richner JM, *et al.* Modified mRNA vaccines protect against Zika virus infection. Cell 2017; 168(6): 1114-1125.e10..

[80] Sette A, Buus S, Grey HM. Method for identifying useful polypeptide vaccines. Google Patents 1993.

[81] Marsian J, Fox H, Bahar MW, *et al.* Plant-made polio type 3 stabilized VLPs-a candidate synthetic polio vaccine. Nat Commun 2017; 8(1): 245.
[http://dx.doi.org/10.1038/s41467-017-00090-w] [PMID: 28811473]

[82] Brennan FR, Dougan G. Non-clinical safety evaluation of novel vaccines and adjuvants:. new products, new strategies. Vaccine 2005; 23(24): 3210-22.

[http://dx.doi.org/10.1016/j.vaccine.2004.11.072] [PMID: 15837222]

[83] Halloran ME, Longini IM, Struchiner CJ. Design and analysis of vaccine studies. Springer 2010; Vol. 18.
[http://dx.doi.org/10.1007/978-0-387-68636-3]

[84] US Food and Drug Administration. Vaccine product approval process 2001.

[85] Wrapp D, Wang N, Corbett KS, *et al.* Cryo-EM structure of the 2019-nCoV spike in the prefusion conformation. Science 2020; 367(6483): 1260-3.
[http://dx.doi.org/10.1126/science.abb2507] [PMID: 32075877]

[86] Walls AC, *et al.* Structure, function, and antigenicity of the SARS-CoV-2 spike glycoprotein. Cell 2020; 181(2): 281-292.e6..
[http://dx.doi.org/10.1016/j.cell.2020.11.032]

[87] Saunders KO. Conceptual approaches to modulating antibody effector functions and circulation half-life. Front Immunol 2019; 10: 1296.
[http://dx.doi.org/10.3389/fimmu.2019.01296] [PMID: 31231397]

[88] Henderson R, Lu M, Zhou Y, *et al.* Disruption of the HIV-1 Envelope allosteric network blocks CD4-induced rearrangements. Nat Commun 2020; 11(1): 520.
[http://dx.doi.org/10.1038/s41467-019-14196-w] [PMID: 31980614]

[89] LaBranche CC, Henderson R, Hsu A, *et al.* Neutralization-guided design of HIV-1 envelope trimers with high affinity for the unmutated common ancestor of CH235 lineage CD4bs broadly neutralizing antibodies. PLoS Pathog 2019; 15(9): e1008026.
[http://dx.doi.org/10.1371/journal.ppat.1008026] [PMID: 31527908]

[90] Murin CD, Wilson IA, Ward AB. Antibody responses to viral infections: a structural perspective across three different enveloped viruses. Nat Microbiol 2019; 4(5): 734-47.
[http://dx.doi.org/10.1038/s41564-019-0392-y] [PMID: 30886356]

[91] Lan J, Ge J, Yu J, *et al.* Structure of the SARS-CoV-2 spike receptor-binding domain bound to the ACE2 receptor. Nature 2020; 581(7807): 215-20.
[http://dx.doi.org/10.1038/s41586-020-2180-5] [PMID: 32225176]

[92] Yuan M, Wu NC, Zhu X, *et al.* A highly conserved cryptic epitope in the receptor binding domains of SARS-CoV-2 and SARS-CoV. Science 2020; 368(6491): 630-3.
[http://dx.doi.org/10.1126/science.abb7269] [PMID: 32245784]

[93] Kwong PD, Mascola JR. Human antibodies that neutralize HIV-1: identification, structures, and B cell ontogenies. Immunity 2012; 37(3): 412-25.
[http://dx.doi.org/10.1016/j.immuni.2012.08.012] [PMID: 22999947]

[94] Sok D, Burton DR. Recent progress in broadly neutralizing antibodies to HIV. Nat Immunol 2018; 19(11): 1179-88.
[http://dx.doi.org/10.1038/s41590-018-0235-7] [PMID: 30333615]

[95] Pardi N, Hogan MJ, Pelc RS, *et al.* Zika virus protection by a single low-dose nucleoside-modified mRNA vaccination. Nature 2017; 543(7644): 248-51.
[http://dx.doi.org/10.1038/nature21428] [PMID: 28151488]

[96] Pollard AJ, Finn A, Curtis N. Non-specific effects of vaccines: plausible and potentially important, but implications uncertain. Arch Dis Child 2017; 102(11): 1077-81.
[http://dx.doi.org/10.1136/archdischild-2015-310282] [PMID: 28501809]

[97] Dayal D, Gupta S. Connecting BCG vaccination and COVID-19: additional data Medrxiv 2020.

[98] Fine P, Eames K, Heymann DL. "Herd immunity": a rough guide. Clin Infect Dis 2011; 52(7): 911-6.
[http://dx.doi.org/10.1093/cid/cir007] [PMID: 21427399]

[99] Quadri-Sheriff M, Hendrix KS, Downs SM, Sturm LA, Zimet GD, Finnell SM. The role of herd immunity in parents' decision to vaccinate children: a systematic review. Pediatrics 2012; 130(3):

522-30.
[http://dx.doi.org/10.1542/peds.2012-0140] [PMID: 22926181]

[100] https://www.biopharmadive.com/news/coronavirus-vaccine-herd-immunity-covid-19/577312/

[101] Randolph HE, Barreiro LB. Herd immunity: understanding COVID-19. Immunity 2020; 52(5): 737-41.
[http://dx.doi.org/10.1016/j.immuni.2020.04.012] [PMID: 32433946]

[102] Amanat F, Krammer F. SARS-CoV-2 vaccines: status report. Immunity 2020; 52(4): 583-9.
[http://dx.doi.org/10.1016/j.immuni.2020.03.007] [PMID: 32259480]

SUBJECT INDEX

A

Kamal Niaz & Muhammad Farrukh Nisar (Eds.)

B

C

D

E

F

G

H

I

J

K

L

M

N

O

P

S

T

U

V

W

X

Z